# Severe Learning Disabilities
## and
# Challenging Behaviours

# Severe Learning Disabilities and Challenging Behaviours

## Designing high quality services

Edited by

*Eric Emerson* MSc, FBPsS, C.Psychol
Deputy Director, Hester Adrian Research Centre,
University of Manchester, UK

*Peter McGill* MPhil, AFBPsS, C.Psychol
Senior Lecturer in the Applied Psychology of Learning Disability,
University of Kent, UK

and

*Jim Mansell* MSc(Econ), AFPsS, C.Psychol
Director of the Centre for the Applied Psychology of Social Care and
Professor of the Applied Psychology of Learning Disability,
University of Kent, UK

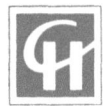

SPRINGER-SCIENCE+BUSINESS MEDIA, B.V.

First edition 1994

© Springer Science+Business Media Dordrecht 1994
Originally published by Chapman & Hall in 1994

Typeset in 10/12 Palatino by Best-Set Typesetters Ltd, Hong Kong

ISBN 978-1-56593-130-5       ISBN 978-1-4899-2961-7 (eBook)
DOI 10.1007/978-1-4899-2961-7

A catalogue record for this book is available from the British Library

Library of Congress Cataloguing-in-Publication data available

 Printed on permanent acid-free text paper, manufactured in accordance
with the proposed ANSI/NISO Z 39.48-199X and ANSI Z 39.48-1984

# Contents

# Contributors

David Allen
Clinical Manager, Intensive Support Service
55 Park Place
Cardiff   CF1 3AT

Chris Cullen
SSMH Chair of Learning Difficulties
Department of Psychology
University of St Andrews
St Andrews, Fife   KY16 9JU

Siobhan de Paiva
Formerly Research Officer
Mental Handicap in Wales Applied Research Unit
55 Park Place
Cardiff   CF1 3AT

Eric Emerson
Deputy Director, Hester Adrian Research Centre
University of Manchester
Manchester   M13 9PL

David Felce
Director, Mental Handicap in Wales Applied Research Unit
55 Park Place
Cardiff   CF1 3AT

Richard Hastings
Department of Psychology
University of Southampton
Southampton   SO9 5NH

Heather Hughes
Assistant Director, Southside Partnership
Scout Hall
Scout Lane
Clapham Old Town
London   SW4

Martin Knapp
Professor of the Economics of Social Care
Personal Social Services Research Unit
University of Kent at Canterbury
Canterbury, Kent   CT2 7LZ

Kathy Lowe
Research Fellow
Mental Handicap in Wales Applied Research Unit
55 Park Place
Cardiff   CF1 3AT

Judith McBrien
Clinical Director
Plymouth Community Services NHS Trust
Cumberland House
Cumberland Road
Devonport
Plymouth, Devon   PL1 4JA

Peter McGill
Senior Lecturer in Applied Psychology of Learning Disability
Centre for the Applied Psychology of Social Care
University of Kent at Canterbury
Canterbury, Kent   CT2 7LZ

Jim Mansell
Professor of Applied Psychology of Learning Disability
Centre for the Applied Psychology of Social Care
University of Kent at Canterbury
Canterbury, Kent   CT2 7LZ

Glynis Murphy
Senior Lecturer in Psychology
Institute of Psychiatry

De Crespigny Park
Denmark Hill
London   SE5 8A5

Hazel Qureshi
Senior Researcher
National Institute of Social Work
5–7 Tavistock Place
London   WC1H 9SS

Sandy Toogood
Team Leader, Intensive Support Team
Broughton Hospital
Broughton
Nr. Chester, Clywd

# Foreword

This is a timely book. The question of how to help people with challenging behaviour – and how to design and manage services so that staff, families and users feel that what should be done is being done – is at the top of the agenda. Failure to deal competently with the issue results in disaffection, poor quality services and a less than optimal quality of life for service users. Moreover, the credibility of services for all people with learning disabilities is intimately connected with how we cope with challenging behaviour, a point made recently by a Department of Health Working Group chaired by Jim Mansell (Department of Health, 1993).

The book is welcome because it draws together what is known about the important questions from a British perspective, although, of course, most of the underlying issues have worldwide relevance. The contributors, while all having a good deal of experience and authority, do not put forward simple portrayals of the problems, nor glib solutions, and this is one of the book's major strengths.

Clarity in the field of challenging behaviour is sometimes elusive. What is presented here forces the reader to confront arguments in a rational and logical fashion.

First we must be clear about the nature of the problem. What constitutes challenging behaviour; how much of it is there? To some extent, much of the behaviour of people with learning disabilities **should** challenge us. The person who sits quietly staring at the television, obeying all instructions from staff or family, presents a challenge to help her to achieve a meaningful life, appropriate skills of assertiveness, and so on. The procedures that we use to help such people reflect on the service as a whole, but it is still important to acknowledge, and quantify, the scale of the challenge posed by those who are aggressive, who offend, who run away, etc.

Once we know about the dimensions of the problem we have to give careful thought to the values and fundamentals which are to inform our interventions. What relation will our services for challenging behaviour have to mainstream services, and what will they tell us about how we value the individuals involved? These are important matters which sometimes force us to look into our own lives. However, values cannot stand in isolation; the days when rhetoric was useful are now gone.

We must develop organizational structures which will support expert help for clients. This means not only having professionals who are proficient at functional assessment, devising sophisticated interventions, paying attention to questions of generalization and maintenance, and so on, but also committed and responsive management to ensure that clients actually receive the service they deserve. How to do this within the real-life constraints with which we have to live is addressed by many contributors.

Another lesson to be taken from this book is that we don't know all the answers. We must continue to be open-minded and flexible, willing to explore new avenues and entertain new ideas. Much of the experience on which the book is based has been gained relatively recently and it is a reasonable supposition that our understanding will develop further during the 1990s.

This is an excellent source book, to give ideas to service planners and providers thinking about meeting the challenge. It will help to address the requirements of the Charter for people with learning disabilities who have challenging behaviour or mental health needs outlined by the Department of Health report (Department of Health, 1993), which includes the injunction: 'Services will strive to continually improve, using the latest research to provide the best treatment, care and support.' (p. 40)

Chris Cullen
St Andrews, August 1992

**Reference**: Department of Health (1993) *Services for People with Learning Disabilities and Challenging Behaviour or Mental Needs: Report of a Project Group* (Chairman: Prof. J.L. Mansell). London: HMSO.

# Preface

In 1985 the South East Thames Regional Health Authority set up the Special Development Team, a project to support the development of community-based services for people with severe learning disabilities and seriously challenging behaviours. It is easy to forget how radical this project seemed at the time. Despite the growing advent of community care these were some of the very people for whom hospitals were still seen as necessary. They were the people that even hospitals had trouble coping with, who often ended up grouped together in special, closed units – hospitals within hospitals.

This book has its origins in that project. Jim Mansell wrote the proposal that led to the setting up of the Special Development Team and later directed the evaluation of the services which were developed. Eric Emerson was the first Team Leader and was succeeded by Peter McGill. One of the original aims of the SDT was to provide advice and information regarding the development of appropriate services for people with severe learning disabilities and challenging behaviours. In many ways this is also the aim of this book, though we are fortunate to have gained the perspectives and experiences of others as well as that of the SDT. As more and more services have been developed, it has become clear that community-based provision for people with challenging behaviour is indeed feasible. Besides the necessary resources, they require, however, two crucial ingredients – the motivation to achieve them and the knowledge to set them up and manage them well. We hope that this book will help provide both. The examples of successful community provision described show that it can be done and show the potential benefits to clients. The discussions of the kinds of practices and supports required demonstrate the complexities involved but, we hope, also suggest how to overcome them.

Given the book's origins, it is most appropriate to address the largest part of our thanks to the clients with whom the SDT worked. Quite apart from their major disabilities, they had spent most of their lives in some of the most deprived conditions to be found in the hospital system. They now had to cope with changed policies about how they should live their lives; their responses and achievements in the face of this new challenge have taught us a great deal. We would also like to thank Sheila Barrett, Fran Beasley, Caroline Bell, Richard Cummings, Michele di Terlizzi, Cliff Hawkins, David Hughes, Heather Hughes, Christine McCool, Guy Offord, Siobhan O'Rourke, June Stein, and Sandy Toogood, all of whom were our colleagues at one time or another with the SDT or its evaluation and contributed greatly to the development of many of the ideas contained in this book. Invaluable secretarial support was provided throughout by Kathy Smith and Yvonne Liebenschutz.

Eric Emerson, Peter McGill and Jim Mansell

September 1992

*Part One*

# The Nature of the Challenge

# 1

# Introduction

*Eric Emerson, David Felce,*
*Peter McGill and Jim Mansell*

In this chapter we will outline the development of community care for people with severe learning disabilities, pointing to the limited progress made with people with challenging behaviour. We will emphasize the importance of comprehensive, high quality services by describing the frequent, extremely adverse consequences of challenging behaviours for individuals and their carers. Finally we will provide a brief overview of the rest of the book.

## The development of community care

The last three decades have witnessed the growth of a veritable catalogue of criticisms of institutional forms of care for people with learning disabilities. Long-stay institutions have been criticized for their excessive size, the segregation of their residents from the outside world, the separation of residents from their family and friends and from the general life of the community, the poverty of their material and social environments, their low staffing levels, the absence of stimulation and of meaningful pursuits for residents, for the development of abnormal systems of care or, in sum, for the degrading and, at times, abusive patterns of relationship characteristic of an institutional culture.

Over the same period, concerns regarding the predicted costs associated with continued institutional provision provided a window of opportunity for planners, managers, professionals and advocates to translate emerging ideas about alternatives into actual practice. As the values and objectives which help shape services have moved away from custodial care to ones which emphasize habilitation, quality of life and normalization, alternative models of community-based provision have begun to be articulated. These alternatives have been broadly defined by the reduced size of their settings, their location within ordinary communities, higher levels of staffing and a redefinition of staff roles to replace the emphasis on health care with aims based upon social care, enabling and support. Community-based services have sought to enable users to experience the patterns of living, learning, working and enjoying their leisure time typical for people of their age in the wider community.

Within the UK, initial reforms centred around the provision of alternative kinds of residential care. Early developments, such as those in Wessex (Felce *et al.*, 1980), sought to provide an intermediate model of domestic community-based provision. However, towards the end of the 1970s, a consensus began to develop that reform needed to be more fundamental. Specifically, it was suggested that ordinary housing should be available for all people who required residential support, an idea which found expression in the King's Fund paper 'An Ordinary Life' (King's Fund, 1980). These ideas were already being put into practice in the second generation of community-based housing projects which sought to provide residential care for all people with severe learning disabilities in ordinary, domestic style housing (e.g., Felce and Toogood, 1988; Humphreys *et al.*, 1987; Mansell *et al.*, 1987).

These fundamental changes in residential provision served to highlight the institutional nature of not only hospital, but also community-based **day care**. Existing 'community-based' services were criticized on the basis of the segregation of users from the surrounding community, the unstimulating and demeaning nature of many of the activities provided and the failure of services to support users to move on to better things. Changing values again helped shape alternative forms of service provision which emphasized the importance of meaningful integration and the provision of support when and where it was needed, and recognized the importance of work in the community at large (King's Fund, 1984).

While the rhetoric accompanying such values now appears well accepted (e.g., Departments of Health and Social Security, Welsh Office, Scottish Office, 1989), the viability of extending the opportunities provided by these alternative models of service provision to **all** people with severe learning disabilities remains contentious. In particular, progress towards providing high quality community-based care for people with severe learning disabilities who also show challenging behaviour has been particularly slow. There appear to be several reasons for this.

As deinstitutionalization and the growth of community-based provision have progressed, people with less severe handicaps and without behavioural difficulties have typically been the first to move, often for financial reasons (e.g., Department of Health, 1989). As a result, the remaining institutional provision is coming to serve an increasingly disabled population. This apparent reluctance of local services to gain experience in serving those with more serious disabilities has itself been used to support arguments for the continuing need to provide institutional services for people with serious disabilities, since either the community itself or local services are perceived as being 'not ready' to support people who challenge services.

A further problem is that both the definition and causation of challenging behaviour are unclear and that potential causes may overlap (Baumeister, 1989). Thus, for example, a common belief within hospital based services is that challenging behaviours primarily result from organic factors or psychiatric dysfunction. This has led to an emphasis on the continuing need for hospitals and the professional competencies associated with psychiatrists and psychiatrically trained nurses. Within such a framework, the environment may be seen as only playing a supporting role in the development of psychiatric disorder and the importance of environmental factors is therefore diminished. One consequence of such a belief system is that adverse comparisons between the social and material environments provided in institutions and community-based provision are seen as less important. Rather, the professional and administrative needs of the staff are considered to be preeminent, especially the potentially adverse effects of decentralization on the efficient organization of treatment and supervision by qualified psychiatric specialists. The importance given to these specialist skills accounts, at least in part, for the continuing call for centralized provision.

In one opposing view, the prevalence of challenging behaviour among people in institutional settings, coupled with analyses of the impoverished nature of life in large institutions, has led some observers to implicate institutional conditions in the causation of challenging behaviour. This has been associated with an expectation or hope that the provision of more normative settings will lead to more usual patterns of activities and interactions which will, in turn, lead to an increase in appropriate behaviour and skills and a concomitant decrease in challenging behaviour. Certainly, the damaging effects of institutionalization have been amply documented (e.g., Zigler and Balla, 1977). In addition, some research has noted the apparent inverse relationship between adaptive and maladaptive behaviour (e.g., Horner, 1980). It has become increasingly clear, however, that simple changes in location, size and the resources allocated to services have, in themselves, little impact upon the prevalence of challenging behaviour. Rather, it is appropriate to see challenging behaviour as the outcome of complex interactions amongst a range of factors – organic, psychiatric, environmental, ecological, historical – some of which will be more important than others in individual cases.

Moreover, as the definition of what constitutes severe challenging behaviour is vague, it is difficult to be convincing when generalizing from individual examples of successful community-based care to what might be feasible for an entire 'class' of people.

Despite these problems the need for different and better services is clear. Long-term institutionalization, the traditional response to the problem posed by seriously challenging behaviour, is no longer an available option in many localities. In addition, as the replacement of hospital settings continues, more people with seriously challenging behaviour are returning to their communities. As a result, local services are increasingly needing to become 'self-sufficient' and to provide services at a local level for all people with learning disabilities, including those with seriously challenging behaviour.

These same local services are already often struggling to provide for the many people with challenging behaviour who continue to live with their families. Qureshi (1990), in summarizing the results of her analysis of services provided to young adults with challenging behaviour living with their parents, concluded that:

> perceived service deficiencies include: day services which may be unsuitable, are not flexibly structured and may even exclude the person entirely; a widespread shortage of short-term and long-term residential facilities in the community; an incapacity to cope with behaviour problems in many existing facilities; a

failure to give parents useful advice on handling behaviour problems at home; insufficient help from social workers and community nurses. (Qureshi, 1990, p.1)

As a result the needs of the service user remain unmet and carers remain faced with a distressing, stressful and (at times) dangerous situation. The pressure in such circumstances to contain the behaviour by increasingly restrictive means is all too obvious.

Often, however, the only available alternatives consist of attempts to 'fix' the individual's challenging behaviour in specialized and geographically remote settings, although access to such specialized treatment facilities is often extremely difficult to arrange. Evidence, albeit largely anecdotal (Newman and Emerson, 1991), also suggests that while such services can be successful in the technical aspects of service provision, for example, the design and implementation of treatment programmes, and as a result achieve marked short-term reductions in the person's challenging behaviour, they also face a number of problems. These include the deleterious effects of congregating together individuals with severe problem behaviour upon user quality of life, staff stress and resulting turnover, and difficulties associated with the person returning to his/her original setting, a move which is itself extremely difficult to arrange and is often associated with reduced levels of programme implementation, increased use of mechanical restraint and failure to sustain treatment gains.

The aim of this book is to provide a resource to planners, managers, professionals and those advocating better services by drawing out some of the key issues and lessons from experience in the field to date. By doing so we hope that future services can avoid some of the problems of the past, for, as we all know, seriously challenging behaviour can blight the lives of service users and those caring for them in a number of ways. They can involve significant risks to the physical well-being of individuals and can lead to users experiencing unacceptable levels of material and social deprivation.

## The personal and social consequences of challenging behaviour

Challenging behaviours can result in direct and indirect threats to the health of service users. Self-injurious behaviour, by definition, can result in damage to the person's health. Indeed, repeated self-injury can lead to secondary infections, permanent malformation of the sites of repeated injury through the development of calcified haematomas, loss of sight or hearing, additional neurological impairments and even death (Mikkelsen, 1986).

In addition, the physical well-being of people with challenging behaviour is often put at risk as a result of the ways in which carers and services respond to them. These unhelpful responses to challenging behaviour are summarized below.

### Physical abuse

Indeed, challenging behaviour is one of the best predictors of who is at risk of being physically abused in institutional settings (Rusch *et al.*, 1986). Maurice and Trudel (1982), for instance, reported that one in 40 ward staff in Montreal institutions indicated that their **typical** response to an episode of self-injury was to hit the client.

### Unnecessary or excess medication

Between 40% and 50% of people who show self-injurious or aggressive behaviour receive psychoactive medication, of which haloperidol, chlorpromazine and thioridazine are the most common (Altmeyer *et al.*, 1987; Oliver *et al.*, 1987; Stone *et al.*, 1989). They are also significantly more likely to be maintained on such medication over time (Chadsey-Rusch and Sprague, 1989). The use of such powerful psychopharmacological agents to control challenging behaviour raises a number of questions given that:

1. there is little methodologically sound evidence that such medication has a **specific** effect in reducing challenging behaviour (Gadow and Poling, 1988);
2. prescription practices for people with learning disabilities and a clearly diagnosed psychiatric illness have been judged to be inappropriate in between 40% and 55% of instances (Bates *et al.*, 1986);
3. drug use in facilities can be substantially reduced through peer review processes with no apparent negative effects (Findholt and Emmett, 1990); and

4. neuroleptic medication has a number of serious side effects including sedation, blurred vision, nausea, dizziness, weight gain, opacities of the cornea, grand mal seizures and a range of extrapyramidal syndromes including parkinsonian syndrome, akathisia, acute dystonic reaction and tardive dyskinesia (Gadow and Poling, 1988).

As Singh and Repp (1989) point out, while the results of drug reduction programmes 'are heartening, they suggest that much of the medication was unnecessary when either originally prescribed or by the time the reduction programme was instituted' (Singh and Repp, 1989, pp. 273–4).

### Physical or mechanical restraint

The use of mechanical restraints and protective devices to manage challenging behaviour, including up to 50% of cases of self-injury (Griffin *et al.*, 1986), gives cause for serious concern given that the use of such procedures can lead to muscular atrophy, demineralization of bones and the shortening of tendons, and result in other injuries during the process of the restraints being applied (Griffin *et al.*, 1986; Richmond *et al.*, 1986; Spreat *et al.*, 1986).

### Deprivation, neglect and abuse

Aside from being placed in jeopardy of physical harm, people with challenging behaviour are at risk of substantial material and social deprivation through being excluded from everyday activities and settings, having their needs neglected and, as noted above, being subjected to abusive practices. Challenging behaviour is a major cause of stress experienced by carers (Quine and Pahl, 1985) and one of the main predictors of whether parents will seek a residential placement for their son or daughter (Tausig, 1985). Services provided to young adults with challenging behaviour living at home with their parents are often insufficient, especially in the area of providing advice or assistance within the parental home to effectively manage episodes of challenging behaviour (Qureshi, 1990). As noted above, people with challenging behaviour are at significantly increased risk of institutionalization and exclusion from community-based services (Lakin *et al.*, 1983; Schalock *et al.*, 1981). Once admitted to institutional care they are likely to spend the bulk of their time in materially deprived surroundings, disengaged from their world and avoided by staff (Emerson *et al.*, 1992; Felce *et al.*, 1985).

People with challenging behaviour are also at risk of having their needs neglected. Most episodes of inappropriate client behaviour occurring in institutions are ignored by staff (Felce *et al.*, 1987), and the low levels of attention which **are** provided are likely to be disproportionately negative in character (Grant and Moores, 1977). People with challenging behaviour are likely to be excluded from day services (Qureshi, 1990), even those provided within institutional settings (Oliver *et al.*, 1987). They are also unlikely to receive specific psychological help for their challenging behaviour (Griffin *et al.*, 1987; Oliver *et al.*, 1987) but are, as noted above, likely to be medicated or restrained. Some of the **socially** undesirable effects of medication and restraint procedures include the general sedative effects of neuroleptic medication (Gadow and Poling, 1988), the impact of mechanical restraints in precluding the person's participation in many everyday activities, and their setting the occasion for reduced levels of interaction with carers (Griffin *et al.*, 1986; Richmond *et al.*, 1986; Spreat *et al.*, 1986). The little evidence that is available also suggests that, at least for frequent or severe self-injury, the psychological interventions which are provided are more than likely to be of a punitive nature. Thus, for example, analysis of the nature of behavioural interventions employed within state institutions in Texas indicates that 30% of treatment programmes implemented for people with frequent self-injury and 66% of programmes for people with severe self-injury are reliant on aversive procedures (Altmeyer *et al.*, 1987). Similarly, Griffin *et al.* (1987) reported that only 33% of children exhibiting self-injurious behaviour in a metropolitan school district had a written formal treatment programme. Of these, 61% contained an aversive component.

## The aims of high-quality services

The personal and social consequences of seriously challenging behaviour stand in stark contrast to the avowed aims of current services for people with learning disabilities. As we have seen, over the past three decades, service aims have come to be explicitly concerned with safeguarding the rights of people with learning disabilities, enhancing their quality of life and providing services that enable users to live as ordinary a life as possible. Normalization in its many forms (Emerson, 1992) has had a significant impact on shaping service objectives in the UK (e.g., Tyne, 1987), North America (e.g., Marlett *et al.*, 1984), Scandinavia (e.g., Bank-Mikkelsen, 1980; Grunewald, 1986), and Australasia (e.g., Anninson and Young, 1980). More recently, these ideas have been explicitly incorporated in the aims of services for people with challenging behaviour (Blunden and Allen, 1987; Emerson *et al.*, 1987).

Blunden and Allen (1987), for example, ground their approach in the 'Ordinary Life' philosophy (King's Fund, 1980) which takes as its starting point that people with learning disabilities and challenging behaviour:

1. have the same human value as anyone else;
2. have a right and a need to live like others in the community;
3. require services which recognize their individuality.

The same authors go on to consider the implications of these values for service objectives in terms of O'Brien's (1987) five 'accomplishments' – aspects of life which services should help people to accomplish. They are:

1. **community presence** – people with learning disabilities have the right to live and spend their time in the community, not segregated in residential, day or leisure facilities which keep them apart from other members of society;
2. **relationships** – living in the community is not enough. People with learning disabilities also need help and encouragement to mix with other non-disabled people in the course of their daily lives;
3. **choice** – people with learning disabilities often have limited power to make choices and look after their own interests. A high quality service will give priority to enhancing the choices available to people and to protecting their human rights generally;
4. **competence** – in order for people with learning disabilities to live a full and rewarding life in their local community, many will require help in experiencing a growing ability to perform useful and meaningful activities with whatever assistance is required;
5. **respect** – people with learning disabilities often have an undeserved bad reputation and are regarded as second-class

citizens. Services can play an important part in helping people to be seen and treated with the same status as other valued members of society.

As we have seen, the reality falls far short of such aims for the vast majority of people with challenging behaviour.

### About this book

As we noted above, the present book represents an attempt to draw out some of the key lessons from experience gained to date in the provision of community-based services for people with severe learning disabilities and challenging behaviour. This is not, however, a 'how to do it' book. To undertake such a venture at our present state of knowledge would be remarkably presumptuous. Rather, we have attempted to bring together a range of contributions which, we hope, will highlight some of the more important issues facing those involved in the development, support, management and purchase of services for people with challenging behaviour.

The book is organized into three sections. Part One contains three further chapters which attempt to set the scene for later analysis and discussion. In Chapter 2, Hazel Qureshi discusses the definition of the term 'challenging behaviour' and draws upon the results of a large epidemiological study and other literature to address some of the important questions relating to the prevalence and persistence of challenging behaviour in people with severe learning disabilities. In the following chapter, Glynis Murphy provides an overview of current knowledge concerning the complex interaction of biological, behavioural and ecological factors which underlie the phenomenon of challenging behaviour. In the final chapter in this section, Jim Mansell, Peter McGill and Eric Emerson discuss some of the organizational and contextual factors determining patterns of service provision and provide a framework within which the complex array of services required to meet the needs of people with challenging behaviour can be identified.

Part Two of the book draws upon descriptions of innovative services which have gained invaluable experience in attempting to put the values embodied in the 'ordinary life' approach into practice for people with challenging behaviour. In Chapter 5, David Felce, Kathy Lowe and Siobhan de Paiva review the experience of the early attempts in Wessex and Cardiff to provide residential accommodation in ordinary houses for all people with severe learning disabilities, including people with challenging behaviour. In the following chapter, Peter McGill, Eric Emerson and Jim Mansell discuss the experience gained by the South East Thames Regional Health Authority's Special Development Team, a project which built on some of the lessons gained in the earlier Wessex projects and attempted to extend them to those people perceived as representing the most serious challenge to services.

Residential care is not, of course, the only aspect of service provision relevant to people with challenging behaviour. The final two chapters in this section review some of the lessons learned from recent approaches to day care and intervention services. In Chapter 7, David Allen describes some of the more innovative approaches to vocational and recreational provision for people with challenging behaviour. Following on from this, Judith McBrien discusses the experiences of the Behavioural Services Team for people with learning disabilities, a peripatetic community-based support and intervention team for people with challenging behaviour.

Part Three contains five chapters which discuss in more detail some of the key issues arising from these, and other, examples of service provision. In particular, these final chapters attempt to identify critical issues for those involved with designing, managing or supporting community-based services for people with challenging behaviour. The first two chapters focus upon issues central to the efficient and effective organization of staff support to people with seriously challenging behaviour. In Chapter 9, Eric Emerson, Richard Hastings and Peter McGill attempt to unpack the complex interrelationships between personal, social and agency values involved in the translation of service ideology into practice. Following on from this, in Chapter 10, Peter McGill and Sandy Toogood provide an organizational framework for considering staff support and client activity within community-based settings.

Chapters 11 and 12 address a number of issues at a wider organizational level. In Chapter 11, Jim Mansell, Heather Hughes and Peter McGill draw upon examples of placement breakdown and other problems in community-based services to identify some of the key organizational tasks important in maintaining and assuring quality. In Chapter 12, Martin Knapp and Jim

Mansell provide a framework for the comprehensive costing of service provision and discuss the relationships between costs and benefits in community care. The section, and the book, is rounded off by Chapter 13, in which Jim Mansell reviews the recent development and nature of current English policy, drawing on the themes emerging in earlier chapters.

## References

Altmeyer, B.K, Locke, B.J., Griffin, J.C., Ricketts, R.W., Williams, D.E., Mason, M. and Stark, M.T. (1987) Treatment strategies for self-injurious behavior in a large service delivery network. *American Journal of Mental Deficiency*, **91**, 333–40.

Anninson, J.E. and Young, W.H.L. (1980) The future forms of residential services for mentally retarded people in Australia – a delphi study. *Australian and New Zealand Journal of Developmental Disabilities*, **6**, 167–80.

Bank-Mikkelsen, N. (1980) Denmark, in *Normalisation, Social Integration and Community Services* (eds R.J. Flynn and K.E. Nitsch). Austin, TX: Pro-Ed, pp. 51–70.

Bates, W., Smeltzer, D. and Arnoczky, S. (1986) Appropriate and inappropriate use of psychotherapeutic medications for institutionalized mentally retarded persons. *American Journal of Mental Deficiency*, **90**, 363–70.

Baumeister, A.A. (1989) Causes of severe maladaptive behavior in persons with severe mental retardation: A review of some hypotheses. Paper presented at the National Institutes of Health, Bethesda, MD.

Blunden, R. and Allen, D. (1987) *Facing the Challenge: An Ordinary Life for People with Learning Difficulties and Challenging Behaviours*. London: King's Fund.

Chadsey-Rusch, J. and Sprague, R.L. (1989) Maladaptive behaviors associated with neuroleptic drug maintenance. *American Journal of Mental Retardation*, **93**, 607–17.

Department of Health (1989) *Needs and Responses: Services for Adults with Mental Handicap who are Mentally Ill, who have Behaviour Problems or who Offend*. London: HMSO.

Departments of Health and Social Security, Welsh Office, Scottish Office (1989) *Caring for People: Community Care in the Next Decade and Beyond*, Cm 849, HMSO, London.

Emerson, E. (1992) What is normalisation?, in *Normalisation: A Reader for the 1990's*, (eds H. Brown and H. Smith). London: Routledge, pp. 1–18.

Emerson, E., Barrett, S., Bell, C., Cummings, R., McCool, C., Toogood, A. and Mansell, J. (1987) *Developing Services for People with Severe Learning Difficulties and Challenging Behaviours*. Canterbury: Institute of Social and Applied Psychology, University of Kent.

Emerson, E., Beasley, F., Offord, G. and Mansell, J. (1992) Specialised housing for people with seriously challenging behaviours. *Journal of Intellectual Disability Research*, **36**, 291–307.

Felce, D. and Toogood, S. (1988) *Close to Home*. Kidderminster: BIMH.

Felce, D., Kushlick, A. and Smith, J. (1980) An overview of the research on alternative residential facilities for the severely mentally handicapped in Wessex. *Advances in Behaviour Research and Therapy*, **3**, 1–4.

Felce, D., Thomas, M., de Kock, U., Saxby, H. and Repp, A. (1985) An ecological comparison of small community based houses and traditional institutions: Physical setting and the use of opportunities. *Behaviour Research and Therapy*, **23**, 337–48.

Felce, D., Saxby, H., de Kock, U., Repp, A., Ager, A. and Blunden, R. (1987) To what behaviors do attending adults respond? A replication. *American Journal of Mental Deficiency*, **91**, 496–504.

Findholt, N.E. and Emmett, C.G. (1990) Impact of interdisciplinary team review on psychotropic drug use with persons who have mental retardation. *Mental Retardation*, **28**, 41–6.

Gadow, K.D. and Poling, A.G. (1988) *Pharmacotherapy and Mental Retardation*. Boston, MA: Little, Brown and Co.

Grant, G.W. and Moores, B. (1977) Resident characteristics and staff behavior in two hospitals for mentally retarded adults. *American Journal of Mental Deficiency*, **82**, 259–65.

Griffin, J.C., Ricketts, R.W. and Williams, D.E. (1986) Reaction to Richmond *et al*.: Propriety of mechanical restraint and protective devices as tertiary techniques, in *Advances in Learning and Behavioural Disabilities*, vol. 5 (ed. K.D. Gadow). London: JAI Press, pp. 109–16.

Griffin, J.C., Ricketts, R.W., Williams, D.E., Locke, B.J., Altmeyer, B.K. and Stark, M.T. (1987) A community survey of self-injurious behavior among developmentally disabled children and adolescents. *Hospital and Community Psychiatry*, **38**, 959–63.

Grunewald, K. (1986) The intellectually handicapped in Sweden – New legislation in a bid for normalisation. *Current Sweden*, **345**, 1–10.

Horner, R.D. (1980) The effects of an environmental 'enrichment' program on the behavior of institutionalized profoundly retarded children. *Journal of Applied Behavior Analysis*, **13**, 473–91.

Humphreys, S., Evans, G. and Todd, S. (1987) *Lifelines: An Account of the Life Experiences of Seven People with a Mental Handicap who used the NIMROD Service*. London: King's Fund Centre.

King's Fund (1980) *An Ordinary Life: Comprehensive Locally-based Residential Services for Mentally Handicapped People*. London: King's Fund Centre.

King's Fund (1984) *An Ordinary Working Life: Vocational Services for People with Mental Handicap*. London: King's Fund Centre.

Lakin, K.C., Hill, B.K., Hauber, F.A., Bruininks, R.H. and Heal, L.W. (1983) New admissions and readmissions to a national sample of public residential facilities. *American Journal of Mental Deficiency*, **88**, 13–20.

Mansell, J., Felce, D., Jenkins, J., de Kock, U. and Toogood, S. (1987) *Developing Staffed Housing for People with Mental Handicaps*. Tunbridge Wells: Costello.

Marlett, N.J., Gall, R. and Wight-Felske, A. (1984) *Dialogue on Disability: A Canadian Perspective*. Calgary: University of Calgary Press.

Maurice, P. and Trudel, G. (1982) Self-injurious behavior: Prevalence and relationships to environmental events, in *Life-Threatening Behavior:*

*Analysis and Intervention* (eds J.H. Hollis and C.E. Meyers). Washington, DC: American Association on Mental Deficiency, pp. 81–103.

Mikkelsen, E.J. (1986) Low dose haloperidol for stereotypic self-injurious behavior in the mentally retarded. *New England Journal of Medicine*, **316**, 398–9.

Newman, I. and Emerson, E. (1991) Specialised treatment units for people with challenging behaviours. *Mental Handicap*, **19**, 113–9.

O'Brien, J. (1987) A guide to life style planning: Using The Activities Catalogue to integrate services and natural support systems, in *The Activities Catalogue: An Alternative Curriculum for Youth and Adults with Severe Disabilities* (eds B. Wilcox and G.T. Bellamy). Baltimore, MD: Paul H. Brookes, pp. 175–89.

Oliver, C., Murphy, G.H. and Corbett, J.A. (1987) Self-injurious behaviour in people with mental handicap: A total population survey. *Journal of Mental Deficiency Research*, **31**, 147–62.

Quine, L. and Pahl, J. (1985) Examining the causes of stress in families with mentally handicapped children. *British Journal of Social Work*, **15**, 501–17.

Qureshi, H. (1990) *Parents Caring for Young Adults with Mental Handicap and Behaviour Problems*. Manchester: Hester Adrian Research Centre.

Richmond, G., Schroeder, S.R. and Bickel, W. (1986) Tertiary prevention of attrition related to self-injurious behaviors, in *Advances in Learning and Behavioral disabilities*, vol. 5 (ed. K.D. Gadow). London: JAI Press, pp. 97–108.

Rusch, R.G., Hall, J.C. and Griffin, H.C. (1986) Abuse provoking characteristics of institutionalized mentally retarded individuals. *American Journal of Mental Deficiency*, **90**, 618–24.

Schalock, R.L., Harper, R.S. and Genung, T. (1981) Community integration of mentally retarded adults: Community placement and program success. *American Journal of Mental Deficiency*, **85**, 478–88.

Singh, N.N. and Repp, A.C. (1989) The behavioural and pharmacological management of problem behaviours in people with mental retardation. *Irish Journal of Psychology*, **9**, 264–85.

Spreat, S., Lipinski, D., Hill, J. and Halpin, M.E. (1986) Safety indices associated with the use of contingent restraint procedures. *Applied Research in Mental Retardation*, **7**, 475–81.

Stone, R.K., Alvarez, W.F., Ellman, G., Hom, A.C. and White, J.F. (1989) Prevalence and prediction of psychotropic drug use in California Developmental Centers. *American Journal of Mental Deficiency*, **93**, 627–32.

Tausig, M. (1985) Factors in family decision making about placement for developmentally disabled adults. *American Journal of Mental Deficiency*, **89**, 352–61.

Tyne, A. (1987) Shaping community services: The impact of an idea, in *Reassessing Community Care* (ed. N. Malin). Beckenham: Croom Helm, pp. 80–96.

Zigler, C. and Balla, D. (1977) Impact of institutional experience on the behavior and development of retarded persons. *American Journal of Mental Deficiency*, **82**, 1–11.

# 2

# The size of the problem

*Hazel Qureshi*

How many people with learning disabilities show challenging behaviour, and what are the characteristics of those who do? On the face of it, these seem to be straightforward questions, which people planning, purchasing or providing services might need to answer. Unfortunately, as anyone who attempts to conduct a counting exercise in relation to challenging behaviour soon discovers, there are a number of obstacles in the way of providing the kind of answers which will stand up to critical scrutiny and be of use from the point of view of services. These problems are rooted in the fact that on an everyday basis the term 'challenging behaviour' is socially defined. Different people, or groups of people, will have different ideas about what is meant by 'challenging'.

The same person, showing the same behaviour, may be seen as challenging by staff in one setting and not by staff in another. Of course, this may be a consequence of environmental differences rather than differences of social definition. For example, a tendency to leave the setting and wander aimlessly nearby may be no problem in a hospital with large grounds in a rural setting, but potentially dangerous in a small staffed house in an inner city with busy roads. However, environmental differences aside, it is clear that differing levels of staff tolerance do mean that different definitions prevail in different settings. In the course of interviews with staff in a range of settings I once spent a considerable amount of time trying to persuade the manager of an Adult Training Centre that setting off the fire alarm deliberately two years previously was not really sufficient in itself to identify someone as showing challenging behaviour. In the same round of interviews, a member of staff in hospital who had been punched in the side of the head by a resident the previous week argued that he should not be identified as challenging because she had been aware of what might happen and had thoughtlessly been standing in the wrong place. Neither example is meant to typify general levels of tolerance in these different settings, but merely to indicate the range which may exist.

In both instances given above, the definition which staff wished to apply conflicted with the definition which I was seeking to apply as part of a research study into the prevalence of challenging behaviour. The kinds of definition which are constructed to be used in research or evaluation studies are known as operational definitions, because they are intended as ways to practically implement, or 'operationalize', particular conceptions of challenging or problem behaviour which are of relevance to the objectives of the study. As we have seen, these conceptions may be at variance with those of front-line staff but may reflect wider academic, clinical or managerial interests. For example managers may be interested in 'people who need additional resources for their care' while a clinical psychologist might wish to identify 'people who might benefit from the application of behavioural or other techniques'.

The likelihood that staff will identify a person as challenging may be influenced by the perceived purpose of the identification. Where additional resources may result there may understandably be an enhanced willingness to identify individuals. On the other hand some staff may be reluctant to label someone as challenging if they believe that this will be stigmatizing to the person concerned. The step from general expressions of interest in particular groups to an operational definition by which they may be identified is by no means straightforward, often because one is trying to draw clear boundaries where none exist. Nevertheless, when interviewing staff to discover the numbers of people who show challenging behaviour, it is clear that some attempt must be made to delineate the boundaries of concern because otherwise the criteria applied will vary, in ways which may seem quite arbitrary, from setting to setting depending on the prevailing expectations and goals of those who are consulted.

### Challenging behaviour and behaviour problems

Most examples of operational definitions come from a tradition of work on 'behaviour problems' or 'behaviour disturbance'. As will be outlined, definitions of 'problem' in these studies cast a wide net in terms of identification, to the extent that it is not unusual to find over half the population of people with learning disabilities identified as showing behaviour problems. From its inception the use of the term 'challenging behaviour' has been intended to focus attention on a much smaller group of individuals, as well as more generally to emphasize that there should be a shift in perspective among service providers away from seeing problems as inherent qualities of people, and towards a focus on services and the ways in which they might respond to behaviour which poses a challenge to the achievement of an ordinary life for people with learning disabilities (Blunden and Allen, 1987). Accepting this considerable difference of emphasis, there is still much which can be learnt from work on behaviour problems and, after discussion of some of the methods of measurement used, a number of relevant findings will be reviewed (for a related discussion, see Chapter 5).

The most usual way of attempting to impose some consistency across settings has been to present staff with a checklist of behaviours considered to be problematic and to ask them to rate each type of behaviour for each person to be assessed. In order to be rated 'symptom-free' on any checklist people have to receive a 'no' rating for every behaviour listed, and this usually means that a great many more people are likely to be rated as showing 'behaviour problems' than would be likely to be seen as showing challenging behaviour. For example, Jacobson (1982), in a study in the USA, used a list of 29 behaviours which were rated according to frequency. In larger institutions, 73% of people were defined as not symptom-free; in community residential facilities, 61%; in family homes, 52%. In the UK Clarke *et al.* (1990) used a checklist of behaviours rated as a severe or mild problem to carers, and as occurring frequently or occasionally. Amongst hospital residents 42% were said to show at least one severe problem at least occasionally; amongst residents of community facilities, 36%; amongst people living in their family home, 41%. Clearly, some indications of severity are needed in order to focus within these studies on a group seen as challenging to services.

Kushlick *et al.* (1973) used a brief list of six types of behaviour: hits out or attacks others; tears up paper, magazines, clothing or damages furniture; extremely overactive, paces up and down restlessly; constantly seeking attention, will not leave adults; continuously injuring self physically, e.g., head banging, picking at sores, beating eyes; antisocial, irresponsible and given to petty offences. Each behaviour could be rated by staff as 'marked', 'lesser' or 'no', with 'marked' defined as behaviour which had occurred within the past month and continued to present serious problems of management.

Holmes *et al.* (1982) expanded this list to 14 behaviours, including additional items such as: objectionable personal habits; screams or makes other disturbing noises; temper tantrums; disturbs others at night; and sexual delinquency. This expanded list forms part of the Disability Assessment Schedule which is administered by interviewers who rate each behaviour for each person as 'severe', 'lesser', 'no' or 'potential'. In this instance the criteria for a 'severe' rating do not include a time window such as 'within the past month', but instead refer to the consequences of the behaviour or the means needed for control: 'Staff have to intervene, or upsets other residents, or marked effect on social atmosphere. Would be unacceptable in public.' These kinds of criteria for severity perhaps give an indication of some of the key dimensions which might be relevant in making a judgement that a given person's behaviour is challenging to services, but in common with all checklist methods there are difficulties in deciding how to aggregate the information about different forms of behaviour so as to distinguish a more challenging group of people among those who are identified.

It is notoriously difficult to achieve high levels of inter-rater reliability using checklists. Perhaps the most comprehensively tested measure of this kind is the Adaptive Behaviour Scale (Nihira *et al.*, 1974) developed for the American Association on Mental Retardation. Part Two of this scale concentrates on what is called Maladaptive Behaviour, and carries checklist measurement to its logical extreme in listing several hundred items of problematic behaviour for staff to rate as occurring not at all, occasionally or frequently. The behaviours are grouped into domains and subdomains for which separate scores are calculated. For example Domain IX – Unacceptable or Eccentric Habits: Sub-domain 29 – Removes or Tears off Own Clothing lists the following items: tears off buttons or zippers; inappropriately removes shoes or socks; undresses at the wrong times; takes off all clothing while on the toilet; tears off own clothing; refuses to wear clothing; other.

Reliability is only measured in relation to domain scores (rather than specific items of behaviour) but, although a single rater will probably be consistent over a period of time, agreement between different raters on many domains is lower than would conventionally be regarded as acceptable for other measures (Isett and Spreat, 1979). The coherence of the domains has been questioned (Leudar *et al.*, 1984), and other criticism has centred on the failure of the scoring system to take account of the relative severity of different behaviours, and the difficulty of interpreting the profiles of Maladaptive Behaviour which result from administration of the scale (Holmes and Batt, 1980; Clements *et al.*, 1980). Nevertheless much subsequent work has drawn on adaptations of the ABS, perhaps involving use of only the more reliable domains, and/or severity weightings devised by other researchers. The availability of information on reliability is an advantage which the ABS has over other measures such as those used in studies already quoted by Jacobson (1982) and Clarke *et al.* (1990) where reliability is not mentioned.

One attempt to deal with difficulties of reliability has been to focus on specific behaviours such as self-injury (for example Griffin *et al.*, 1986; Oliver *et al.*, 1987) or aggression (Harris and Russell, 1989; Reed, 1990). Operational definitions which specify criteria involving tissue damage to self or others and a precise time window, seem to achieve better levels of reliability, and much has been learnt from these studies. Self-injury has been shown to be associated with more severe levels of learning disability, and to be more prevalent in younger age groups. A range of estimates suggest that between 4% and 10% of people with learning disabilities show self-injury, with higher rates of between 10% and 15% in institutions. However, from the point of view of assessing challenging behaviour, studies restricted to a single type of behaviour are substantially limited because the same person may often show many different forms of behaviour which are considered challenging. For example, at least half of those showing self-injury also show other challenging behaviour (Emerson, 1992). These other behaviours may be of greater concern to staff dealing with the person, and behaviours other than self-injury may be the target of any interventions or treatments that are being implemented. This means that it may be difficult to assess service responses or overall service needs from epidemiological studies which focus on one type of behaviour only.

### Selected results from the literature on behaviour problems

It seems to be generally accepted that people with learning disabilities are more likely to show behaviour problems than are comparable members of the population without learning disabilities (Bell and Marlett, 1985; Koller *et al.*, 1982; 1983; Padd and Eyman, 1985). This result has been found using a range of definitions, although the work by Koller and colleagues probably gives a more complex in-depth analysis of differences between people with learning disabilities and matched comparisons than many other studies. In this work, severity and type of behaviour disturbance were rated by the researchers from interviews with parents, and in some cases the young people themselves, and information from agency records. Reliability was checked by a second rater who evaluated a random sample of 30 subjects. Agreement on the type of behaviour disturbance was 100% and weighted Kappa for the severity ratings was 0.87 (Koller *et al.*, 1983).

It was found that the likelihood of showing aggressive behaviour decreased during the post-school period (after age 16) among people with severe learning disabilities, and suggested that this might be a consequence of their later acquisition of appropriate social skills. In the post-school period (age 16–22) Koller *et al.* (1982) reported that there were no significant differences between young men with learning disabilities and their matched comparisons in the proportions who showed physical violence towards others. However young men with learning disabilities were more likely to show antisocial behaviour, largely due to a greater prevalence among those who had mild or moderate rather than severe learning disabilities. Alcohol and drug related problems were found significantly more often among the male comparison subjects. Young women with learning disabilities were more likely to show emotional disturbance than young men, and than their female matched comparisons. They also showed more violent behaviour than matched comparisons, largely because levels of violent behaviour were very low among young women without learning disabilities.

This study found no differences in the proportions of young men and young women who showed behaviour disturbances overall, although other studies have suggested a preponderance of males among those showing behaviour problems (see for example Duker *et al.*, 1986). Differences of definition may well underlie this, since, for example, emotional disturbance may not be defined in other studies as a behaviour problem. Koller *et al.* (1983) observed that these different manifestations of disturbed behaviour might be due to inherent sex differences or they might reflect forms of disturbance customary for males and females and thus be culturally determined. It may be, then, that forms of behaviour disturbance more likely to be displayed by young women are less likely to be viewed as representing a 'problem' or a challenge to services.

It is also generally accepted that certain kinds of behaviour problem are associated with greater likelihood of residence in an institution, rather than in the community. Four major categories of problem discussed in the literature are: physical attacks on others; self-injury; destructive behaviour; other disruptive or socially unacceptable behaviour. The first three of these have been found to discriminate between institutional and community populations (Eyman and Call, 1977). Such a finding could occur either because the presence of these particular behaviours increases the possibility of institutionalization, or because placement in an institution increases the likelihood that such problems will be displayed. The weight of evidence seems to favour the first explanation, which was convincingly supported in a three-year controlled study by Eyman *et al.* (1981). This study compared over 400 young people allocated to community and institutional placements and found considerable stability through time in the presence of behaviour problems, which seemed unaffected by the type of placement. They concluded: 'Whatever maladaptive behaviour exists at time of placement is likely to persist regardless of the client's age group, level of retardation or community vs. institution residence' (Eyman *et al.*, p. 475). Eyman and colleagues were concerned that the persistence of behaviour problems reflected a lack of effective treatment or programming. They wished to caution against an over-optimistic assumption that relocation from institutions would in itself be sufficient to reduce behaviour problems.

Stability over time in the presence of behaviour problems has also been suggested in a follow-up study of 448 people with learning disabilities in the UK (Raynes and Sumpton, 1985). However, a longitudinal study focused on self-injurious behaviour seemed to suggest considerable changes in the population identified over a three-year period (Schroeder *et al.*, 1978). It may be, as

Leudar *et al.* (1984) have indicated, that different forms of problem behaviour exhibit different degrees of longitudinal stability.
Equally, as Emerson (1992) has suggested in relation to self-injury, perhaps more severe forms of problem behaviour are more
likely to persist over time than minor forms. It may also be that
people cease to display one particular type of behaviour but then
begin to show another, so that they would still be identified as
showing 'behaviour problems' despite a change in the form of the
behaviour.

All of these studies have concentrated on prevalence – the
number of cases existing at a particular point in time. In contrast,
the concept of incidence – the number of new cases arising within
a specified time period – has not figured largely in studies of
problem behaviour. This is perhaps unsurprising considering the
difficulties which would be encountered in deciding on criteria
which would identify the 'onset' of problem behaviour, especially
as this may occur at a very early age and only gradually become
evident. In addition, of course, behaviour which is unchanged in
form may **become** challenging to services because of changes in
the person, such as increasing physical strength, or because of
changes in services, such as reduction in staff ratios, or the loss of
staff with special competence. The remainder of this chapter turns
its attention to the question of the prevalence of challenging
behaviour.

### The prevalence of challenging behaviour

What then distinguishes challenging behaviour from behaviour
problems? Hill and Bruininks (1984) showed that only one-third
of incidents of problem behaviour required more than a verbal
response from staff, and suggested that the level of response
required might be useful as a measure of intensity of behaviour.
Nihira and Nihira (1975) found that only 16% of reported maladaptive behaviours were such as to result in jeopardy to health,
safety or general welfare, or the risk of action under the law, thus
indicating that actual or potential consequences may be important. Hollis and Meyers (1982) considered the extreme consequence of 'life-threatening' behaviour. In assessing the degree of
challenge, there is likely to be an interaction between frequency
and intensity. Even if infrequent, the possibility of life-threatening self-injury is likely to pose a challenge. Daily continual dis-

ruption to the activities of others can be very wearing for staff and seriously reduce the quality of life for other people in the setting, even though infrequent episodes may be tolerable. Frequency itself may be difficult to specify precisely because it can be extremely variable, perhaps with intense bouts of challenging behaviour separated by gaps of variable length in which no such behaviour is shown.

### *The study of prevalence of challenging behaviour in the north-west of England*

These considerations influenced the development of an operational definition for a study of people with learning disabilities whose behaviour was such that additional resources were required for their care. This programme of work was undertaken by the Hester Adrian Research Centre, University of Manchester, and funded by the Department of Health. Two aspects of the study will be reported here: first, a set of interviews with senior managers in health, social services and education agencies in seven different Health Districts to investigate policy and practice in relation to people with challenging behaviour; and second, a large-scale epidemiological study designed to discover the numbers and current locations of people in the target group. It was intended that sufficient information would be collected about people identified to make it possible to select out a smaller group whose behaviour was a challenge to services. This latter group were to be defined in relation to reported consequences, frequency, level of control required and type of behaviour.

The study of policy and practice investigated the ways in which people became defined as challenging within services (Routledge, 1990). In open-ended interviews, managers expressed the view that a referral to them as challenging might be a consequence of a person's characteristics and/or of their circumstances (Chapter 10). Many felt that it was possible to make a rule-of-thumb distinction between people whose challenging behaviour was probably service-defined or -maintained, and people whose behaviour might be resistant to changes of social or physical environment. This did not mean that such a distinction would necessarily be obvious in individual cases, but rather reflected a widespread belief that the numbers of people identified as showing challenging behaviour would be substantially reduced if some deficiencies in basic mainstream services could be remedied. Examples of such deficiencies included low levels of staff tolerance and skill, low access to professional support, poor physical environment, lack of stimulating activity, the congregation of clients with a wide range of special needs and inadequate levels of staffing.

Such beliefs lead to some reservations about a strategy for dealing with challenging behaviour which is restricted to an exclusive focus on developing specialist services for delivery to particular individuals (Chapter 4). After all, it would seem to follow that resources devoted to intervention at the system level, such as improved staff training or increased professional support, might be effective in reducing the prevalence of challenging behaviour, although most managers accepted that some specialist services for a small number of particular individuals might still be needed, and these might be required for some people on a long-term basis. Of course, without changing services in the ways suggested and monitoring the results it is not possible to be certain whether these beliefs are accurate, but they do reflect the views of those to whom people are referred as showing 'challenging behaviour' within services.

On an everyday basis the negotiation of the label 'challenging' is a social process. Although there will undoubtedly be some people about whom there is a wide measure of agreement, there will also be others about whom opinions differ across the range of people involved in their care. The person him/herself may also have a view on the matter.

For the study of prevalence, an operational definition was adopted which relied on information from interviews carried out with senior staff in all day and residential service settings within the seven Health Districts, including long-stay hospitals where people from the Districts were residing. The interview concentrated, firstly, on existing special resources within the setting and the individuals for whom these were needed and, secondly, on particular consequences of behaviour problems which had occurred in a given time period. So, for example, one question asked whether the setting had strengthened windows and, if so, for whom these were needed, while another question asked the staff member to identify anyone who had (non-accidentally) broken a window in the past month. Thus people were identified through the consequences of their behaviour in terms of injury to self or others, damage to, or destruction of, their environment, or severe social disruption which affected the quality of life of others. They were also identified if their behaviour was controlled through some feature of their service setting which might avoid or reduce such consequences, for example, strengthened fittings, extra staffing, additional security or segregation.

This initial setting interview provided a limited amount of information about the setting and also produced a preliminary list of individuals about whom further information would be sought. The detailed information included the type, intensity and frequency of difficulties displayed, and the management techniques employed to contain, prevent or reduce problem behaviour in that setting. If the information about behaviour did not confirm the person as a member of the target group they were eliminated from the survey (8% of those initially identified were subsequently dropped from the survey). Across the seven Districts, 701 people were identified, including nine who were not using services but were known to fieldwork teams.

Two exercises were undertaken to check the reliability of the identification process: one in social service settings and one in a long-stay hospital. In both exercises the setting interview was repeated by a different interviewer with a different member of staff in the same setting. The two-stage screening process achieved satisfactory levels of reliability. Cohen's Kappa was estimated as 0.71 in social services settings, 0.62 in hospital settings, both of which are satisfactory levels of agreement (see Qureshi *et al.*, 1989, for full details). Kappa measures the degree to which the observed level of agreement is an improvement over that which would be expected by chance, and is thus generally considered to be superior to simple measures of percentage agreement (Cohen, 1960; Fleiss *et al.*, 1969).

## Defining those showing challenging behaviour

Given the range of information available from the individual schedules it was obviously possible to construct a number of definitions of challenging behaviour. As would be expected the rate of prevalence varied according to the criteria chosen. For example, of those identified, one in three people in hospital were said to at least sometimes require physical intervention by more than one member of staff, while one in four people identified in the community were so rated. This represents 10% of all people screened in hospital and 4% of all people screened in the community. In contrast, 1% of all people in community settings and 2.8% of those in hospital were said to have caused serious injury to themselves or others at some time.

For the majority of the analysis a composite definition of challenging behaviour was adopted which attempted to combine various dimensions, and was based on factors which were associated with high rankings by staff in response to a question about which of the identified individuals were seen by them as most challenging (it was possible for no-one to be ranked as 'most challenging' if staff felt this was appropriate). Factors associated with such a ranking were: injuries to self or others, frequency of behaviour problems, damage to property, placing self in physical danger, disruptive behaviour and level of control required. The criteria given in Table 2.1 attempted to combine type of behaviour and frequency in ways which require the behaviours with less serious consequences to occur more frequently before they are considered challenging.

Forty-two per cent of those initially identified showed behaviour which met these rather broad criteria, representing about 7% of people with learning disabilities overall. People with challenging behaviour formed a higher proportion of the hospital than the community population, with 14% of people who were living in hospital showing challenging behaviour according to this definition, compared with 5% of adults (and 5% of children)

**Table 2.1** Criteria for identifying people with challenging behaviour

---

People were defined as showing challenging behaviour if they:

Had **at some time** caused more than minor injuries to themselves or others, or destroyed their immediate living or working environment

OR

Showed behaviour **at least weekly** which required intervention by more than one member of staff for control, or placed them in physical danger, or caused damage which could not be rectified by immediate care staff, or caused at least an hour's disruption

OR

Caused more than a few minutes disruption **at least daily**

---

**Table 2.2** Gender, age group and residential location of people showing challenging behaviour: total in seven Health Districts (total population 1 540 000

|  | *Men (%)* | *Women (%)* |
|---|---|---|
| Age under 18 |  |  |
| Community facility | 44 | 21 |
| Family home | 56 | 79 |
|  | *n* = 36 | *n* = 14 |
| Age over 18 |  |  |
| Hospital | 57 | 42 |
| Community | 26 | 30 |
| Family home | 17 | 29 |
|  | *n* = 157 | *n* = 84 |

living in the community. Just over half (51%) of all adults in this group were living in hospital and the proportion in hospital rose steadily with increasing age. Eighty per cent of those aged between 30 and 34 lived in hospital compared with only 2% of those aged between 15 and 19. In general, people aged between 15 and 34 were over-represented among those showing challenging behaviour, with 15–19 being the most prominent age group in community settings and 25–29 the most prominent in hospital. Two-thirds of people identified were male, and men were more likely to be placed in hospital than women, and less likely to be living in their family home (Table 2.2).

The children identified were more likely to suffer some physical disability than the adults. Sixteen per cent of children could not walk, even with aids, compared with 4% of adults. Two-thirds of the children and three-quarters of the adults had no difficulty walking. Using figures from the seven Districts it is possible to construct a profile giving the age and location of people showing challenging behaviour in a hypothetical 'average' District, although it should be made clear that such a District did not actually exist among the Districts studied. This profile (Table 2.3), with all figures corrected to whole numbers, shows 42 people in total identified, of whom 10 would be likely to be using services for children. Two people would be in funded placements outside the District.

Even within the seven Districts under study there is consider-

*The size of the problem*

**Table 2.3** Age and location of people showing challenging behaviour in hypothetical average District Health Authority (population 220 000)

|  | *Number* |
|---|---|
| In hospital – adults (18+) | 17 |
| In community |  |
| Age   5–9 | 2 |
| 10–14 | 2 |
| 15–19 | 6 |
| adults (20+) | 13 |
| Placed outside the District | 2 |
| Total | 42 |

able variation around this average picture. The standardized total number of people showing challenging behaviour varied from a low of 31 in the high-status area with a growing population, to a high of 56 in the two inner-city areas. In addition there was considerable variation in the use of hospital placement for adults. The proportion of those identified who were placed in hospital varied between 39% and 80%. The latter District contained two large learning disability hospitals. However, despite these important differences, the greater number of children in the 15–19 age group was almost universal, and the adults always substantially outnumbered the children, although it was usually the case that the majority of adults were in hospital. This suggests that if, as seems likely, hospital admission is more restricted in future, and if the behaviour problems shown by the older children persist over time, there will be a substantial proportionate increase in the number of young adults who require community-based services suitable for people who show challenging behaviour.

Staff were asked to indicate the degree of learning disability for each person. This was categorized as borderline, moderate or severe/profound, with an instruction that the last category meant an IQ of less than 50. In one in eight instances this was recorded as 'not assessed/cannot say'. Of the remainder 71% were classified as severe/profound, 21% moderate and 8% borderline. The importance of the presence of additional disabilities in relation to service use by people with less severe learning disabilities is highlighted by the fact that a majority of the small number of people in the 'borderline' category were said to have a mental illness, whereas only 15% of adults with challenging behaviour overall had a definite diagnosis of mental illness. This last figure represented 16% of people in hospital and 12.6% of people in the community.

Such rates of prevalence of mental illness are not very different from existing estimates of prevalence among the whole population of people with learning disability. For example Jacobson (1982) reported a figure of 12.4% for a general population of people with developmental disability, and Eaton and Menolascino (1982) found 14.3% of a community-based population of people with learning disability were also mentally ill. Thus the findings of the current study do not suggest that people with psychiatric illness are very substantially over-represented among people with challenging behaviour. There are, of course, widely acknowledged difficulties of diagnosis, but it does seem that the vast majority of people with challenging behaviour are not suffering from mental illness. Even if we include cases where staff reported that they suspected mental illness as a possible factor underlying behaviour problems, this only occurred in 6% of cases where such illness had not been formally diagnosed by a psychiatrist. Despite these relatively low levels of mental illness, just over half (52%) of adults showing challenging behaviour were taking antipsychotic drugs. This compares with one in four (27%) who were said by staff to be subject to 'an agreed written behaviour modification programme' (no check was made as to the validity of these responses).

The use of different treatments did vary according to the different types of challenging behaviour rated most serious for the particular individual. As Table 2.4 indicates, drugs were most frequently reported as used in relation to self-injury, although there is considerable doubt about their efficacy (Emerson, 1992). There was considerable overlap between different problem areas. For example, of people who showed self-injury, 70% also made physical attacks on others.

Among children (defined as those under 18) the relative prevalence of different treatment responses is reversed, with 18% said to be taking drugs to control their behaviour and 60% said to be subject to a behaviour modification programme. The distribution of different types of challenging behaviour is similar to that for adults except that children are more likely to be rated as 'poten-

**Table 2.4** Proportions of adults showing challenging behaviour who showed particular types of behaviour and treatment received ($n = 241$)

|  | Type of challenging behaviour | | | |
|  | PA | SI | D | O |
| --- | --- | --- | --- | --- |
| % for whom this was rated one of their most serious management problems | 33 | 23 | 24 | 58 |
| % of above row receiving drugs to control this behaviour | 53 | 73 | 51 | 47 |
| % of first row who had an 'agreed written behaviour modification programme' | 20 | 27 | 28 | 25 |
| % of those identified who showed this behaviour at all | 72 | 54 | 61 | 91 |

PA = physical aggression
SI  = self-injury
D   = destructiveness
O   = other

tially serious but controlled' across all categories of behaviour, and noticeably more likely to have attacks on others rated as one of their most serious areas (42% had this rating compared with 33% of adults).

## Conclusions

How many people show challenging behaviour? It has been argued that senior managers get an end view of a social process of labelling, about which there will be varying degrees of agreement among interested parties. Of course there will undoubtedly be individuals about whom there is a wide measure of social agreement that their behaviour is a challenge to services. However, there will also be others about whom knowledge and opinions differ among different interested parties, among whom may be included both staff and family members, as well as the person in question. In practice, in community-based services it is usually the case that people acquire the label because they are referred to senior managers as posing particular difficulties. On an everyday basis the negotiation of the label 'challenging' is a social process, and although the labelling of individuals may be decried as a possible negative outcome of this process, if this label brings the possibility of additional resources people are likely to feel that the advantages of its use outweigh the disadvantages.

Imposing some consistency of definition across a range of service settings presents many difficulties. Some of these have been illustrated by considering a tradition of work on behaviour problems which, from the point of view of providing information about challenging behaviour, has perhaps sometimes over-emphasized the importance of the forms of behaviour seen as problematic, at the expense of detailed consideration of their actual or possible consequences in individual instances, or the means required for control. Work on behaviour problems, whether general or specific, has provided a number of insights into the question of prevalence and chronicity, although the range of operational definitions has set limits on the comparability of studies.

One epidemiological study which has attempted to address some of these issues has been described, and results indicate that people who show challenging behaviour are more likely to be male, to be over-represented in the age group 15–34 and to be unlikely to be diagnosed as suffering from mental illness. Around one in three show physical attacks on others as one of their most serious management problems but most show more than one form of challenging behaviour. Increasing age increases the likelihood of placement in hospital, although the chances of this vary quite substantially across Health Districts. Among adults with challenging behaviour there is a consistently much greater use of antipsychotic drugs than of behaviour modification, with a majority of those identified using the former. The rates of prevalence derived from this study suggest that a systematic approach to the assessment of the numbers of people in a given District who may have special needs in this respect, should not result in uncovering unmanageably high levels of need, although the socio-economic characteristics of the District and the relative level of use of hospital as opposed to community services will influence the numbers currently using community-based services. The age and location profile of this group at this time underlines the importance of work with young people of school leaving age, if a commitment to keep people with challenging behaviour out of hospital is to become a reality.

## References

Bell, R. and Marlett, N. (1985) Behaviour disturbance in mentally-handicapped and non-mentally handicapped people. *Journal of Practical Approaches to Developmental Handicap*, **10**, 17–22.

Blunden, R. and Allen, D. (eds) (1987) *Facing the Challenge: An Ordinary Life for People with Learning Difficulties and Challenging Behaviour*. London: King's Fund.

Clarke, D.J., Kelley, S., Thinn, K. and Corbett, J.A. (1990) Psychotropic drugs and mental retardation: 1. Disabilities and the prescription of drugs for behaviour and epilepsy in three residential settings. *Journal of Mental Deficiency Research*, **34**, 385–95.

Clements, P., Bost, L.W., DuBois, Y.G. and Turpin, W. (1980) Adaptive Behaviour Scale Part Two: Relative severity of maladaptive behaviour. *American Journal of Mental Deficiency*, **84**, 5, 465–9.

Cohen, J. (1960) A coefficient of agreement for nominal scales. *Educational and Psychological Measurement*, **20**, 37–46.

Duker, P., van Druenen, C., Jol, K. and Oud, H. (1986) Determinants of maladaptive behaviour of institutionalised mentally retarded individuals. *American Journal of Mental Deficiency*, **91**, 51–6.

Eaton, L. and Menolascino, F. (1982) Psychiatric disorders in the mentally retarded: Types, problems and challenges. *American Journal of Psychiatry*, **139**, 1297–303.

Emerson, E. (1992) Self-injurious behaviour: An overview of recent trends in epidemiological and behavioural research. *Mental Handicap Research*, **5**, 49–81.

Eyman, R. and Call, T. (1977) Maladaptive behaviour and community placement of mentally retarded persons. *American Journal of Mental Deficiency*, **82**, 137–44.

Eyman, R., Borthwick, S. and Miller, C. (1981) Trends in maladaptive behaviour of mentally retarded persons placed in community settings and institutional settings. *American Journal of Mental Deficiency*, **85**, 473–7.

Fleiss, J., Cohen, J. and Everitt, B. (1969) Large sample standard errors of Kappa and weighted Kappa. *Psychological Bulletin*, **72**, 323–7.

Griffin, J.C., Williams, D.E., Stark, M.T., Altmeyer, B.K. and Mason, M. (1986) Self-injurious behavior: A state-wide prevalence survey of the extent and circumstances. *Applied Research in Mental Retardation*, **7**, 105–16.

Harris, P. and Russell, O. (1989) *The Prevalence of Aggressive Behaviour Among People with Learning Difficulties in a Single Health District: Interim Report*. Bristol: Norah Fry Research Centre, University of Bristol.

Hill, B. and Bruininks, R. (1984) Maladaptive behaviour of mentally retarded individuals in residential facilities. *American Journal of Mental Deficiency*, **88**, 380–7.

Hollis, J.H. and Meyers, C.E. (1982) *Life-Threatening Behaviour: Analysis and Intervention*. Washington DC: American Association on Mental Deficiency.

Holmes, C.B. and Batt, R. (1980) Is choking others really equivalent to stamping one's feet? An analysis of Adaptive Behaviour Scale items. *Psychological Reports*, **46**, 1277–8.

Holmes, N., Shah, A. and Wing, L. (1982) The Disability Assessment Schedule: A brief screening device for use with the mentally retarded. *Psychological Medicine*, **12**, 879–90.

Isett, R. and Spreat, S. (1979) Test–retest and interrater reliability of the AAMD Adaptive Behaviour Scale. *American Journal of Mental Deficiency*, **84**, 93–5.

Jacobson, J.W. (1982) Problem behaviour and psychiatric impairment within a developmentally disabled population 1:Behaviour frequency. *Applied Research in Mental Retardation*, **3**, 121–39.

Koller, H., Richardson, S., Katz, M. and McLaren, J. (1982) Behaviour disturbance in childhood and the early adult years in populations who were and were not mentally retarded. *Journal of Preventive Psychiatry*, **1**, 453–68.

Koller, H., Richardson, S., Katz, M. and McLaren, J. (1983) Behaviour disturbance since childhood among a 5-year birth cohort of all mentally retarded young adults in a city. *American Journal of Mental Deficiency*, **87**, 386–95.

Kushlick, A., Blunden, R. and Cox, G. (1973) The Wessex Social and Physical Incapacity (SPI) Scale and the Speech, Self Help and Literacy Scale (SSL). *Psychological Medicine*, **3**, 336–78.

Leudar, I., Fraser, W. and Jeeves, M.A. (1984) Behaviour disturbance and mental handicap: Typology and longitudinal trends. *Psychological Medicine*, **14**, 923–35.

Nihira, L. and Nihira, K. (1975) Jeopardy in community placement. *American Journal of Mental Deficiency*, **79**, 538–44.

Nihira, K., Foster, R., Shellhaas, M. and Leland, H. (1974) *AAMD Adaptive Behavior Scale*. Washington, DC: American Association on Mental Deficiency.

Oliver, C., Murphy, G. and Corbett, J. (1987) Self-injurious behaviour in people with mental handicap: A total population study. *Journal of Mental Deficiency Research*, **31**, 147–62.

Padd, W. and Eyman, R. (1985) Mental retardation and aggression: Epidemiologic concerns, and implications for deinstitutionalisation, in *The Education and Training of the Mentally Retarded* (eds A. Ashman and R. Laura). London: Croom Helm, pp. 145–168.

Qureshi, H., Alborz, A. and Kiernan, C. (1989) *Prevalence of Individuals with Mental Handicap who show Severe Problem Behaviour : Preliminary Results. Report to the Department of Health.* Manchester: Hester Adrian Research Centre, University of Manchester.

Raynes, N. and Sumpton, R.A. (1985) *Follow-up Study of 448 People with Mental Handicap. Report to Department of Health.* Manchester: Hester Adrian Research Centre, University of Manchester.

Reed, J. (1990) Identification and description of adults with mental handicaps showing physically aggressive behaviours. *Mental Handicap Research*, **3**, 126–36.

Routledge, M. (1990) *Services for People With a Mental Handicap Whose Behaviour is a Challenge to Services: A Review of the Policy and Service Context in the Seven Districts Covered by the HARC Behaviour Problems Project. Report to Department of Health.* Manchester: Hester Adrian Research Centre, University of Manchester.

Schroeder, S., Schroeder, C., Smith, B. and Dalldorf, J. (1978) Prevalence of self-injurious behaviours in a large state facility for the retarded: A three year follow-up study. *Journal of Autism and Childhood Schizophrenia*, **8**, 261–9.

# 3

# Understanding challenging behaviour

*Glynis Murphy*

A person's challenging behaviour may sometimes seem quite incomprehensible, particularly when the person has few communication skills and is unable to explain anything about their own feelings, wishes or expectations. Nevertheless, a considerable amount is known about the factors which influence the appearance, frequency and intensity of challenging behaviours and it is clear that in many cases a multiplicity of factors may be important. In this chapter, biological, operant and ecological factors will be considered and some tentative models proposed for the understanding of how such factors might interact.

## Biological factors

Severe learning disabilities are largely biological in origin. Seventy per cent of the people with such disabilities have identifiable chromosomal or genetic defects, such as Down's syndrome or Fragile X, while perinatal and postnatal biological factors can be identified for a further 15% of people (Alberman, 1984; Roberts, 1987).

It does not follow, however, that other difficulties, which may covary with learning disabilities, are necessarily biological in origin. A number of well-known epidemiological studies in the 1960s and early 1970s in Aberdeen and the Isle of Wight in the UK and elsewhere (e.g., Kuaii, Hawaii) demonstrated that children with learning disabilities were rated both by their parents and their teachers as showing more behavioural and psychiatric difficulties than other children (Rutter *et al.*, 1970; Werner and Smith, 1977; 1980; Birch *et al.*, 1970; Koller *et al.*, 1982). It appeared that the likelihood of behavioural difficulties generally increased as the severity of the learning disabilities increased and this correlation has been replicated numerous times in a variety of studies of both children and adults. There appeared, however, to be little specific relationship between the degree of learning disability (and hence presumably the degree of brain damage/dysfunction) and the behaviour shown. It was as though increasing degrees of brain dysfunction, which were presumed to underlie the increasing degrees of learning disabilities, simply had the effect of raising the likelihood of a person showing any disturbed or challenging behaviours. It seemed possible, therefore, that either there were specific brain–behaviour links which were masked by the inclusion of all children in a geographical area who had a variety of different kinds of brain dysfunction, or that the links between brain dysfunction and behaviour were indirect (for example, that they were of social origin).

Since then, numerous studies have appeared of the behaviour of children with specific syndromes or diagnoses, for only some of whom the nature of the brain dysfunction is relatively well understood. In general, the specificity of the links between the behaviour observed and the medical diagnosis or the neurobiological disturbances known have been disappointing. A few examples will suffice to demonstrate the findings in this area.

The most common single cause of severe learning disabilities is Down's syndrome. This chromosomal defect accounts for approximately one-third of all cases of severe learning disabilities (Alberman, 1984) and yet careful longitudinal studies of cohorts of children with Down's syndrome have failed to identify much in the way of behaviour disturbance when compared with other children with learning disabilities (Carr, 1988; Gath and Gumley, 1987). This may seem surprising in view of the fact that at least some of the biochemical consequences of the extra chromosome 21 are known, e.g., a raised level of intracellular superoxide dismutase, which is thought to produce an increase in cellular oxidative processes with a resultant disturbance in neurotransmitters (Clements, 1987). Later in life, challenging behaviours may appear as part of the clinical signs of Alzheimer's disease (Oliver and Holland, 1986) but these behaviours are not specific to Down's syndrome. The dementia is probably a result of the presence of the gene for familial Alzheimer's disease on chromosome 21 (Holland, 1991).

In contrast, Fragile X, a much more recently identified genetic disorder which accounts for probably less than 10% of all cases of severe learning disabilities amongst boys (and fewer amongst girls), is said to be linked to particularly high rates of attention deficit, hyperkinesis and 'autistic-like' behaviour, such as stereotypies and echolalia (Borghgraef *et al.*, 1990). The underlying brain dysfunction in Fragile X syndrome is not well understood but the syndrome is commonly considered to be a good example of how brain dysfunction and behavioural disturbance may be linked. It is sobering to note, however, that in Borghgraef's study, hyperkinetic behaviour, for example, was observed in 29% of those boys with Fragile X and 16% of a control group of boys matched for social class and degree of learning disabilities. It could not, therefore, be said that the presumed neurobiological conditions following from Fragile X are necessary and sufficient conditions for the appearance of this (or any other) behaviour.

To take another example where the neurobiology is better understood, phenylketonuria is an inherited condition (occurring in one per 10 000 children in the UK) in which the conversion of phenylalanine to tyrosine is impaired and low-phenylalanine diets can prevent severe learning disabilities (Smith, I., 1985). There are known disturbances to neurotransmitter levels and these include reduced neurotransmitter amine synthesis when plasma phenylalanine concentrations are high. The behavioural concomitants of phenylketonuria in a study by the UK register included increased rates of 'neurotic' deviance, even after IQ had been taken into account, amongst children (Stevenson *et al.*, 1979) and it has been demonstrated that these were correlated with the children's blood phenylalanine levels (Smith and Beasley, 1989; Smith *et al.*, 1988) and hence presumably their neurotransmitter levels. The behaviours are also shown, however, by children without the disorder (Stevenson *et al.*, 1979), so that again it is difficult to argue precisely what form any brain–behaviour link might take.

There are only two known conditions which can be biologically defined and which always lead to a specific behavioural difficulty: Lesch–Nyhan syndrome and Prader–Willi syndrome. The former is a very rare X-linked inheritable condition (occurring in approximately one in 380 000 births) in which there is an abnormal gene on the X chromosome, a deficit in a particular enzyme (hypoxanthine guanine phosphoribosyltransferase or HGRPT enzyme) and resultant spasticity, choreoathetosis and a variable degree of learning disability (Crawhill *et al.*, 1972; Christie *et al.*, 1982). In the largest sample of people with Lesch–Nyhan syndrome described, it has been reported that all of them showed self-injurious behaviour, specifically hand-biting, with some also showing lip-biting and other forms of self-injury, the behaviour appearing by around two years of age (Christie *et al.*, 1982).

There is no certainty with respect to the manner of the link between the gene, the enzyme deficit and self-injury but alterations in neurotransmitter receptors and possible dopamine receptor supersensitivity have been reported and may be crucial (Oliver and Head, 1990). It is important to note, however, that in a total population survey of people with learning disabilities who self-injured, only four out of the 596 people identified suffered from Lesch–Nyhan syndrome (Oliver *et al.*, 1987). It is thus a sufficient but by no means a necessary condition for the appearance of self-injurious behaviours.

Prader–Willi syndrome is also a rare condition (affecting approximately one in 14 000 children) associated with learning disabilities, short stature and obesity. Abnormalities of chromosome 15 are common but not invariable and the link between this and the behavioural phenotype is not understood. During childhood and adulthood, people with Prader–Willi syndrome invariably overeat and their parents and/or carers frequently have to resort to locking food away. Research into their eating behaviour has suggested that it may result from a failure of appetite control or satiety, their continued feelings of hunger leading to theft of food and gross overeating with its concomitant health risks and the prejudicial social consequences of being grossly overweight (Blundell, 1990; Holland, 1991).

It appears then that these (Lesch–Nyhan and Prader–Willi) are the only two biologically definable syndromes which appear to constitute sufficient conditions for the appearance of particular challenging behaviours. There are no syndromes known which are necessary conditions for particular challenging behaviours. In other words, for any particular challenging behaviour there is never a single biological syndrome which can be defined, as far as is currently known.

Perhaps we should also ask whether there are any known neurobiological or neurophysiological factors which might cut across syndromes, which are necessary and/or sufficient for the appearance of challenging behaviour. For example, do particular known neurotransmitter disturbances or neurophysiological events always lead to particular challenging behaviours?

For many years, it has been asserted that there is a link between epilepsy, a condition known to be common in learning disabilities, and challenging behaviours, particularly aggression. A particular form of epilepsy, temporal lobe epilepsy, is well-established as frequently but not invariably associated with aggressive outbursts (Lindsay *et al.*, 1979). Moreover, there are reports of aggressive outbursts coinciding with ictal activity in the amygdala and elsewhere, and several cases of people becoming aggressive following cysts in the amygdala or close by, whose aggressive behaviour disappeared following neurosurgery (Fenwick, 1986). Fenwick comments, however, that ictal aggression is rare and that by no means all the people with temporal lobe epilepsy have a history of aggressive behaviour. He concludes that epileptic discharges in particular areas of the brain should only be seen as one, possible, very rare, cause of aggressive behaviour and that apparent correlations between aggression and epilepsy in general are probably a function of other uncontrolled factors in poorly designed studies.

With respect to neurotransmitter disturbances, there are relatively few which have been unequivocally established as having any clear relationship to challenging behaviour. There is some evidence that disturbances in serotonin are linked to aggressive behaviour in animals but little convincing evidence of this in human beings. Moreover, the specificity of the links in animals are questionable since serotonin is a neurotransmitter which has also been implicated in disturbances of sleep, eating, mood and a variety of behaviours (Herbert, in press).

Perhaps one of the most specific links between neurotransmitters and challenging behaviour is that between endorphins and self-injury. Endorphins are endogenous opiates which are released at times of pain and stress in human beings. They produce analgesic and probably also euphoric effects, and have been shown to be raised in people who repeatedly cut themselves (Coid *et al.*, 1983). Opiate antagonists such as naloxone and naltrexone, when given to people who self-injure, have the effect of reducing the frequency and/or intensity of the self-injurious behaviour and it is thought that they may act by blocking the analgesic/euphoric effects of the endorphins (Oliver and Head, 1990). On their own, endorphins cannot account for the appearance of self-injury but they may be able to contribute to explanations of the maintenance of chronic self-injurious behaviour, particularly in combination with other biological and social factors (Oliver and Head, 1990).

Finally, some consideration needs to be given to the issue of whether people with psychiatric disorders as well as learning disabilities have an increased likelihood of displaying challenging behaviours (see also Chapter 2) and, if so, why this might be. The term 'psychiatric disorders' includes the so-called 'neurotic' disorders, which are probably learnt behaviours and a variety of other disorders which are almost certainly biological in origin (e.g., autism and the psychoses, such as schizophrenia). Some psychiatrists have argued that people with (biologically-based) psychiatric disorders are more likely than other people with learning disabilities to show challenging behaviours in general. This issue is an extremely complicated one and the arguments put in favour of a link between serious psychiatric and behaviour disorders are often tautological, since the 'abnormal' behaviour taken as a sign of a psychiatric disorder is often also taken as evidence that those with psychiatric disorders tend to show higher rates of 'abnormal' behaviour. This is a particular problem where people have severe/profound learning disabilities and are unable to communicate their inner experiences or feelings, since careful psychiatric diagnosis depends on precisely this. In such circumstances, psychiatric diagnoses are at best unreliable and at worst unhelpful labels.

In studies which have employed standard measures to examine rates of psychiatric disorder and challenging behaviour in people with varied degrees of learning disabilities there have been contradictory results, some showing considerable overlap (Sturmey and Ley, 1990; Jacobson, 1982) and some little overlap (Fraser *et al.*, 1986). There are only a few studies which have employed truly 'independent' indicators of psychiatric disorders in severely disabled people. The best of these, by Wing and colleagues, has suggested that social impairment, as a facet of autism, may be associated with an increased likelihood of challenging behaviours (Wing, 1981).

For people with mild learning disabilities who can communicate their feelings and beliefs it is, however, possible to diagnose mental illness accurately and, while this may at times co-exist with challenging behaviour, the two are not necessarily causally related, though they may sometimes be (Holland and Murphy, 1990).

In conclusion, it appears that a variety of conditions are associated with increased rates of challenging behaviour. These conditions include learning disabilities themselves (most challenging behaviours becoming more common as the degree of disability increases), epilepsy, Fragile-X and possibly autism and other mental illnesses. The neurobiological basis of many of these conditions is quite unknown and, even where it is beginning to be understood, the links between the neurobiology and behaviour remain obscure. Only two conditions are clearly sufficient to produce particular forms of challenging behaviour: Lesch–Nyhan syndrome and Prader–Willi syndrome. In these cases, it seems likely that direct causal pathways may be established in the next few years. However, for the remaining conditions, it appears that, since the conditions are neither necessary nor sufficient for the appearance of challenging behaviours, any links will be multifactorial and/or indirect.

## Operant factors

It has been clear for many years that challenging behaviour can be learnt and that this is just as true for children and adults with learning disabilities as it is for those without learning disabilities. Operant learning theory is particularly important in considerations of how children and adults with severe learning disabilities acquire challenging behaviours. Social learning theory is likely to be less important since modelling and vicarious learning are often not part of the repertoires of people with severe and profound learning disabilities (Clements, 1987).

In principle, challenging behaviours may be considered to be operant behaviours learnt in one of two ways: by positive reinforcement (presentation of rewards) or negative reinforcement (removal of aversive stimuli). Much of the research on operant learning is based on animal learning and the process of such learning may be described by the following model, where A stands for antecedents, B for behaviour and C for consequences:

$$A \rightarrow B \rightarrow C$$

When the consequences (C) of a behaviour are reinforcing, the likelihood of the behaviour recurring in the presence of the antecedents (A) increases in a way which can be predicted by the reinforcement schedule (Blackman, 1974; Walker, 1987). If the consequences are not reinforcing, the behaviour tends to extinguish. Positive and negative reinforcers are unequivocally defined by their effect and may be primary or secondary in nature. Primary reinforcers are those associated with biological needs (e.g., food and drink). Secondary reinforcers (e.g., wages) are those stimuli which come to exert reinforcing effects as a result of their pairing with primary reinforcers. Whether social stimuli are primary reinforcers and whether all primary reinforcers are related to biological needs are controversial points (Walker, 1987) but, generally, positive reinforcers can be considered to include rewarding events, such as social praise, food and drink, and negative reinforcers usually remove aversive stimuli (i.e., those which the person would escape or avoid), such as excessively difficult tasks, noisy or cold environments.

Precisely what stimuli act as positive or negative reinforcers depends on the client him/herself: for many autistic people, for example, social praise may not be reinforcing and social closeness may be aversive; for people with a very profound hearing loss music may not be reinforcing but vibration might be; for people unable to chew food, chocolate biscuits may not be reinforcing but chocolate milkshakes may be. There is considerable evidence that individual preferences for different positive reinforcers can be extreme, very specific and quite enduring (Murphy, 1982). The same may well be true for aversive stimuli (Gaylord-Ross, 1982).

The effectiveness of all reinforcers is dependent upon short-term satiation and deprivation effects. If someone is satiated with food, for example, it is unlikely to act as a reinforcer (until some time later). On the other hand, if someone is deprived of a reinforcer, such as social attention (e.g., because they are living in an under-staffed environment), then it may act as a very powerful reinforcer, until such a time as the person is satiated.

Antecedent stimuli may come to set off behaviours if those behaviours have been consistently reinforced in the past, in the presence of the antecedent stimuli. So, for example, if a particular family member (e.g., the father) reinforces a particular behaviour, but other family members (e.g., mother, siblings) do not, then that behaviour will come to occur in the presence of the father but not of the mother and siblings and the father could be said to be the discriminative stimulus for the behaviour.

In addition, some changes in the environment make certain behaviours more likely to occur even though these conditions are not discriminative stimuli (i.e., have not been specifically associated with reinforcers in the past). For example, the presentation of difficult tasks may raise the likelihood of an escape response, whether or not such responses have been reinforced in the past. Such environmental conditions are known as establishing operations (Michael, 1982; see also Chapter 10) and they can include deprivation states. For many behaviours, there may also be more general conditions which make the behaviours more likely to occur and these are referred to as setting conditions. They differ from establishing operations in that they have a broader and less specific effect on behaviour (Michael, 1982).

The other important aspect of operant learning is that of the schedules of reinforcement. Reinforcers can be provided after every response (continuous reinforcement) or after a fixed number of responses (fixed ratio schedule), a variable number of responses (variable ratio schedule), a fixed length of time (fixed interval schedule) or variable length of time (variable interval schedule). The different schedules have different effects on response rates. Continuous schedules produce the fastest initial learning though, once established, behaviours which only receive occasional reinforcement are most resistant to extinction (the partial reinforcement effect) and this is often a very important factor in the maintenance of chronic challenging behaviour.

The importance of positive social reinforcement in the maintenance of challenging behaviours among people with learning disabilities has been demonstrated in numerous studies. Lovaas *et al.* (1965), for example, showed that if carers responded to a child's self-injurious behaviour (SIB) by warm, caring social responses his SIB increased. Similarly, Carr and MacDowell (1980) found that parental comments to their son every time he scratched his face led to an increase in scratching. Equally, responding to aggressive behaviour (slapping) with social comments was demonstrated to increase the frequency of slapping in a young man with learning disabilities (Martin and Foxx, 1973). In both of these last two studies, it was also shown that non-presentation of the presumed reinforcer (social attention) led to a reduction in the self-scratching (Carr and MacDowell, 1980) and in the aggression (Martin and Foxx, 1973) of the clients concerned.

It is more difficult to discover examples of people showing challenging behaviours which have been reinforced by non-social stimuli, such as sensory stimuli or tangible events. However, there are descriptions of children and adults who showed challenging behaviours which appeared to be reinforced by the sensation produced or by the provision of drinks or food given by adults contingent on their behaviour (Rincover, 1978; Durand and Crimmins, 1988; Smith, M.D., 1985).

Evidence also exists that challenging behaviours may be learnt as escape/avoidance behaviours which are reinforced by the termination of aversive stimuli, i.e. by a process of negative reinforcement. For example, Carr *et al.* (1976) showed that presenting demands increased the frequency of self-injury in a young boy and it seemed likely that the behaviour had been reinforced in the past by the cessation of demands subsequent to his self-injury. Similarly, Carr and others have demonstrated that other challenging behaviours also appear in the presence of demands, for example, aggression (Carr *et al.*, 1980), tantrums (Carr and Newsom, 1985) and stereotyped behaviour (Durand and Carr, 1983, quoted in Carr and Durand, 1985b). It was proposed by Carr and colleagues that these behaviours had been reinforced in the past by removal of the demands contingent on the challenging behaviour. As might be predicted, certain reinforcement schedules produced characteristic patterns of responding and procedures which involved the provision of escape from the demands (e.g., 'time out') resulted in increased responding (Carr and Durand, 1985b). Moreover, stimuli which signalled the end or the removal of a task appeared to act as 'safety signals' and were followed by a rapid cessation of responding (Carr and Durand, 1985b). Reducing the difficulty of tasks has also been shown to reduce the challenging behaviour, presumably by reducing the 'aversiveness' of the task (Gaylord-Ross, 1982).

Examples of aversive stimuli other than demands are less well documented. Presumably, loud noise, cold and being attacked by others may all be aversive stimuli and may act as establishing operations for escape behaviours, and the escape behaviours may increase if as a consequence the aversive situation ceases or is removed. Interestingly, Oliver *et al.* (in press) have demonstrated that for some people close social contact appears to be aversive, sets the occasion for self-injurious behaviour and has in all probability been reinforced in the past by the consequence of social distancing.

During the 1960s and 1970s a vast number of research studies were published, particularly in journals such as the *Journal of Applied Behavior Analysis*, demonstrating that challenging behaviours could also be unlearnt, i.e., that operant principles could be employed to reduce challenging behaviours by, for example, stimulus control, extinction, differential reinforcement of other appropriate behaviours, time-out from positive reinforcement and other punishment techniques (Murphy and Oliver, 1987). In the 1980s there was a growing emphasis on constructional approaches which aimed to build competencies rather than merely to eliminate challenging behaviour (Goldiamond, 1974; Cullen and Partridge, 1981) and on selecting the least restrictive alternatives (Rapoff *et al.*, 1980; Donnellan *et al.*, 1988).

The increased understanding of the possible roles of various social, tangible and sensory stimuli as reinforcers maintaining challenging behaviours has also led to a renaissance of interest in functional analysis since it was clear that making an incorrect assumption about the reinforcers maintaining a behaviour could lead to unsuccessful treatment (Murphy and Oliver, 1987). Early on in behavioural treatment research, it was frequently asserted that a functional analysis was necessary prior to treatment, i.e., that the function of the various stimuli should be clarified before embarking on treatment (Kiernan, 1973; Owens and Ashcroft, 1982). In practice, though, scant attention was paid to such an analysis, apart from the use of standard ABC charts (e.g., Murphy, 1987).

More recently, however, a number of possible methods of functional analysis have emerged, including questionnaire measures, use of analogue conditions and naturalistic observations. These will be illustrated with reference to self-injurious behaviour, for which some of the methods were first developed, because of their importance in aiding the understanding of challenging behaviour.

In 1982, Iwata and colleagues described a way of analysing the function of people's self-injurious behaviour by observing the effect of repeated brief exposure to a standard set of settings, 'analogue conditions', designed to mimic conditions which might occur naturally (Iwata *et al.*, 1982). In the 'social disapproval' condition, the children or young adults, all of whom had severe/ profound learning disabilities, were provided with self-occupational equipment by an adult who remained present and interacted with them (expressed social disapproval) only if they displayed self-injurious behaviour. In the 'academic demand' condition, the clients were seated at a table with the adult, who asked them to complete a task which was known to be quite difficult for them. Successful responding, with or without prompts, was followed by social praise and self-injury was followed by brief removal of the task. In the 'alone' condition, the client was in the room alone, without staff or equipment and in the 'unstructured play' condition, the clients were given self-occupational equipment, self-injury was ignored and the adult present reinforced appropriate behaviour with social praise. The settings were designed to mimic conditions in which SIB was attention-maintained (social disapproval condition) or reinforced by escape from demands (demand condition) or reinforced by sensory feedback (alone condition). The unstructured play condition was a control/comparison setting.

The results demonstrated that, for four of the nine children, SIB was highest in the alone condition, suggesting that their SIB had the function of self-stimulation in barren conditions. For two children, their SIB was highest in the demand condition, suggesting that their SIB had the function of escaping from demands. One child showed highest rates of SIB in the social disapproval condition, suggesting attention-maintained SIB, and two showed similar levels of SIB in all conditions. The significance of the study was that it allowed a better understanding of the operant function of the children's self-injurious behaviour and hence permitted logical treatment plans to be developed. In contrast, the application of behavioural treatment plans in an absence of any understanding of the function of the behaviour may well fail (Murphy and Oliver, 1987).

Since then, the use of analogue conditions as a method of a functional analysis has become widely accepted, although minor disputes have arisen over the precise form of the conditions, the need for observing collateral behaviours and the best ways of interpreting the eventual data (Oliver, 1991a, b; Oliver *et al.*, in press).

In addition, some questionnaires or rating scales for deriving function have been developed (Durand and Crimmins, 1988; 1991) and some sophisticated techniques for interpreting function from naturalistic observations have appeared (Burgess, 1987). The advantages and disadvantages of these different techniques for determining the function of behaviour have been described by Oliver (1991a) and Durand and Crimmins (1991). The only study to date to have compared the outcome for a group of clients using all three different methods has shown poor agreement across methods (Oliver, 1991b). Methods for determining the operant function of challenging behaviours are thus clearly in their infancy.

Before leaving the issue of the role of operant factors in challenging behaviours, there is one further recent development which requires explanation. Children's and adults' challenging behaviours often have an effect on their social world. For example, when a child with learning disabilities engages in a bout of head-hitting, the carers or parents who observe this frequently conclude that (s)he is unhappy or uncomfortable or needs something but is unable to ask because of communication deficits. They may therefore go over to the child and offer comfort or food or drink or they may stop doing a task or action, feeling it is upsetting the child. Their own behaviour will be negatively reinforced if the child then stops self-injuring (presuming they find his/her self-injury aversive). The child and carers or parents may thus fall into what Oliver has termed the SIB trap, may be locked into a system of 'control and counter-control' (Oliver, 1991b) and the child's SIB will increase in frequency just as the parents' action will also increase in frequency. From the carer's or parent's view, the child's SIB has acted as a form of communicative act, or what Bates (1976) would term a protoimperative or protodeclarative act, resembling the early communicative act of crying in a young baby (Bell and Ainsworth, 1972). The same argument holds for other challenging behaviours of course and for adults as well as children with learning disabilities.

Within a constructional approach, therefore, it is possible to argue that the best way to tackle such behaviour might be to teach the client more appropriate communicative responses (Carr and Durand, 1985b) and Carr and Durand have attempted precisely this with autistic children showing challenging behaviour (Carr and Durand, 1985a). They demonstrated that it was possible to teach verbal requests to match the function of the children's challenging behaviour (derived by analogue conditions) and that this then resulted in a reduction of challenging behaviours without other interventions being necessary. The problem of teaching similar non-verbal responses to less able children and adults with severe learning disabilities and no demonstrable language is immense. However, some initial studies of this approach, involving differential reinforcement of communicative behaviour or functional communication training, with non-verbal adults, have appeared (Durand and Kishi, 1987; Steege *et al.*, 1990).

In summary, operant factors clearly have an important role in the maintenance of challenging behaviour. Recent developments in the field have shown that operant learning is sufficient to maintain a variety of challenging behaviours and that functional analysis may assist carers and parents in understanding such behaviour (and designing logical treatment plans). Challenging behaviours can often be seen as early forms of communication between the individual with learning disabilities and others and, while this may not be goal-directed on the part of the client, it may be helpful to view the behaviours as communicative and to consider the possibility of developing other more appropriate ways of communicating as a way of reducing the challenging behaviour.

### Ecological factors

Human ecology is the study of the interaction of people with their environment or, as Bronfenbrenner (1979) put it, with respect to development:

> The ecology of human development involves the scientific study of the progressive, mutual accommodation between an active, growing human being and the changing properties of the immediate settings in which the developing person lives, as this process is affected by relations between these settings and by the larger contexts in which the settings are embedded. (Bronfenbrenner, 1979, p. 21)

Bronfenbrenner divided the environment into microsystems ('the pattern of activities, roles and interpersonal relations experienced by the developing person in a given setting with particular physical and material characteristics', Bronfenbrenner, 1979, p. 22), mesosystems (the interrelations between two or more settings such as school, family and neighbourhood), exosystems (settings outside the mesosystems but affecting them or being affected by them) and macrosystems (systems at the subcultural or cultural level). He saw the systems as nested within one another and considered important changes within people's lives to be ecological transitions (from one setting or one role to another).

The impact of Western thought and culture (the macrosystem) on the lives of people with learning disabilities is obviously enormous and the ideas of normalization or social role valorization (Nirje, 1969; Wolfensberger, 1980a; 1983) were intended to alter the macrosystem (Chapter 9). So far they have only resulted in widespread changes to the microsystems and mesosystems in which people reside and to their daily activities, perhaps because of the enthusiasm with which the ideas have been taught to community-based carers. The ideas have had relatively little impact on the attitudes and beliefs of people with no direct contact with individuals with learning disabilities. Consideration of ecological factors in relation to challenging behaviour will therefore be restricted to two issues at the microsystem and mesosystem level with direct relevance to understanding challenging behaviour: firstly, the effects of early family life on the development of such behaviour; and secondly, the effects of the changes in residential placement from institution to community home that have been so much a part of recent experience for people with learning disabilities.

One strand in the argument that ecological factors are of importance in understanding challenging behaviours comes from research into parenting and family life. A variety of measures of home life and parenting have been developed and it has become clear that particular aspects of family life predict particular difficulties in the children.

Caldwell and colleagues (Bradley and Caldwell, 1976; Bradley, 1985), for example, developed a measure called the HOME inventory (Home Observation for Measurement of the Environment) which examined six aspects of home life for infants: maternal responsivity, maternal acceptance, environmental organization, provision and variety of toys, maternal involvement with the child and variety of daily stimulation. They demonstrated that the child's ability at four and a half years was very strongly correlated with the HOME scores at six months and a variety of other similar results have been obtained by other researchers using the HOME inventory. Similarly, Nihira and colleagues have shown that higher levels of educational stimulation on their measure of home environment predicted intellectual development in children with learning disabilities (Nihira *et al.*, 1980; 1985).

In contrast, it appears that challenging behaviours are predicted by conflict, disorganization and discontinuity in the home, at least for children without severe learning disabilities. Richardson *et al.* (1985), for example, examined the rates of behaviour disturbance amongst young adults with and without mild learning disabilities in Aberdeen. They found that the frequency of behaviour disturbance increased for both groups as conditions of upbringing measured over the first 15 years of life became more unstable (i.e. when upbringing was rated as more discontinuous, discordant or disorganized and/or more characterized by neglect). Nihira *et al.* (1980) reported similar findings for children with learning disabilities, with increased ratings of disorganization and conflict at home being linked to increased challenging behaviour, while Werner and Smith (1980) found much the same in their Kuaii study, with poor parental emotional support and understanding predicting less improvement in behavioural difficulties during adolescence.

Many of these studies have been undertaken with large geographical samples of children, some of whom have developed learning disabilities while most have not and some of whom have shown challenging behaviours while most have not. It seems clear from the studies that poverty alone does not lead to learning disabilities or challenging behaviours. Rather, it requires poor intellectual/educational stimulation to produce mild learning disabilities and disorganized, conflictual and unresponsive parenting to produce challenging behaviours. Where all of these characteristics apply within a family then both mild learning disabilities and challenging behaviours are likely in the children. However, this is not necessarily true for severe learning disabilities, which are of largely biological origin. It may be that the same features of family life tend to produce challenging behaviour in children with severe learning disabilities as with mild learning disabilities but as yet there are no research studies which bear directly on this issue.

The birth of a child who is likely to develop learning disabilities (for example, a child with Down's syndrome) also has an effect on the family, with many parents going through stages of shock, denial and adaptation (Carr, 1985). Later on, families may cope with the task of bringing up a child with added difficulties extremely well but there is undoubtedly an extra burden of caregiving (estimated in one study as an average of seven hours' care a day) and an increased restriction particularly in the lives of the mothers, who are often less able than other mothers to obtain paid work outside the home (Carr, 1985, 1988). The intellectual ability of the child does not appear to be an important factor in family adaptation but the presence of challenging behaviours in the child, social isolation in the parents and family adversity in general (e.g., being a single parent, having unsuitable housing, having health problems in other family members) all make it more likely that the mother in the family will feel highly stressed (Quine and Pahl, 1985). This in turn makes depression (in the mothers) and alterations in mother–child interactions more likely, which may further exacerbate any challenging behaviours in the child. The effects of the child with learning disabilities on the family and of the family on the child are thus bidirectional and complex (Crnic *et al.*, 1983; Nihira *et al.*, 1985).

People who show challenging behaviour are known to be most at risk of admission and re-admission to hospital and they are usually the last to be discharged (Sutter *et al.*, 1980). Hospital environments are characterized by institution-oriented practices, relatively low staffing levels and poor environmental standards (King *et al.*, 1971; Raynes *et al.*, 1979) as well as low levels of staff–client engagement (Felce *et al.*, 1986). Moreover, they tend to provide 'closed' environments, with clients rarely visiting parts of the general community and tending to have few visitors from outside.

In the 1960s and 1970s, institutions were heavily criticized by both sociologists (e.g., Goffman, 1961) and by psychologists (e.g., Tizard, 1974), for a number of these features. The subsequent advent of the normalization movement, 'the use of culturally valued means in order to enable people to live culturally valued lives' (Nirje, 1969; Wolfensberger, 1980a), caused people increasingly to question the appropriateness of institutional life for those who engaged in challenging behaviour. Certainly, it seemed unlikely that those remaining housed within institutions would achieve any of O'Brien's five objectives of choice, competence, community presence, participation and respect (O'Brien, 1987). Moreover, they could not adopt valued social roles within institutions, something which Wolfensberger (1983) considered was the most important goal for people with disabilities.

The ideas of normalization/social role valorization certainly have some importance in the understanding of challenging behaviour. It is a common observation that people with a long history of such behaviour are often disliked within a service and treated with less respect than other clients. This may well have effects on their self-esteem and on the appearance of challenging behaviour. It seems unlikely, however, even if they had valued social roles, that the challenging behaviours (e.g., physical or sexual assaults) of some people would ever become valued in themselves (cf. Wolfensberger, 1980b).

A growing number of research projects in the UK and elsewhere have examined the effects of deinstitutionalization on people's quality of life, skills and behaviour. It is agreed that, in general, moves into the community are accompanied by improvements in the direction of normalization in the physical environment and increases in community presence for residents, except when the new residential placement is simply a small hospital-type unit (Shah and Holmes, 1987). Some evidence exists of increases in adaptive skills though this is certainly not invariable (Allen, 1989). It also appears that major increases in people's engagement in constructive activities are possible but not inevitable when they move from institutions to community homes (Felce *et al.*, 1986; Allen, 1989; Mansell and Beasley, 1990; see also Chapter 6). Certainly, neither increases in engagement nor adaptive behaviours will result simply from increases in staffing levels (Landesman-Dwyer, 1981) and both Landesman and others have argued that there is enormous variation in community placements both within them, for different residents and between them (Landesman and Butterfield, 1987).

The implications of deinstitutionalization and normalization/SRV for the understanding of challenging behaviour are multiple and complex. Firstly, it is clear that high engagement levels and skill development are almost never possible in hospital environments for people with severe learning disabilities, so that it has to be concluded that institutions are unlikely to reduce challenging behaviours because of increased adaptive behaviours. On the other hand, challenging behaviours may decline in community settings as adaptive behaviours and engagement levels increase (e.g., Bratt and Johnston, 1988) but this is not inevitable (as might indeed be predicted from an understanding of the operant factors involved). People whose challenging behaviours have the function of avoiding/escaping from demands, for example, would be expected to show an increase in challenging behaviours if demands increase, as is likely in a community setting, whereas those whose behaviours have self-stimulatory functions might be expected to show decreases in challenging behaviours (for related discussions, see Chapters 5 and 6).

Secondly, it has to be said that, although Wolfensberger asserts that deviant behaviour is the result of social devaluation, this may be an ideological position rather than a scientific one, since there is little evidence to date to demonstrate that simply providing people with more valued social roles necessarily reduces their challenging behaviour.

## Towards-an integrated view

In the understanding of challenging behaviour, there is a tendency towards polarization which works against real understanding. Wolfensberger (1980a, p. 12), for example, views the medical model and therefore presumably the biological model as not only unhelpful but as definitely harmful, because of its devaluing and segregating effects. Equally, Throne (1975), Mesibov (1990) and others have criticized normalization for being simplistic, idealistic and unrealistic. Meanwhile, those who adhere to models of learning theory are at times rejecting of biological models and *vice versa*.

It has been argued here that biological factors may contribute to the appearance of challenging behaviours in people with learning disabilities but, although they may be occasionally seen as sufficient (for example, in Lesch–Nyhan and Prader–Willi syndrome) they are never necessarily present for particular challenging behaviours. Equally, it was argued that operant learning could be shown to be a sufficient cause for challenging behaviours but was not invariably a necessary factor. It appeared too that ecological factors might be important in understanding challenging behaviours although again they were not necessarily always present. There are, then, three sets of factors, all of which may be important and the difficulty is to see how to develop an integrated view.

Firstly, it has to be recognized that the different views about the genesis and maintenance of challenging behaviours are not in-compatible. There are, for example, demonstrations of effective operant/behavioural treatments for the reduction of self-injuri-ous behaviour in people with Lesch–Nyhan syndrome (Bull and LaVecchio, 1978). Equally, it has been argued that behavioural views are by no means incompatible with those of normalization (Emerson and McGill, 1989; Kiernan, 1991) and there are a num-ber of examples of services where the ecological and the operant views have been integrated (Emerson, 1990; see also Chapter 6).

Secondly, although it would be possible to view certain charac-teristics as predispositions or 'risk factors' (e.g., organic factors), this would probably lead to an over-simplification in that it might imply that those factors operated first and then other factors followed. While this may be the case at times, it is much more likely that the interactions between the factors are dynamic rather than static, so that the interactions between factors may be bi-directional, continuous and progressive.

Figure 3.1 illustrates the way in which the various factors might interact for a child with epilepsy while Figures 3.2 and 3.3 show how the factors might interact for a child with Prader–Willi syn-drome. The examples are based on clinical cases but will not, of course, be true for all children with epilepsy or Prader–Willi syndrome. The first case is intended to illustrate a situation in which organic factors play a relatively small initial role in the eventual appearance of challenging behaviour (aggression), the major factors being the parental expectations, set up within the micro- and mesosystems by a mistaken GP, and the operant learning which followed. The second example shows how organic factors can have a more enduring relevance to the appearance of challenging behaviour, which in this case involved tantrums and family arguments over food and stealing of food outside the home. Social factors were important at a micro-, meso-, exo- and macrosystem level and operant learning was also an intricate part of the difficulties.

Similar models can be found for other challenging behaviours in Oliver and Head (1990), Clare *et al.* (in press), Murphy (in press), together with discussions of intervention effectiveness.

In the first example, an apparently healthy baby boy led to no worries until, at the age of two and a half years, the child began to have epileptic seizures sometimes in the day and sometimes at night. This was associated with a loss of the child's early language

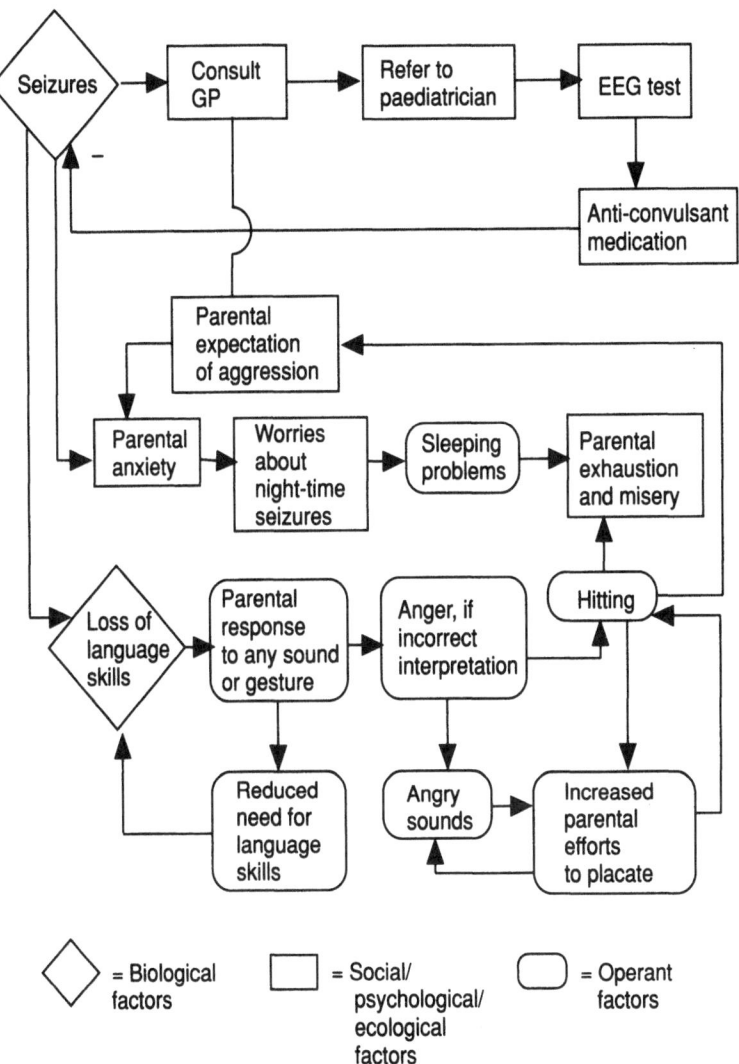

**Figure 3.1** Biological, social/psychological/ecological and operant factors in the life of a boy with epilepsy.

and caused immense parental anxiety. The GP explained to the parents that most seizures could be controlled by anticonvulsants but that the child was likely to have an 'epileptic personality' (the latter being a myth). The GP said to the parents that this meant the

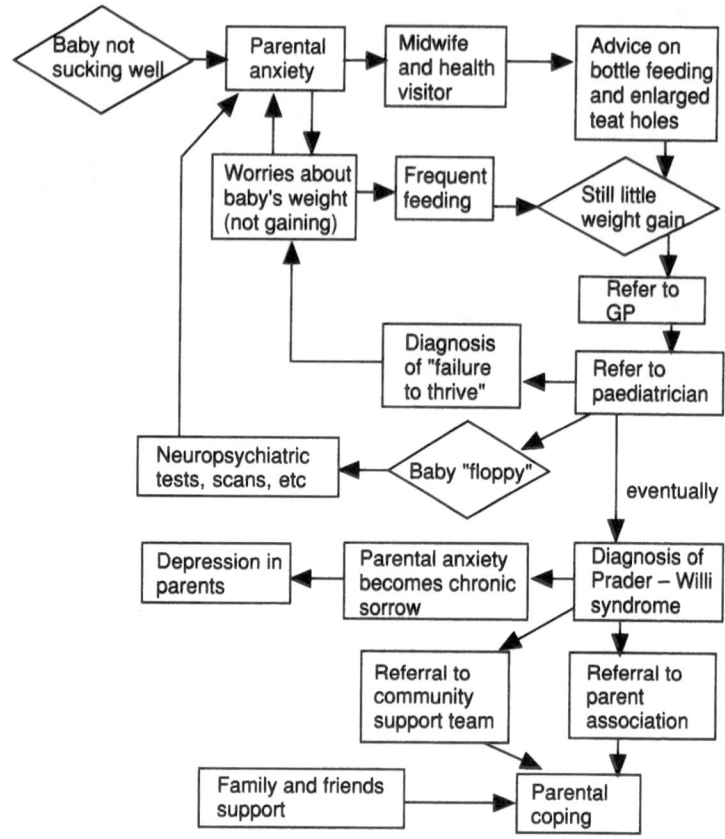

**Figure 3.2**   Biological, social/psychological/ecological and operant factors in the life of a young person with Prader–Willi syndrome. The early years.

boy would be more irritable than most children and liable to temper outbursts and aggression later on. He referred the family to a paediatrician who arranged an EEG, confirmed that the seizures were epileptic and started the boy on anticonvulsant therapy. Due to the long waiting time in the hospital, the need for an EEG and the consultant paediatrician's lengthy list, the appointment was brief and the paediatrician omitted to dispel any myths which the parents held about epilepsy.

The loss of language was frustrating and stressful for the parents (and the boy). They tried to anticipate their son's needs and

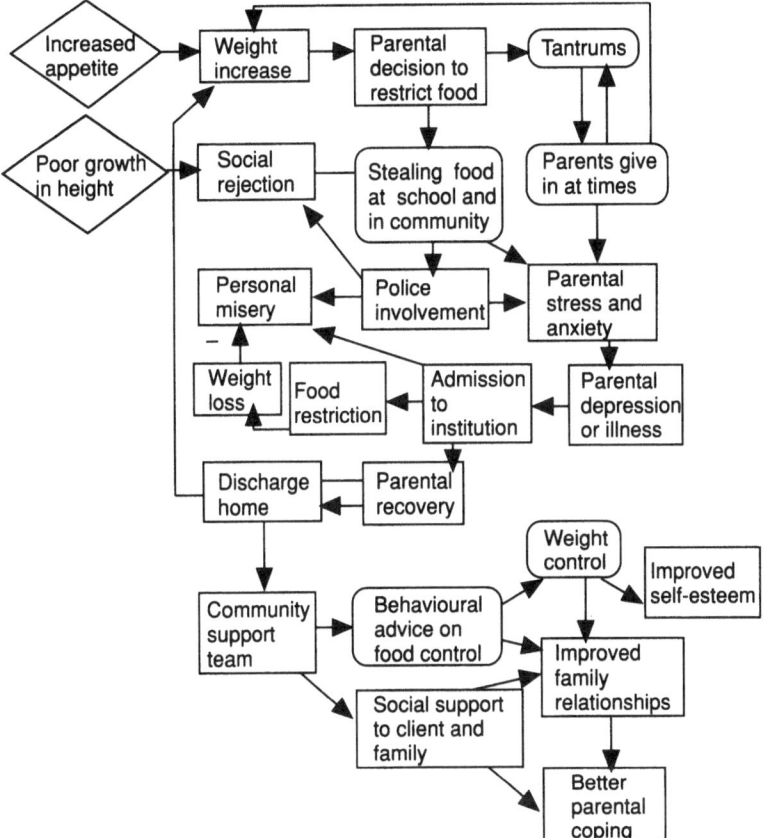

**Figure 3.3** Biological, social/psychological/ecological and operant factors in the life of a young person with Prader–Willi syndrome. Later years.

to react to any sounds he made by trying to find him what he wanted. Angry noises simply made the parents try harder to guess 'what he really means' and to pacify the child. The boy learnt that most of his needs could be met without the use of language. When he requested a fifth biscuit one day just before lunch and his mother refused he hit her and she gave him the biscuit 'because it must be so frustrating for him, he doesn't understand'. The boy's aggressive behaviour was thus reinforced and became more likely to recur. The parents saw this simply as the fulfilment of the GP's prophecy.

Meanwhile, their worry that he might have fits at night that would go undetected led them to allow him into their bed at night. However, the boy was a light sleeper and the outcome was exhausted parents with a non-existent sex-life. Without good social support, the most probable outcome is a depressed mother, a stressed and disenchanted father, who may leave the family, and an increasingly aggressive little boy. The need for a community-based support team to provide behavioural advice, speech therapy and a nursery place at least is clear. In the absence of such an intervention, it seems likely that the boy will eventually start school but be excluded as an aggressive boy and be at risk of ending up in an institution when his parents can no longer cope.

In the second example, of a child with Prader–Willi syndrome, parental worry and anxiety began with the birth of a baby girl who was unable to suck well but appeared otherwise healthy. The parents consulted the midwife and then the health visitor. They were advised to give up breast feeding and try bottle feeding, using teats with enlarged holes. As the baby still had trouble sucking, the family consulted the GP, who diagnosed possible failure to thrive and referred the family to the local paediatrician. This did not lead immediately to diagnosis (since Prader–Willi syndrome is difficult to diagnose) and, as the parents were still anxious about the child, a lack of clear diagnosis (and hence no clear prognosis) simply increased their anxiety. Even when a diagnosis was made, the gloomy prognosis led to some reduction in parental anxiety but feelings of chronic sorrow instead. If this were combined with poor social support (e.g., a lack of confidants) and/or the presence of other children under five years and/or other social risk factors (poverty, poor housing, unemployment) then depression in the parents would be likely. With better social support from friends or relatives or from a parent support group or community support team, parental depression might be averted. The support team might help the family to work with the child to help her learn cognitive, social and self-help skills (e.g., by enrolment on a Portage programme). This might reduce the probable developmental delay, which would otherwise be likely to increase parental anxieties about their child's future.

Later on, as increased appetite led the child to eat more, the parents became worried by the child's weight increase and tried to restrict her food intake, first by suggestion and then by locking cupboards and refrigerators. The child reacted with tantrums because she was, presumably, feeling a real hunger. This distressed the parents, who occasionally gave in on the basis that the child seemed 'really' hungry. This reinforced the tantrums and eventually the resultant increase in the frequency of this and other related behaviours, such as stealing food while at school/out in the community, led to such levels of parental stress and depression (e.g., after police involvement) that the child was admitted to an institution for a period. Strict control of food intake here led to weight loss, while the absence of the child at home allowed some parental recovery, though the child was unhappy away from home. The child was then discharged home but the cycle was likely to begin again, unless an intervention was made available from a local support team. Increasingly, as the child became a teenager and eventually an adult, she was treated as 'abnormal' by others and socially rejected, particularly by people who did not know her, because she was very short and overweight. She developed a desire to be slimmer and to look 'normal' but her appetite made this very difficult. This, combined with a probable social isolation, particularly when she left school, might also put her at risk of becoming depressed, though continued assistance from a local support team might be able to avert this.

### Summary

Biological, operant and ecological factors in the development and maintenance of challenging behaviours are all of importance. Specific syndromes are sometimes sufficient to produce particular challenging behaviours but there are no known behaviours which are invariably linked to biological conditions. Biological or organic factors can therefore be seen as sometimes sufficient but not as necessary for the appearance of challenging behaviour. Very often, even when biological factors can be identified, they may be difficult to ameliorate.

Operant factors have also been demonstrated to be sufficient to produce and maintain challenging behaviours. Both positive and negative reinforcement are important and an understanding of establishing operations, discriminative stimuli and schedules of reinforcement is essential to elucidating how challenging behaviours may develop and how they may be eliminated. Recent emphasis on determining the function of a person's behaviour and on constructional solutions has improved the likelihood of efficacy in behavioural assessment and intervention with challenging behaviours.

Finally, ecological views of learning disabilities can be seen as relevant to the development of challenging behaviour at the micro-, meso-, exo- and macrosystem levels. Two important areas of ecological influence, early family life and later residential setting, are reviewed with respect to their probable influence on challenging behaviours.

For those working with children or adults with challenging behaviours, the most difficult task may be to develop an integrated view of how biological, operant and ecological factors interact. Two case examples are given which illustrate how such integrated models may be developed for individuals to provide starting points for the understanding of their needs and the planned amelioration of their challenging behaviour.

## References

Alberman, E. (1984) Epidemiological aspects of severe mental retardation, in *Scientific Studies in Mental Retardation* (eds F. Dobbing, A.D.B. Clarke, J.A. Corbett, J. Hogg and R.O. Robinson). London: Royal Society of Medicine, pp. 3–23.

Allen, D. (1989) The effects of deinstitutionalization on people with mental handicaps. *Mental Handicap Research*, 2, 18–37.

Bates, E. (1976) *Language and Context*. New York: Academic Press.

Bell, S.M. and Ainsworth, M.D.S. (1972) Infant crying and maternal responsiveness. *Child Development*, 43, 1171–90.

Birch, H., Richardson, S.A., Baird, D., Horobin, G. and Illsley, R (1970) *Mental Subnormality in the Community: A Clinical Epidemiological Study*. Baltimore, MD: Williams and Wilkins.

Blackman, D (1974) *Operant Conditioning: An Experimental Analysis of Behaviour*. London: Methuen.

Blundell, J.E. (1990) Appetite disturbance and the problems of overweight. *Drugs Supplement*, 39, 1–19.

Borghgraef, M., Fryns, J.P., Van den Bergh, R., Ryck, K. and Van den Berghe, H. (1990) The post-pubertal Fra (X) male: A study of the intelligence and the psychological profile of 17 Fra (X) boys, in *Key Issues in Mental Retardation Research* (ed. W.I. Fraser). London: Routledge, pp. 94–105.

Bradley, R. (1985) The HOME inventory: Rationale and research, in *Recent Research in Developmental Psychopathology* (ed. J.E. Stevenson). Oxford: Pergamon Press, pp. 191–201.

Bradley, R. and Caldwell, B. (1976) The relationship of infants' home environments to mental test performance at fifty-four months: A follow-up study. *Child Development*, **47**, 1171–74.

Bratt, A. and Johnston, R. (1988) Changes in life style for young adults with profound handicaps following discharge from hospital care into a 'second generation' housing project. *Mental Handicap Research*, **1**, 49–74.

Bronfenbrenner, U. (1979) *The Ecology of Human Development*. Cambridge, MA: Harvard University Press.

Bull, M. and LaVecchio, F (1978) Behaviour therapy for a child with Lesch–Nyhan Syndrome. *Developmental Medicine and Child Neurology*, **20**, 368–75.

Burgess, A. (1987) *Functional Analysis of Self-injurious Behaviour using Direct Observations: A Comparison with Interview and Analogue Methods.* Unpublished MSc Thesis, University of Surrey.

Carr, E.G. and Durand, V.M. (1985a) Reducing behavior problems through functional communication training. *Journal of Applied Behavior Analysis*, **18**, 111–26.

Carr, E.G. and Durand, V.M. (1985b) The social communicative basis of severe behaviour problems in children, in *Theoretical Issues in Behaviour Therapy* (eds S. Reiss and R. Bootzin). New York: Academic Press, pp. 219–54.

Carr, E.G. and McDowell, J.J. (1980) Social control of self-injurious behavior of organic etiology. *Behavior Therapy*, **11**, 402–9.

Carr, E.G. and Newsom, C.D. (1985) Demand-related tantrums: Conceptualisation and treatment. *Behavior Modification*, **9**, 403–26.

Carr, E.G., Newsom, C.D. and Binkoff, J.A. (1976) Stimulus control of self-destructive behavior in a psychotic child. *Journal of Abnormal Child Psychology*, **4**, 139–53.

Carr, E.G., Newsom, C.D. and Binkoff, J.A. (1980) Escape as a factor in the aggressive behavior of two retarded children. *Journal of Applied Behavior Analysis*, **13**, 101–17.

Carr, J. (1985) The effect on the family of a severely mentally handicapped child, in *Mental Deficiency: The Changing Outlook* (eds A.M. Clarke, A.D.B. Clarke and J.M. Berg). London: Methuen, pp. 512–548.

Carr, J. (1988) Six weeks to twenty-one years old: A longitudinal study of children with Down's Syndrome and their families. *Journal of Child Psychology and Psychiatry*, **29**, 407–31.

Clare, I.C.H., Murphy, G.H., Cox, D. and Chaplin, E.H. (in press) Assessment and treatment of firesetting: A single case investigation using a cognitive-behavioural model. *Criminal Behaviour and Mental Health*.

Clements, J. (1987) *Severe Learning Disability and Psychological Handicap*. Chichester: John Wiley and Sons.

Christie, R., Bay, C., Kaufman, I.A., Bakay, B., Borden, M. and Nyhan, W.L. (1982) Lesch–Nyhan disease: clinical experience with nineteen patients. *Developmental Medicine and Child Neurology*, **24**, 293–306.

Coid, J., Allolio, B. and Rees, L.H. (1983) Raised plasma metenkephalin in patients who habitually mutilate themselves. *Lancet*, **2**, 545–6.

Crawhill, J.C., Henderson, J.F. and Kelly, W.N. (1972) Diagnosis and treatment of the Lesch–Nyhan Syndrome. *Paediatric Research*, **6**, 504–13.

Crnic, K.A., Friedrick, W.N. and Greenberg, M.T. (1983) Adaptation of families with mentally retarded children: A model of stress, coping and family ecology. *American Journal of Mental Deficiency*, **88**, 125–38.

Cullen, C. and Partridge, K. (1981) The constructional approach: A way of using different data. *Apex: Journal of the British Institute of Mental Handicap*, **8**, 135–6.

Donnellan, A.M., LaVigna, G.W., Negri-Shoultz, N. and Fassbender, L.L. (1988) *Progress Without Punishment*. New York: Teachers College Press.

Durand, V.M. and Crimmins, D.B. (1988) Identifying the variables maintaining self-injurious behaviour. *Journal of Autism and Developmental Disorders*, **18**, 99–117.

Durand, V.M. and Crimmins, D.B. (1991) Teaching functionally equivalent responses as an intervention for challenging behaviour, in *The Challenge of Severe Mental Handicap: A Behaviour Analytic Approach* (ed. B. Remington). Chichester: John Wiley and Sons, pp. 71–95.

Durand, V.M. and Kishi, G. (1987) Reducing severe behavior problems among persons with dual sensory impairments: An evaluation of a technical assistance model. *Journal of the Association for Persons with Severe Handicaps*, **12**, 2–10.

Emerson, E. (1990) Designing individualised community-based placements as an alternative to institutions for people with severe mental handicap and severe problem behaviour, in *Key Issues in Mental Retardation Research* (ed. W.I. Fraser). London: Routledge, pp. 395–404.

Emerson, E. and McGill, P. (1989) Normalisation and applied behaviour analysis: Values and technology in services for people with learning difficulties. *Behavioural Psychotherapy*, **17**, 101–17.

Felce, D., De Kock, U. and Repp, A. (1986) An eco-behavioral analysis of small community based houses and traditional large hospitals for severely and profoundly mentally handicapped adults. *Applied Research in Mental Retardation*, **7**, 393–408.

Fenwick, P (1986) Aggression and epilepsy, in *Aspects of Epilepsy and Psychiatry* (eds M.R. Trimble and T.G. Bolwig). Chichester: John Wiley and Sons, pp.31–60.

Fraser, W.I., Leudar, I., Gray, J. and Campbell, I. (1986) Psychiatric and behaviour disturbance in mental handicap. *Journal of Mental Deficiency Research*, **30**, 49–57.

Gath, A. and Gumley, D. (1987) Retarded children and their siblings. *Journal of Child Psychology and Psychiatry*, **28**, 715–30.

Gaylord-Ross, R.J. (1982) Curricular considerations in treating behavior problems of severely handicapped students, in *Advances in Learning and Behavioral Disabilities*, vol 1 (eds K.D. Gadow and I. Bialer). Greenwich, CT: JAI Press, pp.193–224.

Goffman, E. (1961) *Asylums*. Harmondsworth: Penguin Books.

Goldiamond, I. (1974) Towards a constructional approach to social problems. *Behaviorism*, **2**, 1–84.

Herbert, J. (in press) The neurodendocrinology of aggression, in *The Science and Psychiatry of Violence* (ed. C. Thompson). Oxford: Butterworth-Heinemann.

Holland, A.J. (1991) Learning disability and psychiatric/behavioural disorders: a genetic perspective, in *The New Genetics of Mental Illness* (eds P. McGuffin and R. Murray). Oxford: Butterworth-Heinemann, pp. 245–58.

Holland, T. and Murphy, G. (1990) Behavioural and psychiatric disorder in adults with mild learning difficulties. *International Review of Psychiatry*, **2**, 117–36.

Iwata, B.A, Dorsey, M.F., Slifer, K.J., Bauman, K.E. and Richman, G.S. (1982) Towards a functional analysis of self-injury. *Analysis and Intervention in Developmental Disabilities*, **2**, 3–20.

Jacobson, J.W. (1982) Problem behavior and psychiatric impairment within a developmentally disabled population I: Behavior frequency. *Applied Research in Mental Retardation*, **3**, 121–39.

Kiernan, C.C. (1973) Functional analysis, in *Assessment for Learning in the Mentally Handicapped* (ed. P. Mittler). London: Churchill, pp. 263–91.

Kiernan, C. (1991) Professional ethics: Behaviour analysis and normalisation, in *The Challenge of Severe Mental Handicap: A Behaviour Analytic Approach* (ed. B. Remington). Chichester: John Wiley and Sons, pp. 369–392.

King, R., Raynes, N. and Tizard, J. (1971) *Patterns of Residential Care: Sociological Studies in Institutions for Handicapped Children*. London: Routledge and Kegan Paul.

Koller, H., Richardson, S.A., Katz, M. and McLaren, J. (1982) Behaviour disturbance in childhood and the early adults years in populations who were and were not mentally retarded. *Journal of Preventive Psychiatry*, **1**, 453–68.

Landesman, S. and Butterfield, E.C. (1987) Normalization and deinstitutionalization of mentally retarded individuals: Controversy and facts. *American Psychologist*, **42**, 809–16.

Landesman-Dwyer, S. (1981) Living in the community. *American Journal of Mental Deficiency*, **86**, 223–34.

Lindsay, J., Ounstead, C. and Richards, P. (1979) Long-term outcome in children with temporal lobe seizures. *Developmental Medicine and Child Neurology*, **21**, 630–6.

Lovaas, O.I., Freitag, G., Gold, V.J. and Kassorla, I.C. (1965) Experimental studies in childhood schizophrenia: Analysis of self-destructive behavior. *Journal of Experimental Child Psychology*, **2**, 67–84.

Mansell, J. and Beasley, F. (1990) Severe mental handicap and problem behaviour: Evaluating transfer from institutions to community care, in *Key Issues in Mental Retardation Research* (ed. W. Fraser). London: Routledge, pp. 405–14.

Martin, P.L. and Foxx, R.M. (1973) Victim control of the aggression of an institutionalized retardate. *Journal of Behavior Therapy and Experimental Psychiatry*, **4**, 161–5.

Mesibov, G.B. (1990) Normalisation and its relevance today. *Journal of Autism and Developmental Disorders*, **20**, 379–90.

Michael, J. (1982) Distinguishing between discriminative and motivational functions of stimuli. *Journal of Experimental Analysis of Behavior*, **37**, 149–55.

Murphy, G. (1982) Sensory reinforcement in the autistic and mentally handicapped child: A review. *Journal of Autism and Developmental Disorders*, **12**, 265–78.

Murphy, G. (1987) Direct observation as an assessment tool in functional analysis and treatment, in *Assessment in Mental Handicap: A Guide to Assessment Practices, Tests and Checklists* (eds J. Hogg and N.V. Raynes). London: Croom Helm, pp. 190–238.

Murphy, G. (in press) The treatment of challenging behaviour in people with learning difficulties, in *The Science and Psychiatry of Violence* (ed. C. Thompson). Oxford: Butterworth-Heinemann.

Murphy, G. and Oliver, C. (1987) Decreasing undesirable behaviours, in *Behaviour Modification for People with Mental Handicaps*, 2nd edn (eds W. Yule and J. Carr). London: Croom Helm, pp. 102–42.

Nihira, K., Meyers, C.E. and Mink, I.T. (1980) Home environment, family adjustment and the development of retarded children. *Applied Research in Mental Retardation*, **1**, 5–24.

Nihira, K., Mink, I.T. and Meyers, C.E. (1985) Home environment and development of slow learning adolescents: Reciprocal relations. *Developmental Psychology*, **21**, 784–94.

Nirje, B. (1969) The normalisation principle and its human management implications, in *Changing Patterns in Residential Services for the Mentally Retarded* (eds R. Kugel and W. Wofensberger). Washington, DC: Government Printing Office, pp. 179–95.

O'Brien, J. (1987) A guide to life-style planning: Using The Activities Catalog to integrate services and natural support systems, in *A Comprehensive Guide to the Activities Catalogue: An Alternative Curriculum for Youth and Adults with Severe Disabilities* (eds G.T.Bellamy and B. Wilcox). Baltimore, MD: Paul H. Brookes, pp. 175–89.

Oliver, C. (1991a) The application of analogue methodology to the functional analysis of challenging behaviour, in *The Challenge of Severe Mental Handicap: A Behaviour Analytic Approach*, (ed. B. Remington). Chichester: John Wiley and Sons, pp. 97–118.

Oliver, C. (1991b) *Self-injurious Behaviour in People with Mental Handicap: Prevalence, Individual Characteristics and Functional Analysis*. Unpublished PhD Thesis, University of London.

Oliver, C. and Head, D. (1990) Self-injurious behaviour in people with learning difficulties: Determinants and interventions. *International Review of Psychiatry*, **2**, 101–16.

Oliver, C. and Holland, A.J. (1986) Down's Syndrome and Alzheimer's Disease: A review. *Psychological Medicine*, **16**, 307–22.

Oliver, C., Murphy, G. and Corbett, J.A. (1987) Self-injurious behaviour in people with mental handicap: A total population study. *Journal of Mental Deficiency Research*, **31**, 147–62.

Oliver, C., Crayton, L., Murphy, G. and Corbett, J. (in press) Self-injurious behaviour in Retts Syndrome: Interactions between features of Retts Syndrome and operant conditioning. *Journal of Autism and Developmental Disorders*.

Owens, R.G. and Ashcroft, J.B. (1982) Functional analysis in applied psychology. *British Journal of Clinical Psychology*, **21**, 181–9.

Quine, L. and Pahl, J. (1985) Examining the causes of stress in families with severely mentally handicapped children. *British Journal of Social Work*, **15**, 501–17.

Rapoff, M.A., Altman, K. and Christophersen, E.R. (1980) Suppression of self-injurious behaviour: Determining the least restrictive alternative. *Journal of Mental Deficiency Research*, **24**, 37–46.

Raynes, N., Pratt, M. and Roses, S. (1979) *Organisational Structure and the Care of the Mentally Retarded*. London: Croom Helm.

Richardson, S., Koller, H. and Katz, M. (1985) Relationship of upbringing to later behavior disturbance of mildly mentally retarded young people. *American Journal of Mental Deficiency*, **89**, 1–8.

Rincover, A. (1978) Sensory extinction: a procedure for eliminating self-stimulatory behavior in developmentally disabled children. *Journal of Abnormal Child Psychology*, **6**, 229–310.

Roberts, D.F. (1987) Population genetics of mental handicap, in *Prevention of Mental Handicap: A World View* (eds G. Hosking and G. Murphy). London: Royal Society of Medicine, pp. 9–20.

Rutter, M. Tizard, J. and Whitmore, K. (1970) *Education, Health and Behaviour*. London: Longmans.

Shah, A. and Holmes, N. (1987) Locally-based residential services for mentally handicapped adults: A comparative study. *Psychological Medicine*, **17**, 763–74.

Smith, I. (1985) The hyperphenylalaninaemias, in *Genetic and Metabolic Disease* (eds J.K. Lloyd and C.R. Scriver). London: Butterworths International Medical Reviews, pp.166–209.

Smith, I. and Beasley, M. (1989) Intelligence and behaviour in children with early treated phenylketonuria. *European Journal of Clinical Nutrition*, **43**, 1–5.

Smith, I., Beasley, M.G., Wolff, O.H. and Ades, A.E. (1988) Behaviour disturbance in 8-year old children with early treated phenylketonuria. *Journal of Paediatrics*, **12**, 403–8.

Smith, M.D. (1985) Managing the aggressive and self-injurious behavior of adults disabled by autism. *Journal of the Association for Persons with Severe Handicaps*, **10**, 228–32.

Steege, M.W., Wacker, D.P., Cigrand, K.C., Berg, W.K., Novak, C.G., Reimers, T.M., Sasso, G.M. and DeRaad, A. (1990) Use of negative reinforcement in the treatment of self-injurious behavior. *Journal of Applied Behavior Analysis*, **23**, 459–67.

Stevenson, J.E., Hawcroft, J., Lobascher, M., Smith, I., Wolff, O.H. and Graham, P.J. (1979) Behavioural deviance in children with early treated phenylketonuria. *Archives of Disease in Childhood*, **54**, 14–8.

Sturmey, P. and Ley, T. (1990) The Psychopathology Instrument for Mentally Retarded Adults: Internal consistencies and relationship to behaviour problems. *British Journal of Psychiatry*, **156**, 428–30.

Sutter, P., Mayeda, T., Call, J., Yanagi, G. and Yee, S. (1980) Comparison of successful and unsuccessful community-placed mentally retarded persons. *American Journal of Mental Deficiency*, **85**, 262–7.

Throne, J.M. (1975) Normalisation through the normalisation principle: Right ends, wrong means. *Mental Retardation*, **13**, 23–5.

Tizard, J. (1974) Services and the evaluation of services, in *Mental Deficiency: The Changing Outlook*, 3rd edn (eds A.M. Clarke and A.D.B. Clarke). London: Methuen, pp. 840–56.

Walker, S. (1987) *Animal Learning: An Introduction*. London: Routledge and Kegan Paul.

Werner, E.E. and Smith, R.S. (1977) *Kuaii's Children Come of Age*. Honolulu, HI: University Press of Hawaii.

Werner, E.E. and Smith, R.S. (1980) An epidemiologic perspective on some antecedents and consequences of childhood mental health problems and learning disabilities, in *Annual Progress in Child Psychiatry and Development* (eds S. Chess and A. Thomas). New York: Brunner/Mazel, pp. 133–47.

Wing, L. (1981) Language, social and cognitive impairments in autism and severe mental retardation. *Journal of Autism and Developmental Disorders*, **11**, 31–44.

Wolfensberger, W. (1980a) The definition of normalisation: update, problems, disagreements and misunderstandings, in *Normalization, Social Integration and Community Services* (eds R.J. Flynn and K.E. Nitsch). Baltimore, MD: University Park Press, pp. 71–115.

Wolfensberger, W. (1980b) Research, empiricism and the principle of normalization, in *Normalization, Social Integration and Community Services* (eds R.J. Flynn and K.E. Nitsch). Baltimore, MD: University Park Press, pp. 117–129.

Wolfensberger, W. (1983) Social role valorisation: A proposed new term for the principle of normalisation. *Mental Retardation*, **21**, 234–9.

# 4

# Conceptualizing service provision

*Jim Mansell, Peter McGill and Eric Emerson*

The rapid growth of staffed housing as a replacement for institutional care in hospitals and hostels has offered many people with severe learning disabilities a better life in the community: nearer to family members, in better accommodation, with more staff and more individualized care. But the opportunities created by the staffed housing model are often only beginning to be realized. Some people, especially those with challenging behaviour, have exchanged long hours of boredom and isolation in hospital for more of the same in the community.

Whereas American studies have more or less consistently reported overall improvements, British experience is more mixed. American research has focused mainly on gains in adaptive behaviour, measured by asking staff to complete a rating scale (Nihira *et al.*, 1974; Conroy and Bradley 1985) before and after resettlement. Significant gains have been found in a number of studies (see reviews of the deinstitutionalization literature by Haney (1988) and Allen (1989)) and these, together with improvements in user and family satisfaction and other aspects of service delivery, have led some authors to conclude that the debate over residential care options is now settled conclusively in favour of housing-based community services (Conroy and Feinstein, 1990). British studies have made less use of measures of skill acquisition (e.g., Felce *et al.*, 1986b; Lowe and de Paiva, 1990), though even here results are mixed, with one study showing no improvement (Beswick, 1992). They have favoured observational measures of client involvement in meaningful activity (Durward and

Whatmore, 1976; Repp and Felce, 1990; Beasley *et al.*, 1989).

Despite some very good results from demonstration projects in the UK (Mansell *et al.*, 1984; Felce *et al.*, 1986a; Felce and Repp, 1992; Mansell and Beasley, in press; see also Chapter 6), second-generation projects have reported mixed results. Rawlings (1985a, b) reported higher levels of engagement in meaningful activity in three residential homes than in three hospital wards, and Hewson and Walker (1992) found levels comparable with the first-generation projects in a post-test only study. But other studies report no significant change, or comparable levels to hospital care (Bratt and Johnston, 1988; Joyce, 1988; Evans *et al.*, 1985; Hughes and Mansell, 1990). Even in the demonstration projects, good results may be difficult to sustain (Mansell and Beasley, in press).

Although most other aspects of service quality have been found to be better in staffed housing, the persistence of low levels of service user involvement in meaningful activity and low levels of staff–client interaction in some services represents a failure to fully realize the opportunities created by the abandonment of institutions.

There is not yet much data about day services, but what little there is suggests that similar problems of the quality of service offered to users arise (Pettipher and Mansell, in press) and that similar approaches can be used to explore the relationship between service organization and client experience (Dalgliesh and Matthews, 1980; 1981). The radical alternative to traditional day centres is supported employment, where there is good evidence from demonstration projects of the feasibility of the model, aspects of organization and the outcomes achieved for service users (Bellamy *et al.*, 1979; 1988; Rusch, 1986); but similar issues may arise with widespread replication of the demonstration projects.

As pointed out elsewhere in this volume, problems in the quality of residential and day services are likely to differentially affect people with challenging behaviour; they are more likely to be 'unpopular patients', to be at risk of neglect and abuse, and to have less chance of securing, and most chance of losing, placement in the community. The interpretation placed on challenging behaviour here (see also Chapter 1) is that it is the product of a range of individual and environmental factors. In a sense, therefore, challenging behaviour represents a special vulnerability to weaknesses of, or problems in, the management of the care environment.

The nature of the problems implies that it is the way in which staff work with service users, rather than the way staffed housing is set up, that is responsible. Better family and community contact probably reflects the location of new services rather than any great sophistication in staff performance and, similarly, greater individualization is likely to be mainly a product of small group size. Whether service users, especially those with additional problems of communication or challenging behaviour, are enabled to take part in a wide range of interesting household and community activities depends not only on the physical resources of the setting but crucially on the quality of face-to-face interaction between service users and staff (McCord, 1982; Rice and Rosen, 1991).

Yet it is in precisely this area that management is typically weakest. The prevailing approach is usually one that identifies the caring task as essentially unskilled (see, for example, paragraph 35 of the 1988 Griffiths Report), that emphasizes training in philosophy and principles rather than working practices (e.g., see Hughes and Mansell, 1990), and that sets up services in a flurry of excitement and interest before moving on to new projects, leaving the staff and service users to make their future as best they can. In residential services, perhaps this is because managers simplistically conceptualize the environment as a family, which the (overwhelmingly female) workforce is expected to make work; perhaps it also reflects the lack of a clear alternative model (or, in the jargon of normalization, a 'culturally valued analogue') for a group of adults living together collectively, with support from a team of staff (a point made over 20 years ago by Townsend (1974) when discussing the lack of clarity about the then-favoured hostel model).

Work is therefore needed to think through the model of community-based services, to clarify how staff should work together to meet the needs of the people they serve and what kinds of organization they should adopt to do so. This needs to be done partly at the level of the placement (the staffed house or flat, the job or course), but it is also required at the level of the service system, to integrate the placement within the wider network of other services and the rest of the service-providing organization.

The first part of this chapter addresses the organization of the care environment, arguing for a model which conceptualizes the placement as a production system, in which the product is the quality of lifestyle experienced by the person(s) served. This is a theme taken up in Chapter 10. The second part of the chapter addresses the relationship between the placement and the culture of the service and its implications for the maintenance of quality over time, arguing for an integration of participative management approaches with clearer direction and leadership (see also Chapter 9). Finally, the chapter addresses the organization of the service system, arguing that some problems experienced in individual settings are the product of deficiencies elsewhere in services which need to be attended to at service system level. This is also taken up again later, in Chapter 11. The argument in this chapter focuses mainly on staffed housing, reflecting the greater experience with this kind of service in the UK than with supported employment or integrated education. Nevertheless many of the issues discussed will also apply to other care environments.

## The organization of the care environment

The body of knowledge about how care environments for people with learning disabilities work is derived largely from studies of institutions and their alternatives.

The general picture emerging from studies of institutions in the 1960s was of very inflexible environments, in which there was actually very little for residents to do – at once a fixed and an empty life. As Morris (1969) described it in her study of learning disability hospitals in England and Wales:

> Without any shadow of doubt, and with the exception of the exclusively high grade wards and hostel patients, the great majority spent their day sitting, interspersed with eating. Only in very few wards . . . did we find nurses helping patients with individual or group **leisure** activities; nurses were usually cleaning either the wards or the patients, helping to prepare meals, cutting or washing hair, dressing or undressing patients or feeding them. When they were not so occupied nurses tended to sit or stand around talking to each other rather than to the patients. (Morris, 1969, p. 169)

In services, the first advance on this was the introduction of individual habilitation planning: a structure which specified for each person the therapeutic work they needed, together with a plan for its delivery. In the UK, individual programme planning and its variants have become an important part of service provision, but it is in the USA, where such plans are often legally required and enforceable, that they have had the greatest impact on the organization of group care environments.

The point of interest here is that the effect of **individualized** prescription has been to neglect the group dimension. So, for example, staff in the group care environment distinguish clearly between someone being 'in program', when they are participating in an activity specified in their individual plan, and 'out of program', when they are not. A major goal then becomes increasing the proportion of time that the person spends 'in program'.

However desirable entirely individual services might be, they are not likely to be feasible for most people because of the cost of the staff help needed. So for this reason the group dimension is important. But even more important than this is the recognition that large parts of life and work are conducted in groups, even if not in groups defined entirely as disabled. Those who organize the workplace, the neighbourhood or the school are organizing for people collectively and an entirely individualized approach would be inadequate.

In services, Hart and Risley (1976) first pointed this out in their work in infant day care centres. They argued that the programmatic elements of care actually took up a relatively small part of the day and that the service users could spend large amounts of time waiting for their turn within activities and waiting between activities. In a series of studies (e.g., Doke and Risley, 1972; LeLaurin and Risley, 1972; Quilitch and Risley, 1973; Twardosz *et al.*, 1974) Risley and his colleagues showed how the group care environment could be reorganized to reduce waiting time and increase client participation by changing aspects of staff deployment and performance. This work was introduced to services in the UK mainly by Kushlick (1975a, b; 1976) and by Porterfield *et al.* (1980), whose replication of the 'room manager' procedure in a day care special unit led to a number of further studies (Porterfield and Blunden, 1979; McBrien and Weightman, 1980; Mansell *et al.*, 1982; Crisp and Sturmey, 1984; 1988). In learning disability, a further rationale for this kind of approach is that a major goal of services should be enhanced competence rather than just enhanced skills: that engaging constructively with other people and the materials and tasks of everyday life is more important than just amassing skills, which might in any case be lost if not used (Mansell *et al.*, 1987, pp. 197–200).

These studies involve conceptualizing the key dependent variable as the level of engagement or participation throughout the day, rather than more narrowly as skill acquisition. The development of the idea of normalization has provided a framework within which this essentially behavioural perspective can be located, so that Bellamy and his colleagues, for example, offer a definition of lifestyle as the key outcome by which services should be judged, in which they include the extent of participation in activity in the care environment and the community, as well as other issues like the individuals' social network or the extent to which they control their lives (Bellamy *et al.*, 1986).

This broader perspective on the outcomes the care environment should achieve has been matched by considering a wider range of independent variables. These have included the environmental context (small community-based settings rather than institutions); the physical organization of the environment and the numbers of people together; the deployment of staff; their interaction with service users and the kind of activities in which client participation is sought.

In contrast to the kind of services studied by Morris in the mid-1960s, therefore, the model services of the 1980s were characterized by attempts to construct a set of staff procedures which make most use of the opportunities presented by the socially and materially enriched environments provided by supported housing, employment and education services. In the USA, this approach is best represented by the work of Bellamy, Horner, Wilcox and their colleagues in the Specialized Training Program at the University of Oregon. Using a behaviour analytic approach, Bellamy and his colleagues developed a model sheltered workshop for people with severe and profound learning disabilities which involved detailed prescriptions for how staff should organize work so that individuals could do it productively, as well as for running the workshop as a small business, later extending the technology to supported employment in individual jobs (Bellamy *et al.*, 1979; 1988). Wilcox and Bellamy (1982) took a similar approach to designing integrated high-school programs and in residential care, Newton *et al.* (1988) and Horner and O'Neill (1992) have developed model staffed housing programs, the latter focusing particularly on people with challenging behaviour.

In the UK, a similar approach was taken by Mansell *et al.* (1987) in Andover, and more recently in the Special Development Team project (Chapter 6).

The metaphor in all these projects is that the house or work or school placement can be thought of as a production system – as a kind of machine (Figure 4.1). The product the service 'makes' is the lifestyle experienced by the service user, and the task of the innovator is to construct a service which can deliver this outcome. The assumption is that poor-quality care environments, once adequately resourced, do not have mechanisms for working effectively with service users. The focus is therefore initially on inventing organizational arrangements and procedures (like the room manager procedure or opportunity planning) which effectively enable service users to make use of the opportunities provided by the service location and setting (see also Chapter 10). Once more than a few such arrangements are worked out, they have to be effectively coordinated, which means not only making them consistent one with another (so that, for example, the priorities staff attend to in incidental teaching are those identified in the individual programme plan) but also balancing the work involved in keeping all the elements working (for example not spending so much resource on individual programme planning that there is no time left for organized activities at the group level).

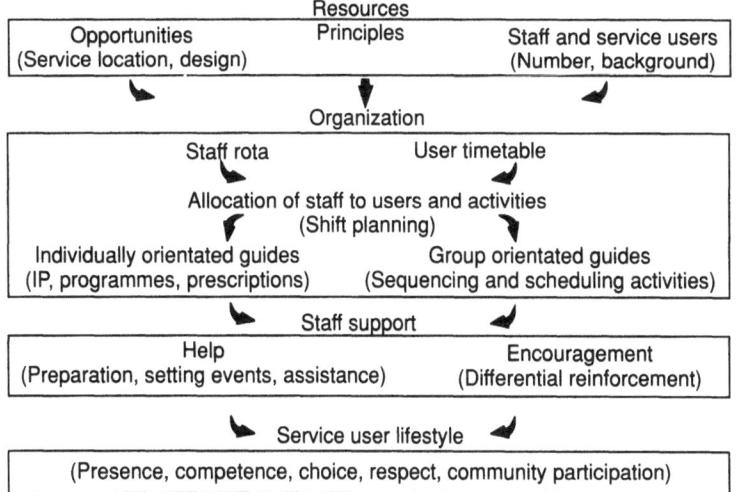

**Figure 4.1**   The production of service user lifestyles.

The strength of this approach is evident in the results achieved by the demonstration projects concerned. No other projects reported in the literature have achieved such good results. But viewing the service as a machine for the production of lifestyle has also brought disadvantages. First, it is not easy to identify the best procedures or methods of working, because the variability of results achieved by the same methods exceeds the variability between methods. There is therefore ample scope for investing effort in procedures which have less than optimal effectiveness. Felce (1989) has argued that applied researchers should not be distracted from the task of building and replicating effective services by the need to unravel the individual effects of particular components of services (because this would be difficult and time-consuming), but even accepting this there are likely to be problems where procedures are too cumbersome to be used in practice.

The second disadvantage of the machine metaphor is even more important. The implicit assumption in much intervention research has been that poor-quality environments exist because of lack of resources, knowledge and skills; that in a sense they are empty, and therefore ready and waiting for innovation. As anyone involved in intervention soon finds out, the way services are organized is rarely accidental; it is usually the product of quite clearly identifiable demands in the wider environment. The way a service works before intervention is therefore functional for someone, and intervention produces resistance to change, together with problems of poor maintenance and generalization.

Conceptualizing the care environment as a production system is important, but it is not enough. It is important because managers need to determine the kinds of staff performance that produce the outcomes desired by service users and their advocates and the kinds of management that support good work by staff, rather than relying on accident or attitudes to produce the results. It is not enough because introducing these ways of working will mean displacing other ways of working which already have roots in the situation.

## The culture of the service

The common experience is that good new services are fragile and rarely survive. As the innovators move on, the service becomes more and more fragile to external pressures and either reverts gradually to the same level of performance as other local services or collapses completely.

This problem has spawned a large literature addressing the ways in which improved performance can be maintained after the initial intervention. At first, the dominant approach was to replace the control exercised by the innovator in the beginning with control exercised by managers. Thus, there have been many studies involving supervision of staff performance and employing many techniques with which supervisors could attempt to reward good performance (see for example Reid *et al.*, 1989).

There has been a growing dissatisfaction with this approach. In particular, the introduction of monitoring by supervisory staff may inadvertently teach staff to respond more to management than to the needs of the individual people they serve. It is already clear that client behaviour (or needs) exerts relatively little influence on how staff implement individual programmes (Woods and Cullen, 1983). Building supervision hierarchies may not help make staff more responsive to clients. For example, in a study designed to teach a group of hospital staff to run an 'activity period' for one hour each week day with a small group of young people with severe and profound learning disabilities, Coles and Blunden (1981) implemented a 'monitoring hierarchy' to keep the intervention running (this was needed even though the intervention produced demonstrable benefits to clients). The nurse responsible for running the activity period made a weekly report to his/her line manager. The line manager made a weekly report to his/her line manager (one of the hospital management team) and, in addition, made a fortnightly check on what the nurse was actually doing in the activity period. The hospital manager made a monthly report to the hospital management team. Although successful (in getting the one-hour activity period to run) this seems an extraordinary amount of effort needed to get staff to provide the young people they cared for with some toys and attention, and it suggests that staff at each level were required to respond more to those in the level above them than to the needs of the people served or the staff who cared for them.

Staff are also likely to associate closer management attention with punishment, so that they begin to conceal the problems they face and to sharpen up on the issues they believe are attended to even if they are less important or relevant. For example, Bible and

Sneed (1976) covertly observed staff work with clients in a learn-ing disability hospital during a visit by an accreditation team. They found a 256% increase in the amount of time staff worked with the people served during the visit, with an immediate rever-sal to the original level once the accreditation team had gone. Repp and Barton (1980) compared licensed and unlicensed resi-dential facilities for people with learning disabilities, and con-cluded that

> The data show that there is little difference and this result has two implications: (a) that various standards and guidelines may not be getting at the heart of the matter when . . . based on building constructions, on objectives written in (individual educational plans) and on many other areas to the exclusion of direct observation; and (b) that a unit or facility may be licensed even when it is not providing active habilitation. (Repp and Barton, 1980, p. 339)

One response to this problem has been 'positive monitoring', in which management attention is made contingent on achievement rather than non-achievement of good practice (Risley and Favell, 1979). In practice, these studies do not demonstrate that manage-ment attention is actually reinforcing, and (in the UK at least) are likely to conflict with the individual experience of staff in every other area of their life, so that staff remain sceptical and continue to act defensively.

In commerce and industry these problems have led to interest in greater attempts to obtain worker commitment to the produc-tion process, using methods of devolved goal-setting and man-agement, exemplified by the idea of the 'quality circle' (Mohr and Mohr, 1983). These approaches have been adopted in services for people with learning disabilities. For example, Burgio *et al.* (1983) described a project in which the staff team were enabled to set their own goals, agree on measures to achieve them, check their own performance and give each other feedback. Another ex-ample, described by Boles and Bible (1978), used a checklist of goals (called the 'student service index') and involved giving staff immediate feedback on their performance. As the items on the index were achieved, the list was revised to include more ambi-tious goals. This example illustrates how the goals set early in the project may be very modest, but that as people experience the success of achieving these goals they can set more and more ambitious targets for their own performance. In this way, the problem that unrealistic goals encourage staff to conceal real levels of performance may be overcome.

These examples also indicate the importance of management practice consistent with promoting quality. If staff are encouraged to set goals for improving their service, it is important that managers respond to these decisions – that they reinforce the acts of raising issues, discussing them, setting goals and so on. If every time staff identify an issue they want to do something about they are met with prevarication, discouragement or refusal they will learn that it is not worth their while to bother. The kind of support needed will include giving staff money, resources, skills (through training) and expertise (through access to advice), and making this contingent on the success of previous attempts rather than on their failure.

There are however some potential problems with this participative management approach where it is developed not so much in the spirit of 'we, the managers will support you moving in the directions we and you approve of' but of 'who knows what is supposed to happen in these services – so you can decide on your own'. Where staff are left to manage themselves they may become isolated and inward-looking and their norms and values may drift away from those of the wider community. As Handy (1985) says

> The overall risk with autonomous work groups is that they will come to set norms and objectives that do not match those of the organization . . . although the reported studies always describe studies where there is a synchronization of group and organization goals, there is clearly a possibility that the groups might misappropriate the trust and relaxation of control. (Handy, 1985, pp. 333–4)

Services for people with learning disabilities have already experienced this phenomenon in the back wards of the large hospitals (Jones *et al.*, 1975). Exactly the same problem could arise in the scattered staff teams supporting people with severe and profound learning disabilities in staffed housing, where young, ideologically committed staff challenge what they see as the ill-thought-out policies of managers (e.g., Mansell and Beasley, 1989) or where staff are simply cut adrift from management (see for example the discussion in Orlowska, 1992).

Thus, participative management is not a substitute for clear leadership. But whereas the focus in studies such as that by Coles and Blunden is on management control to ensure staff adherence to externally defined procedures, the participative management model implies that leadership is responsive to staff definitions of the goals to be followed. This is important because external prescriptions are sometimes quite impracticable. Consider, for example, the work, referred to earlier, carried out over several years in the late 1970s on the 'room manager' procedure. This apparently showed that dramatic increases in participation in activity by people with severe and profound learning disabilities could be achieved with a staff ratio of 1:10 or 1:15 people (Porterfield *et al.*, 1980; Mansell *et al.*, 1982). But the real lesson of these studies was the utter futility of trying to occupy people for long periods with pre-school toys in environments where there was no purpose to increased activity or competence on the part of the people with learning disabilities served.

The implications of work on the problem of maintenance are, therefore, that innovators need to see the services in which they intervene as already existing cultures with which they have to work, rather than as open space in which to build afresh. There are obvious parallels here with the change in perspective in clinical work with people who present challenging behaviour, away from 'cookbook' applications of predetermined interventions towards more careful assessment of the functional relationships which already exist. Hoskin and Mansell (1989), for example, offer a framework for 'quality enhancement' through which staff assess their own performance in working with service users, the support they need and what they actually get from managers and professionals and then establish what are, in effect, contracts for support (interest, enthusiasm, resources, help) to enable them to sustain their own goal-setting and quality improvement process (Figure 4.2).

### The service system

An important characteristic of those services which have shown good outcomes for clients is that they have been set up as pilot or demonstration projects, carefully monitored and protected. Often this has been necessary to get the project established in the first place.

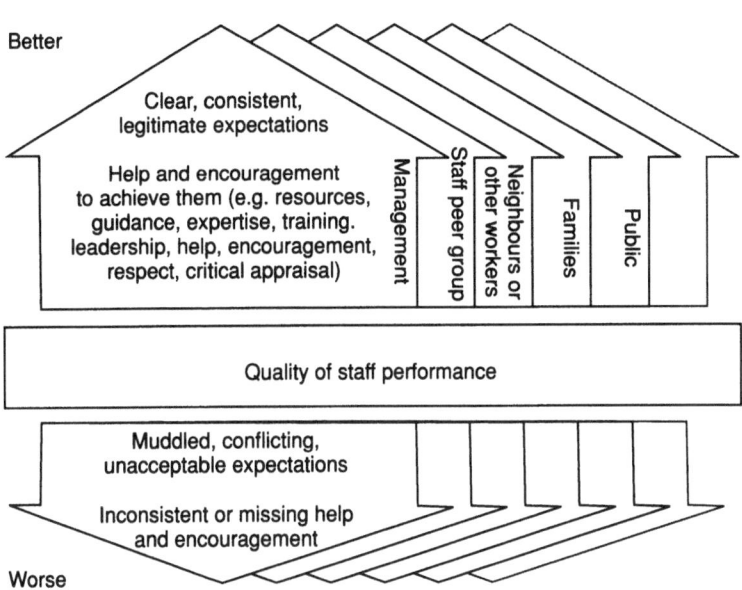

**Figure 4.2** Conditions which enhance or weaken staff performance.

Pilot projects withdraw from the wider organization behind specially constructed barriers, so that they can develop new ways of working unhindered by mainstream processes. This protection is functional for a while. It allows good practice to grow and develop. It is a strategy which one also sees in the voluntary sector. But at the end of the day, as writers on quite different kinds of organizations have noted (Leavitt *et al.*, 1989), it is often a flawed strategy because the world passes the pilot project by. The wider service system continues unchanged, either not noticing the innovation in its midst or resenting it for the resources and acclaim it attracts. When the pilot project is vulnerable (e.g., when there is staff turnover) the wider system seeps under the barricades and washes away the foundations.

It is this which largely explains the poor survival of pilot projects and the constant drift back to custodial care practices. For demonstration projects to succeed, simultaneous attention has to be given to working through the implications of new program models at service system level. Far from withdrawing, the demonstration project needs to engage with the wider service system if it is to succeed, so that awareness and dissemination of new practices and arrangements occurs from the outset (even though this may mean challenging some cherished ways earlier than would otherwise be the case).

This practice of 'defensive isolation' is also seen in second-generation projects, where the gap between management and staff grows so that both withdraw from effective dialogue about the way the service works. Where this happens, as in the example described in Chapter 11, a problem presents itself for service managers responsible for the whole system of local services. At **service system level** a crucial outcome is comprehensiveness – that everyone in need should be served. If the network of service placements are isolated one from another, each is more fragile and within the whole network of services there can be no certainty that the capacity will exist to meet everyone's needs. In the study reported in Chapter 11, the service was experiencing rapidly arising and unpredictable crises in houses leading to placement breakdown and reinstitutionalization, coupled with increasing staff turnover and failure to replenish staff numbers. The problems experienced in individual houses seemed remote from managers, who saw the whole service system as verging on complete breakdown.

In this and other similar situations the fragility of community services and their lack of resilience when tested by problems of challenging behaviour is striking. Challenging behaviour represents the 'test case' for service competence: the point at which most services (institutional as well as community-based models) are weakest and most likely to break down.

Conceptualizing service provision does not therefore only consist in defining the best available models of residential, work, education or other services: it requires a view of how these services should be integrated into a comprehensive local service. In relation to challenging behaviour, the goal is to ensure that all placements provide support in ways which minimize its occurrence, and also to maintain enough placements which have the resilience and capability to cope with what challenges do occur. We have found it helpful to identify four subsystems of activity which appear to be required at service system level. The four subsystems are (1) prevention, (2) early detection, (3) crisis management and (4) specialized long-term support (Figure 4.3).

| Prevention | Early detection |
|---|---|
| Enriched environments at home and work<br><br>Staff organized to provide appropriate help and encouragement to promote adaptive behaviour | Seeing potential problems as they first emerge<br><br>Looking for early signs of placement breakdown in "successful" placements |

| Crisis management | Specialized long-term support |
|---|---|
| Contingency plans that provide more help, not removal<br><br>Respite in and out of home<br><br>Skilled intervention<br><br>Access to new homes and jobs | Sophisticated, individualized help in good places to live and work<br><br>Very high levels of technical and emotional support to staff |

**Figure 4.3**    Four subsystems required to manage challenging behaviour.

### Prevention

The prevention subsystem is required because of the relationship between specialized services for people with challenging behaviour and mainstream services. Since many people have challenging behaviour in their repertoire and since people with challenging behaviour are most likely to be squeezed out of mainstream supported housing, it is essential to organize mainstream services so that they can manage moderate levels of challenge over long periods, and at least not make matters worse.

This entails providing enriched environments at home and at work, in the way described in Chapter 10, so that there are stimulating opportunities for client involvement and growth in independence; and organizing staff to provide help and encouragement (i.e. managing setting events, prompts, assistance and differential reinforcement) to make the most of the opportunities the setting provides. It also requires that challenging behaviour that does occur is appropriately managed at the time, using a 'reactive strategy' (LaVigna *et al.*, 1989) which is effective but nevertheless consistent with the longer-term treatment of the challenging behaviour.

Within the whole service, this approach needs to be followed to ensure the provision of some homes providing a great deal of this kind of structure as well as houses providing less, so that the capacity exists to serve people with widely differing needs for structure and support. But even this is not enough, since the needs of individuals will change over time, sometimes quickly. If the service system includes only a small number of placements which can provide very carefully organized and individualized support, service users are likely to end up being moved into them (i.e. they will become the specialist 'challenging behaviour houses'). Rather, many placements (or, to put it another way, many staff teams) need to have the capacity to vary the amount of structure in response to the needs of individual residents.

The prevention subsystem, therefore, concerns the recruitment, training and management of staff to ensure that well-organized and responsive support is provided in the housing, work or education placements provided. As already discussed, this entails a well-worked out specification of what is needed at the placement level – a clear model which people can understand and follow. Beyond this, the task is primarily to construct arrangements which will work across the service: a recruitment strategy that fills posts quickly with the right kind of people; training that reaches everyone at the start, that produces real hands-on competence and that is carried through into and reinforced in practice; and management that provides leadership and direction based on good information about services and clear commitment to principles.

### Early detection

With many individuals vulnerable to ineptly organized support, early detection is important to locate and identify problems before they become intractable through habit or before they develop into crises. Where a service has invested time and effort and has (1) identified what features of placement organization increase the chances of challenging behaviour, (2) worked with staff and managers to shape up ways of providing support that minimize the challenge, and (3) provided teaching, counselling or treatment for the service user to increase his/her ability to cope with variations in the placement, it is clearly important that this investment should not be wasted. For some service users there will be a direct and immediate relationship between placement organization and challenging behaviour: if the organization wavers, challenging behaviour will increase. In these cases it will be obvious that the service has to provide more or less precisely the package that works for that person.

In a way, though, there is a greater risk when problems do **not** immediately occur: when 'success' of carefully worked out interventions leads to their relaxation (**decay**), and there is no obvious impact on the service user. What may happen in these cases is that over time the staff team become less practised, less skilled, at delivering what is needed so that the situation becomes more vulnerable. Then, when arrangements are tested by some minor crisis, the staff team are not able to recover the skilled performance needed in time and the service user presents a major challenge again. It is particularly because of this scenario that a crucial area of activity in any service system is the early detection of placement decay and breakdown.

The early detection subsystem therefore consists of the ways in which the managers of the whole system check that placements are maintaining their capability to work with service users when they present a special challenge. Partly these ways will consist of information about staff performance at placement level (e.g., sample information about levels of client engagement in meaningful activity, how challenging behaviour is managed, how staff and users interact) and about staff training and turnover across the whole service (e.g., what proportion of staff have had various kinds of training, what exit interviews reveal about reasons for termination). Just as important as information, though, is a culture which uses it; in which the way staff support service users, and managers and professionals support staff, is everybody's business, rather than a private matter. This entails open communication, in which senior staff are talking to clients and staff so that they know what life is like at the front-line ('management by walking about' still has much to commend it).

### Crisis management

The third subsystem is that concerned with crisis management. Here the central issue is that newly developed community services often seem to have been set up on the assumption that everything will go right; when things go wrong, panic or cover-up become too likely responses. If procedures do not exist to guide action in the most difficult circumstances, it is perhaps not surprising that the organization's responses should be less than optimal. For example, in the study by Hughes and Mansell (1990) (Chapter 11) when staff were brought together to talk through typical crises and how the service responded to them, one example given was of a fire in a house, serious enough to call out the Fire Brigade, but which the house leader had not felt necessary to report to his own manager. Also in this service, weekend crises in placements were usually met by emergency admission to a private institutional placement – sometimes before the Care Group Director even knew about it. In these cases the problem was not just procedural but reflected the lack of options available to the service.

Effective crisis management arrangements will therefore entail a range of service options: the option of providing respite care in the house (by putting in extra staff, skills and support, by giving other residents a break elsewhere); respite care out of house (a short-term adult placement, a place in an otherwise vacant flat or house, a place in a local short-term care facility, a break or holiday); the provision of effective treatment (but not using this as the excuse for exclusion and institutionalization); and, if need be, finding a new placement to replace the one that has broken down. Providing these options locally will entail keeping some places in reserve (necessary anyway to cope with sudden needs for service resulting from family crises) and/or retaining some skilled people prepared to provide an adult placement in an emergency.

Having these resources available is important but it is only part of effective crisis management arrangements. Just as important are procedures to identify the emerging crisis and deal with it. These include procedures for clearly identifying who can make what kinds of decision (and what has to be referred on) but, most of all, must include plans to build up resources on the assumption that the problem will get worse and will take longer to resolve. The most important requirement of services is that they should be able to **retrieve** crises; to manage them while they occur and to steadily bring the situation back to one in which the problems can be tackled over the longer term. This will mean garnering the resources to cope for weeks or months rather than days, so that 'crisis management' becomes more a question of the 'long haul' than the 'quick fix'. In particular this will mean putting in more expert and managerial time to ensure that the placement uses extra resources to put back in place arrangements which enable the service user to stay (rather than expecting staff in the situation to cope with the stress of working through it as well as the extra work involved in getting out of it). It will also mean making contingency plans which look beyond the next step, so that if the situation gets worse the resources (intellectual and practical) are on hand to cope (rather than trying one thing and then giving up).

### Specialized long-term support

The fourth subsystem is that providing specialized long-term support. This recognizes that some people need very carefully designed and managed support for ever, because of the chronicity and severity of the problems they face. In such homes (or supported jobs or courses), staff will need much higher levels of technical skill, for example in working with people who have problems of severe self-injury or aggression to others. In addition, staff and residents will have greater needs for emotional support, so that counselling and group-work skills will need to be constantly available. To some extent the specialized nature of these services will set them apart from others, because of the extra support needed; but if the 'mainstream' community services are provided by staff who understand the need for a range of levels of structure and organization the gap between them and the specialized placements will not be so great. When specialized placements need extra support they will be able to call on a more skilled pool of staff elsewhere in the service and there will be greater understanding of (and perhaps willingness to appreciate) the work involved; similarly, the specialized support subsystem is potentially a source of expertise in direct-care work with service users, in management and in training.

### Conclusion

In so far as community services fail to achieve marked improvement in quality of life for the people they serve, when compared to less expensive institutional care, they will continue to be vulnerable to cost-cutting measures. In the UK, the gap between what was achieved in the first demonstration projects and what appears to be happening in second-generation services is striking. The evidence is that the quality of life experienced by some people is in important respects not much improved, and that the services themselves are fragile.

This presents a special problem for people who have challenging behaviour, because they are particularly vulnerable to inadequacies in the way services are organized. They are the most likely to be excluded from community services.

The key to improving services, once community-based models have been selected so that the best opportunities are provided, is the way front-line staff work with the people they serve. Far from being of little relevance to managers, whose task finishes with the establishment of the placement, this is actually their central continuing responsibility. This chapter has argued that to tackle this responsibility requires a new conceptualization of services based on the demonstration projects and recent experience with community services. At the level of the placement (the staffed house, supported job or course) it requires treating the placement as a production system whose product is the lifestyle lived by service users, in which the elements of the placement are explicitly planned and managed to achieve this end. In terms of how the placement relates to the wider service culture, it requires a recognition of the already existing relationships between staff, attention to their empowerment and commitment and the construction of a 'support community' of managers and others, whose actions help rather than hinder the enhancement of quality over time.

It is not possible to work only at the level of the particular placement because the whole network or system of services has to serve everyone, and this requires interdependence and complementarity. The problems addressed here are largely problems of the transition from small-scale services, in which only one or two houses exist in an area and there is much enthusiasm and commitment, to large-scale systems of 20 or 30 houses. Once service systems on this scale come into being, they experience common 'organizational growing pains' (Flamholz, 1989) which need to be addressed at the systemic level. The model offered here identifies subsystems of activity which need to be present to preserve the system's capability to meet the needs of people with challenging behaviour.

The greatest challenge for any innovation lies at this point: in the move from the first exemplars to widespread implementation.

Over the next few years, those individuals leading the development of learning disability services face a choice. Either they will develop the infrastructure needed to deliver and sustain good services or they will produce pale imitations, even new institutions in the community. The people who will suffer most if this happens are those who have challenging behaviour.

## References

Allen, D. (1989) The effects of deinstitutionalisation on people with mental handicaps: A review. *Mental Handicap Research*, 2, 18–37.

Beasley, F., Hewson, S. and Mansell, J. (1989) *MTS: Handbook for Observers*. Canterbury: Centre for the Applied Psychology of Social Care, University of Kent.

Bellamy, G.T., Horner, R.H. and Inman, D.P. (1979) *Vocational Habilitation of Severely Retarded Adults: A Direct Service Technology*. Baltimore, MD: University Park Press.

Bellamy, G.T., Newton, J.S., LeBaron, N.M. and Horner, R.H. (1986) *Toward Lifestyle Accountability in Residential Services for Persons with Mental Retardation*. Eugene, OR: Specialized Training Program.

Bellamy, G.T., Rhodes, L.E., Mank, D.M. and Albin, J.M. (1988) *Supported Employment: A Community Implementation Guide*. Baltimore, MD: Paul H. Brookes.

Beswick, J. (1992) *An Evaluation of the Effects on Quality of Life Outcome Measures for People with Learning Difficulties (Mental Handicap) of Changes in the Living Situation from Hospitals to Community Environments*. Unpublished PhD Thesis, University of Manchester.

Bible, G.H. and Sneed, T.J. (1976) Some effects of an accreditation survey on program completion at a state institution. *Mental Retardation*, 14, 14–5.

Boles, S.M. and Bible, G.H. (1978) The student service index, in *Current Behavioral Trends for the Developmentally Disabled* (ed. M.S. Berkler). Baltimore, MD: University Park Press, pp. 153–95.

Bratt, A. and Johnston, R. (1988) Changes in lifestyle for young adults with profound handicaps following discharge from hospital care into a 'second generation' housing project. *Mental Handicap Research*, 1, 49–74.

Burgio, L.D., Whitman, T.L. and Reid, D.H. (1983) A participative management approach to improving direct care staff performance in an institutional setting. *Journal of Applied Behavior Analysis*, 16, 37–53.

Coles, E. and Blunden, R. (1981) Maintaining new procedures using feedback to staff, a hierarchical reporting system and a multi-disciplinary management group. *Journal of Organisational Behavior Management*, 3, 19–33.

Conroy, J.W. and Bradley, V.T. (1985) *The Pennhurst Longitudinal Study: A Report of Five Years of Research and Analysis*. Philadelphia, PA, and Boston, MA: Temple University Developmental Disabilities Centre and Human Services Research Institute.

Conroy, J.W. and Feinstein, C.S. (1990) A new way of thinking about quality, in *Quality Assurance for Individuals with Developmental Disabilities* (eds V.J. Bradley and H.A. Bersani). Baltimore, MD: Paul H. Brookes, pp. 263–78.

Crisp, A. and Sturmey, P. (1984) Organising staff to promote purposeful activity in a setting for mentally handicapped adults: An evaluation of alternative strategies – small groups and room management. *Behavioural Psychotherapy*, **12**, 281–99.

Crisp, A.G. and Sturmey, P. (1988) The promotion of purposeful activity in micro-environments for people with a mental handicap. *Advances in Behaviour Research and Therapy*, **10**, 7–23.

Dalgleish, M. and Matthews, R. (1980) Some effects of environmental design on the quality of day care for severely mentally handicapped adults. *British Journal of Mental Subnormality*, **26**, 94–102.

Dalgleish, M. and Matthews, R. (1981) Some effects of staffing levels and group size on the quality of day care for severely mentally handicapped adults. *British Journal of Mental Subnormality*, **27**, 30–5.

Doke, L.A. and Risley, T.R. (1972) The organisation of day-care environments: Required vs. optional activities. *Journal of Applied Behavior Analysis*, **5**, 405–20.

Durward, L. and Whatmore, R. (1976) Testing measures of the quality of residential care: A pilot study. *Behaviour Research and Therapy*, **14**, 149–57.

Evans, G., Todd, S., Blunden, R., Porterfield, J. and Ager, A. (1985) *A New Style of Life: The Impact of Moving into an Ordinary House on the Lives of People with a Mental Handicap*. Cardiff: Mental Handicap in Wales Applied Research Unit.

Felce, D. (1989) Necessary and sufficient conditions for high quality residential services (letter). *Mental Handicap Research*, **2**, 108–9.

Felce, D. and Repp, A. (1992) The behavioral and social ecology of community houses. *Research in Developmental Disabilities*, **13**, 27–42.

Felce, D., de Kock, U. and Repp, A. (1986a) An ecobehavioral analysis of small community-based houses and traditional large hospitals for severely and profoundly mentally handicapped adults. *Applied Research in Mental Retardation*, **7**, 393–408.

Felce, D., de Kock, U., Thomas, M. and Saxby, H. (1986b) Change in adaptive behaviour of severely and profoundly mentally handicapped adults in different residential settings. *British Journal of Psychology*, **77**, 489–501.

Flamholz, E.G. (1989) Managing the stages of organizational growth, in *Readings in Managerial Psychology* (eds H.J. Leavitt, L.R. Pondy and D.M. Boje). Chicago, IL: University of Chicago Press, pp. 705–19.

Griffiths, R. (1988) *Community Care: Agenda for Action*. London: HMSO.

Handy, C.B. (1985) *Understanding Organisations*. Harmondsworth: Penguin Books.

Haney, J.I. (1988) Empirical support for deinstitutionalization, in *Integration of Developmentally Disabled Individuals in the Community* (eds L.W. Heal, J.I. Haney and A.R.N. Amado). Baltimore, MD: Paul H.

Brookes, pp. 37–58.

Hart, B. and Risley, T.R. (1976) Environmental programming: Implications for the severely handicapped, in *Early Intervention for the Severely Handicapped: Programming and Accountability* (eds H.J. Prehms and S.J. Deitz). Eugene, OR: University of Oregon.

Hewson, S. and Walker, J. (1992) The use of evaluation in the development of a staffed residential service for adults with mental handicap. *Mental Handicap Research*, **5**, 188–203.

Horner, R.H. and O'Neill, R. (1992) *Oregon Community Support: A two year analysis of community support for 11 people with histories of severe problem behaviour.* Paper presented at Association for Behavior Analysis Annual Convention, San Francisco, CA.

Hoskin, S. and Mansell, J. (1989) *What Matters Most: Quality Assurance for Front-line Staff.* Bexhill-on-Sea: South East Thames Regional Health Authority.

Hughes, H.M. and Mansell, J. (1990) *Consultation to Camberwell Health Authority Learning Difficulties Care Group: Evaluation Report.* Canterbury: Centre for the Applied Psychology of Social Care, University of Kent.

Jones, K., Brown, J., Cunningham, W.J., Roberts, J. and Williams, P. (1975) *Opening the Door: A Study of New Policies for the Mentally Handicapped.* London: Routledge and Kegan Paul.

Joyce, T.A. (1988) *Individual and Environmental Determinants of Normalisation-related Outcomes for Mentally Handicapped People Living in Hospital, Hostels and Staffed Houses.* Unpublished PhD Thesis, University of London United Medical and Dental Schools.

Kushlick, A. (1975a) Improving the services for the mentally handicapped, in *Behaviour Modification with the Severely Retarded* (eds C.C. Kiernan and F. P. Woodford).Amsterdam: Associated Scientific Publishers, pp. 263–93.

Kushlick, A. (1975b) The rehabilitation or habilitation of severely or profoundly retarded people. *Bulletin of the New York Academy of Medicine*, **51**, 143–61.

Kushlick, A. (1976) Wessex, England, in *Changing Patterns in Residential Services for the Mentally Retarded* (eds R.B. Kugel and A. Shearer). Washington, DC: President's Committee on Mental Retardation, pp. 297–311.

LaVigna, G.W., Willis, T.J. and Donellan, A.M. (1989) The role of positive programming in behavioral treatment, in *The Treatment of Severe Behavior Disorders* (ed. E. Cipani). Washington, DC: American Association on Mental Retardation, pp. 59–83.

Leavitt, H.J., Dill, W.R. and Eyring, H.B. (1989) Strategies for survival: How organizations cope with their worlds, in *Readings in Managerial Psychology* (eds H.J. Leavitt, L.R. Pondy and D.M. Boje). Chicago, IL: University of Chicago Press, pp. 722–32.

LeLaurin, K. and Risley, T.R. (1972) The organisation of day-care environments: 'Zone' vs. 'man-to-man' staff assignments. *Journal of Applied Behavior Analysis*, **5**, 225–32.

Lowe, K. and de Paiva, S. (1990) *The Evaluation of NIMROD, a Community*

*Based Service for People with Mental Handicap: Changes in Clients' Skill Levels and Usage.* Cardiff: Mental Handicap in Wales Applied Research Unit.

McBrien, J. and Weightman, J. (1980) The effect of room management procedures on engagement of profoundly handicapped children. *British Journal of Mental Subnormality,* **26,** 38–53.

McCord, W.T. (1982) From theory to reality: obstacles to the implementation of the normalization principle in human services. *Mental Retardation,* **20,** 247–53.

Mansell, J. and Beasley, F. (1989) Small staffed homes for the severely mentally handicapped: Strengths and weaknesses, in *Current Approaches: Mental Retardation* (eds V. Cowie and V.J. Harten-Ash). Southampton: Duphar Laboratories Limited, pp. 26–34.

Mansell, J. and Beasley, F. (in press) Small staffed houses for people with a severe mental handicap and challenging behaviour. *British Journal of Social Work,* (in press).

Mansell, J., Felce, D., de Kock, U. and Jenkins, J. (1982) Increasing purposeful activity of severely and profoundly mentally handicapped adults. *Behaviour Research and Therapy,* **20,** 593–604.

Mansell, J., Jenkins, J., Felce, D. and de Kock, U. (1984) Measuring the activity of severely and profoundly mentally handicapped adults in ordinary housing. *Behaviour Research and Therapy,* **22,** 23–9.

Mansell, J., Felce, D., Jenkins, J., de Kock, U. and Toogood, S. (1987) *Developing Staffed Housing for People with Mental Handicaps.* Tunbridge Wells: Costello.

Mohr, W.L. and Mohr, H. (1983) *Quality Circles: Changing Images of People at Work.* Reading, MA: Addison-Wesley.

Morris, P. (1969) *Put Away.* London: Routledge and Kegan Paul.

Newton, J.S., Romer, M., Bellamy, G.T., Horner, R.H. and Boles, S.M. (1988) *Neighbourhood Living Project: Tenant Support Operations Manual.* Eugene, OR: Center on Human Development.

Nihira, K., Foster, R., Shellhaas, M. and Leland, H. (1974) *AAMD Adaptive Behavior Scale.* Washington, DC: American Association on Mental Deficiency.

Orlowska, D.M.I. (1992) *An Ecobehavioural Perspective on the Performance of Direct Care Staff in Facilities for People with Learning Difficulties.* Unpublished PhD Thesis, University of Kent at Canterbury.

Pettipher, C. and Mansell, J. (in press) Engagement in meaningful activity in day centres: An exploratory study. *Mental Handicap Research,* (in press).

Porterfield, J. and Blunden, R. (1979) *Establishing Activity Periods in Special Needs Rooms within Adult Training Centres: A Replication Study.* Cardiff: Mental Handicap in Wales Applied Research Unit.

Porterfield, J., Blunden, R. and Blewitt, E. (1980) Improving environments for profoundly handicapped adults: Using prompts and social attention to maintain high group engagement. *Behavior Modification,* **4,** 225–41.

Quilitch, H.R. and Risley, T.R. (1973) The effects of play materials on social play. *Journal of Applied Behavior Analysis*, **6**, 573–8.

Rawlings, S. (1985a) Behaviour and skills of severely retarded adults in hospitals and small residential homes. *British Journal of Psychiatry*, **146**, 358–60.

Rawlings, S. (1985b) Life-styles of severely retarded non-communicating adults in hospitals and small residential homes. *British Journal of Social Work*, **15**, 281–93.

Reid, D.H., Parsons, M.B. and Green, C.W. (1989) *Staff Management in Human Services: Behavioral Research and Application*. Springfield, IL: Charles C. Thomas.

Repp, A.C. and Barton, L.E. (1980) Naturalistic observations of institutionalised retarded persons: A comparison of licensure decisions and behavioural observations. *Journal of Applied Behavior Analysis*, **13**, 333–41.

Repp, A.C. and Felce, D. (1990) A microcomputer system used for evaluative and experimental behavioural research in mental handicap. *Mental Handicap Research*, **3**, 21–32.

Rice, D.M. and Rosen, M. (1991) Direct-care staff: A neglected priority. *Mental Retardation*, **29**, iii–iv.

Risley, T.R. and Favell, J. (1979) Constructing a living environment in an institution, in *Behavioral Systems for the Developmentally Disabled: II – Institutional, Clinic and Community Environments* (ed. L.A. Hamerlynck). New York: Brunner/Mazel, pp. 3–24.

Rusch, F.R. (ed.) (1986) *Competitive Employment: Issues and Strategies*. Baltimore, MD: Paul H. Brookes.

Townsend, P. (1974) The political sociology of mental handicap – A case-study of failure in policy, in *The Social Minority* (ed. P. Townsend). London: Allen Lane, pp. 196–209.

Twardosz, S., Cataldo, M.F. and Risley, T.R. (1974) Open environment design for infant and toddler day care. *Journal of Applied Behavior Analysis*, **7**, 529–46.

Wilcox, B. and Bellamy, G.T. (1982) *Design of High School Programs for Severely Handicapped Students*. Baltimore, MD: Paul H. Brookes.

Woods, P.A. and Cullen, C. (1983) Determinants of staff behaviour in long-term care. *Behavioural Psychotherapy*, **11**, 4–17.

*Part Two*

---

# Service Options

# 5

# Ordinary housing for people with severe learning disabilities and challenging behaviours

*David Felce, Kathy Lowe and Siobhan de Paiva*

Many individuals with learning disabilities and challenging behaviours have lived and continue to live in traditional hospitals. The presence of such behaviours is commonly cited among the reasons for admission or readmission to institutional services (Pagel and Whitling, 1978; Sternlicht and Deutsch, 1972; Campbell *et al.*, 1982; Sherman, 1988; Sutter *et al.*, 1980; Hemming, 1982). As a consequence, the prevalence of severe challenging behaviour is higher in residential than community populations (Department of Health and Social Security and Welsh Office, 1971; Department of Health and Social Security, 1972; Harris and Russell, 1989; Kushlick and Cox, 1973; Oliver *et al.*, 1987; see also Chapter 2). Moreover, the fact that challenging behaviour occurs in community settings and is a primary cause of community placement breakdown does contribute to the view that there is a continuing need for traditional specialist services. People with challenging behaviour have typically not been included in the moves to community services to date as the rundown of traditional hospitals has progressed (Department of Health, 1989).

Despite the growth in acceptance of an 'Ordinary Life' model of service (King's Fund, 1980), ordinary housing services for people with severe learning disabilities and challenging behaviour have remained contentious. Whatever the merits of the respective posi-

tions, the lack of consensus between and within influential professional and other groupings has probably contributed to the continuing uncertainty characterizing national and local policies (see
also Chapter 13). Differences on the correct course of action seem
to have generated inaction. Experience of providing ordinary
housing services comprehensively to all adults with severe learning disability (with or without challenging behaviours) is, therefore, relatively meagre. However, as reduction in institutional
size proceeds to eventual closure, we are reaching the point when
the future options need to be determined and developed successfully. This chapter aims to make a contribution to this endeavour
by reviewing two community-based residential services which
have tested the water and, in doing so, have been the subject of
extensive research.

In 1981, the first houses were opened by the NIMROD service
in Cardiff and by Winchester Health Authority in Andover. Both
schemes are important and relevant to the current purpose because they set out to provide comprehensively for adults with
severe learning disabilities who required a residential service,
whether or not they had challenging behaviours. People with
challenging behaviours were not the exclusive focus of concern
but were not to be excluded. Moreover, both schemes adopted a
rigorous demographic basis to determine service availability. The
fact that each development aimed to provide for a comprehensive
demographic sample helps overcome some of the problems of
generalizing experience from one area to another.

## Definition of challenging behaviours in people with severe or profound learning disabilities

The term 'challenging behaviour' has come into usage recently,
replacing previous terms such as problem behaviour or
behaviour disorder, to reflect a view that the problem is not a
property of the behaving person but arises from how the
behaviour is perceived, tolerated or managed by other people.
The degree of challenge depends not only on the nature of the
behaviour but also on the abilities of carers and others to respond
to the behaviour to ameliorate or discourage it or to lessen its
impact. This creates a problem in arriving at a clear definition of
challenging behaviour: specifying behavioural topography is not
enough (Chapter 2).

However, previous terms were not in themselves more precise. Kushlick *et al.* (1973) described a short rating scale in which 'severe behaviour disorder' was defined by either aggression, self-injury or extreme overactivity at a marked frequency, by destructiveness and attention seeking both at a marked frequency, or by one of the latter at a marked frequency with the four other categories listed at a lesser frequency. Although well used in its original or slightly amended forms (e.g., Department of Health and Social Security, 1972; Caddell and Woods, 1984; National Development Team for Mentally Handicapped People, 1985), the definition of severe behaviour disorder embodied in the scale was by no means authoritative. For example, Wing and Gould (1979) amplified the list of behaviour problems included in their Handicaps, Behaviour and Skills Schedule and its short form, the Disability Assessment Schedule (Holmes *et al.*, 1982). Not surprisingly, they found a higher prevalence of behaviour disorder compared to surveys using the Kushlick, Blunden and Cox classification.

Part Two of the Adaptive Behavior Scale (ABS) (Nihira *et al.*, 1974) contains a list of 44 behaviour problem categories, not all of which would necessarily be viewed as severely challenging. In order to investigate which were, MacDonald and Barton (1986) designed a study to ascertain how direct-care staff viewed the relative severities of the 44 categories. They found that five behaviours were always viewed as severe problems, at whatever frequency they occurred. These were Physical Violence, Damage to Other's Property, Damage to Public Property, Self-injury and Substance Abuse. In addition, Damage to Personal Property, Violent Temper, Ignores Regulations, Impudent Attitude, Runs Away, Steals, Lies or Cheats, Removes Clothing, Inappropriate Masturbation, Exposes Body, Homosexual Tendencies, and Sexually Inappropriate Behaviour were rated as severe problems if they occurred frequently.

There is only partial overlap between MacDonald and Barton's findings and the Kushlick, Blunden and Cox categorization of severe behaviour disorder. There is, however, much greater overlap with the Disability Assessment Schedule (DAS). Table 5.1 shows the correspondence between DAS categories and ABS Part Two items classified according to their ratings in the MacDonald and Barton study as constituting either a severe or moderate challenge. Three behaviour categories used in the DAS (Night

**Table 5.1** Correspondence between the DAS and ABS Part Two behaviour problem items basing the categorization of severity on the results of MacDonald and Barton (1986)

| DAS | ABS | |
| --- | --- | --- |
| Physical aggression | Physical violence | Considered as severely challenging behaviours if marked or severe |
| Self-injury | Self-abuse | |
| Destructiveness | Damage to others' property<br>Damage to public property | |
| | Damage to personal property | Considered as severely challenging behaviours if marked |
| Temper tantrums | Violent temper | |
| Wanders off | Runs away | |
| Anti-social | Steals, lies, cheats (untrustworthy) | |
| | Masturbates | |
| Inappropriate sexual | Exposes body<br>Homosexual tendencies<br>Sexually inappropriate | |
| Objectionable personal habits | Removes clothing<br>Unacceptable oral habits<br>Strange/eccentric habits | Considered as moderately challenging behaviours if marked |
| Attention-seeking | Demands attention | |
| Overactivity | Hyperactive | |
| Disturbing noises | Disturbing speech | |
| Stereotyped behaviour | Stereotyped behaviour | |

Disturbance, Scatters or Throws Objects Around Aimlessly and Other) could not be paired with a counterpart from the ABS. The remaining 12 items provide a good basis for describing major categories of maladaptive behaviour, which, by reference to the MacDonald and Barton results, we can classify as either severely or moderately challenging. DAS assessments were available for all NIMROD and Andover residents so we have adopted the schema set out in Table 5.1 for the description of their behaviour.

### The NIMROD and Andover developments

Towards the end of the 1970s, plans began to be implemented in Cardiff to provide a jointly funded comprehensive community-based service, called NIMROD, to all people with learning disabilities in a defined territory of approximately 60 000 total population. At the same time, a more limited development was beginning in Winchester Health Authority with the aim of providing a comprehensive service to all adults with the most severe or profound learning disabilities who required residential care. The initial phase of this development was centred on the town of Andover and the surrounding countryside which fell within Test Valley Social Services Area, a territory which, coincidentally, also comprised approximately 60 000 total population. In both the NIMROD and the Andover projects, a staffed residential service was to be made available using ordinary community housing. The majority of the initial residents were expected to be people resettled from existing residential institutions, but both schemes were also designed to serve individuals in need who were currently living in family homes.

The NIMROD territory, situated in the west of the City of Cardiff (Welsh Office, 1978), was selected to typify the city as a whole, taking into account factors such as population distribution, natural community boundaries, housing types, socio-economic characteristics, availability of local community amenities and distribution of health and social services facilities. One important criterion in the selection of the territory was that the area did not have a concentration of facilities already within its boundaries, and that boundary divisions caused no unnecessary difficulties in co-ordination with existing services. The area was sub-divided into four distinct areas, or 'communities', of similar population size. The boundaries of all the communities closely followed existing electoral wards and natural boundaries, such as major roads, railway lines and rivers. The NIMROD service was introduced into the four communities sequentially over a two-and-a-half year period, between 1981 and 1983.

The service was designed to serve all people with a learning disability living in or, for those in residential care, originating from the catchment area. The identification of clients was undertaken by NIMROD personnel. A written approach was made to all learning disability agencies within South Glamorgan and to all learning disability hospitals throughout Wales and England. Extensive cross-checking of service records and the electoral register was undertaken to obtain a comprehensive client list. In addition, NIMROD personnel had access to the results of a prevalence survey of the city conducted by the researchers. Geographical location of each client's family home and current or previous receipt of learning disability services were the major criteria used to establish eligibility. No-one was excluded on the basis of severity of disability. However, a 'too able' checklist was developed to establish an upper cut-off limit for use with people whose diagnosis was unclear and who had not used any learning disability facility (Lowe and de Paiva, 1989). The boundaries of the four communities were precisely adhered to: where boundary lines cut through roads, only the addresses which fell within the catchment area were included.

NIMROD incorporated a range of components to provide a comprehensive service to clients, which included individual planning, keyworkers, staffed houses, supported group homes, domiciliary support, social work and psychology services, a volunteer scheme and family-based respite care (Lowe and de Paiva, 1989). The focus here is on the staffed residential component. All accommodation provided was in ordinary housing, mainly large terraces for groups of between four and six residents. Five houses were established: each had a team of seven and a half whole-time-equivalent care staff, including one senior. Residents attended conventional day services and staff rotas were organized to ensure that two or three staff were on duty early mornings, late afternoons and evenings on weekdays and throughout the day at weekends, while night time cover was provided by waking night staff. Three flats were also established, supported by one team of care staff, incorporating sleeping-in night staff.

Staff duties were prescribed in a series of detailed procedural guides. Client development was a major focus within the houses, and each resident had a designated 'training day'. As well as administrative and household tasks, staff responsibilities included working directly with residents during their training days on skill-related goals set at individual plan meetings. Staff were also directed to encourage residents' active participation in the day-to-day running of the house. The house seniors were responsible for monitoring the operation of the houses and for individual care staff reviews. The houses were overseen by community care managers, one of whom was appointed to each community, who held overall responsibility for all NIMROD services in their area.

A total of 125 clients were identified as eligible to receive NIMROD services at baseline: 62 living in traditional forms of residential care and 63 in the family home. Of the former 62, 22 were subsequently transferred to NIMROD staffed accommodation. No significant differences in clients' characteristics, as measured by the Social and Physical Incapacity (SPI), and Speech, Self Help and Literacy (SSL) Scales (Kushlick *et al.*, 1973), and by the Quality of Social Interaction (QSI) Scale (Holmes *et al.*, 1982), were evident between the group transferring to NIMROD accommodation and the total group of eligible clients, indicating no bias in the selection of those for transfer. Twelve of the 22 residents were male. Resident ages ranged from 20 to 80 years (mean age 45 years). According to the SPI and SSL Scales, the vast majority could walk (95%) and were continent (86%). Almost half had speech (45%) and were competent in the skills of feeding, washing and dressing (41%). Around a quarter were rated as severely behaviour disordered (27%) and 14% were literate. According to the QSI Scale, nearly two-thirds were said to interact appropriately to varying degrees, while a third were said to be socially impaired.

The Andover territory was approximately one-third of Winchester and Central Hampshire Health District and included a moderately-sized market town (30 000 total population) and its rural hinterland. The territory was defined by Health and Social Services Area boundaries. The outlying rural areas were well linked to the town by a number of arterial roads centring on Andover. The territory was subdivided to provide distinct catchment areas for each of two houses provided. The houses were provided by the health authority and opened in November 1981 and April 1983.

The houses were designed to serve all adults of 'health service dependency', who required a residential service and who had current next-of-kin living in either of the two catchment areas. In line with the divided responsibilities of health and social services agencies to provide residential care (Department of Health and Social Security and Welsh Office, 1971), Winchester District had agreed with its local authority counterpart to make provision for adults with the most severe learning disabilities. Operationally, eligibility was defined by address of next-of-kin and by behavioural criteria. The houses served adults with a local claim requiring residential care who were either Non-Ambulant, or had Severe Behaviour Disorder, or were Severely Incontinent Only or, if Continent, Ambulant and with No Severe Behaviour Disorder, were unable to feed, wash and dress independently (No Self-Help), using the above terms as defined by Kushlick *et al.* (1973). Within this eligibility spectrum, the service was to be comprehensive; no-one was to be excluded because they were too handicapped or behaviourally difficult.

In order to obtain a full identification of eligible clients, three search procedures were followed.

1.  A listing was obtained from the Wessex Register, which had a historical file dating back to the survey undertaken in 1963, of all adults in residential care with next-of-kin in the defined territory.
2.  A new survey was conducted by the Register, on behalf of the researchers, of everyone in residential care within Wessex and contiguous counties to identify people with current ties to the territory.
3.  A list was made of people currently attending services in the territory, including trainees at the local Adult Training Centre and leavers from the Special School.

New SPI/SSL Scale ratings were completed to check the behavioural criteria. Eligible clients were then identified in terms of those who were already in residential services and met the criteria. For those living at home, who met the required criteria, families were contacted and offered the service; a number either took the immediate opportunity for their child to move on or said that this was something which they would see occurring in the next few years.

The housing service has been extensively described elsewhere (e.g., Mansell *et al.*, 1987; Felce, 1989). In brief, each house had eight places, some of which were initially reserved to offer short-term care or to provide for the later admission of people living with their families. Accommodation was in ordinary housing extended to provide some ground-floor bedrooms, and furnished and equipped to meet private domestic standards. Eleven whole-time-equivalent staff, including one senior and one deputy, provided 24-hour support. This was sufficient to allocate two or three staff from early morning to late evening seven days per week and one waking night staff. Rotas were designed to allow staff to attend a two and a half hour weekly meeting together. Staff followed structured procedures for individual programme planning, individual teaching, providing specific individualized opportunities for activity each day, supporting resident participation in the domestic routine generally and for organizing household and community activity each day. Ways of monitoring resident activity (both in the house and outside), their social and family contacts and their development over time were embedded within these procedures (see Mansell *et al.*, 1987; Felce, 1989; 1991 for further details; see also Chapter 10).

Twenty-seven adults were identified who had next-of-kin in the research territory, had a severe learning disability and met the behavioural disability criteria. Of these, 13 people were already in residential care. Ten of this group moved into the houses on their opening. The three who remained in their previously available residential situation did so for reasons independent of their behaviour or severity of handicap: one because her parents were adamant that she should not return to live locally and it took several years to reverse their decision; one because his father had more than one address and his existing placement was close to another of his father's homes; and one because he was already resident in a local authority hostel locally. In addition to those being resettled from existing settings, four people initially living in their family homes were admitted to the ordinary housing services during the research period. A total of 14 adults therefore lived in the two houses during this time. Their behavioural characteristics were representative of the total identified sample. According to the SPI/SSL Scales, all were Ambulant, seven (50%) had Severe Behaviour Disorder, one (7%) was Severely Incontinent Only and six (43%) were rated as CAN but No Self Help. In terms of the SSL Scale alone, one person was rated as having Self

**Table 5.2** Reported behaviour problems at baseline for those who moved from hospital into NIMROD accommodation

| | Individual staffed house residents who moved from hospital | | | | | | | | | | | | | | | | | | | | | |
|---|---|---|---|---|---|---|---|---|---|---|---|---|---|---|---|---|---|---|---|---|---|---|
| | 1 | 2 | 3 | 4 | 5 | 6 | 7 | 8 | 9 | 10 | 11 | 12 | 13 | 14 | 15 | 16 | 17 | 18 | 19 | 20 | 21 | 22 |
| *Severely challenging behaviours** | | | | | | | | | | | | | | | | | | | | | | |
| Physical aggression | – | – | – | ✓ | – | – | – | ✓ | ✓ | ✓ | ✓ | – | – | – | ✓ | – | – | – | ✓ | – | – | ✓ |
| Destructiveness | – | ✓ | – | – | – | – | ✓ | ✓ | ✓ | ✓ | – | – | – | – | ✓ | ✓ | – | – | – | – | ✓ | ✓ |
| Self-injury | – | – | – | ✓ | – | – | ✓ | ✓ | ✓ | ✓ | – | ✓ | – | – | ✓ | – | – | ✓ | – | – | – | ✓ |
| Temper tantrums | – | – | – | ✓ | – | ✓ | – | ✓ | ✓ | – | ✓ | – | – | – | ✓ | – | – | – | – | ✓ | – | – |
| Wandering off | – | – | – | ✓ | – | – | – | – | – | – | – | – | – | – | – | – | – | – | – | – | – | – |
| Anti-social | – | – | – | – | – | – | – | – | – | – | – | – | – | – | – | – | – | – | – | – | – | – |
| Inappropriate sexual | – | – | – | – | – | – | – | – | – | – | – | – | – | – | – | – | – | – | – | – | – | – |
| *Moderately challenging behaviours* | | | | | | | | | | | | | | | | | | | | | | |
| Overactivity | – | – | – | ✓ | – | – | – | – | – | – | – | – | – | – | ✓ | – | – | – | – | – | ✓ | – |
| Attention seeking | – | – | – | ✓ | – | – | – | – | – | – | – | – | – | – | ✓ | – | – | – | – | – | – | – |
| Disturbing noises | – | – | – | – | – | – | – | – | – | – | ✓ | – | – | – | – | – | – | – | ✓ | – | – | – |
| Objectionable personal habits | – | ✓ | ✓ | ✓ | ✓ | ✓ | – | – | – | – | – | – | – | – | – | – | – | ✓ | ✓ | – | – | – |
| Stereotypies | – | – | ✓ | ✓ | ✓ | – | – | – | – | ✓ | – | – | – | – | ✓ | – | – | – | – | – | – | – |

* Physical aggression, destructiveness and self-injury at marked or lesser frequency; remaining behaviours in both categories at marked frequency

Help Only, four as having Speech Only and the remaining nine (64%) as having No Speech, Self Help or Literacy. Five were assessed as having the triad of social impairments and seven as being socially impaired (Wing and Gould, 1979). Three adults had been transferred to the houses directly from locked hospital wards where, between them, they had spent about 70 years.

## The presence of challenging behaviour

Tables 5.2 and 5.3 show the presence of challenging behaviour for each resident of the NIMROD and Andover houses included in the research. The data are taken from DAS assessments prior to admission using the classification of severely or moderately challenging behaviour from MacDonald and Barton (1986) as discussed earlier.

Fourteen people (64%) who moved to NIMROD accommodation were rated as presenting behaviours which could be classified as severely challenging. Eight were rated as having physical aggression, five were destructive, eight self-injurious, three had temper tantrums, three caused problems because of wandering off and three had other antisocial behaviours. Four residents were rated as having two severely challenging behaviours, two were

**Table 5.3** Reported behaviour problems at baseline for those who moved into the Andover houses

| | Individual staffed house residents | | | | | | | | | | | | | |
| | 1 | 2 | 3 | 4 | 5 | 6 | 7 | 8 | 9 | 10 | 11 | 12 | 13 | 14 |
|---|---|---|---|---|---|---|---|---|---|---|---|---|---|---|
| *Severely challenging behaviours** | | | | | | | | | | | | | | |
| Physical aggression | ✔ | ✔ | – | – | ✔ | – | – | – | – | – | ✔ | ✔ | ✔ | – |
| Destructiveness | ✔ | ✔ | – | – | ✔ | – | ✔ | – | – | – | – | – | – | – |
| Self-injury | – | ✔ | ✔ | – | ✔ | ✔ | ✔ | – | – | ✔ | – | – | – | – |
| Temper tantrums | – | – | ✔ | – | ✔ | – | ✔ | – | – | – | ✔ | – | – | – |
| Wandering Off | ✔ | – | – | – | – | – | – | – | – | – | – | – | – | – |
| Anti-social | – | – | – | – | – | – | – | – | – | – | – | – | – | – |
| Inappropriate sexual | – | – | – | – | – | – | – | – | – | – | – | ✔ | – | – |
| | | | | | | | | | | | | | | |
| *Moderately challenging behaviours* | | | | | | | | | | | | | | |
| Overactivity | ✔ | – | – | – | – | – | ✔ | – | – | – | – | ✔ | – | – |
| Attention seeking | ✔ | – | – | – | – | – | – | – | – | – | – | – | – | – |
| Disturbing noises | – | ✔ | – | – | ✔ | – | ✔ | – | – | – | ✔ | – | – | – |
| Objectionable personal habits | ✔ | – | – | – | – | – | ✔ | – | ✔ | ✔ | – | – | – | – |
| Stereotypies | ✔ | ✔ | – | – | ✔ | – | ✔ | – | – | ✔ | – | ✔ | – | – |

* Physical aggression, destructiveness and self-injury at marked or lesser frequency; remaining behaviours in both categories at marked frequency

rated as having three and two as having five. In addition, moderately challenging behaviours of overactivity, attention seeking, making disturbing noises, having objectionable personal habits or engaging in stereotypic behaviour were variously reported for 11 residents. Only five people (23%) were rated as having neither severely nor moderately challenging behaviour. The residents classified as having at least one severely challenging behaviour had, on average, 3.0 severely or moderately challenging behaviours each (range, 1–8).

Coincidentally, a similar proportion of the people (nine, 64%) who moved to the Andover houses were rated as presenting behaviours which could be classified as severely challenging. Six were rated as having physical aggression, four were destructive, six self-injurious, four had temper tantrums, one caused problems because of wandering off and one had inappropriate sexual behaviour. Four residents were rated as having two severely challenging behaviours, three were rated as having three and one as having four. In addition, moderately challenging behaviours of overactivity, attention seeking, making disturbing noises, having objectionable personal habits or engaging in stereotypic behaviour were variously reported for eight residents. Only four people (28%) were rated as having neither severely nor moderately challenging behaviour, although a fifth had only one problem behaviour classified here as presenting a moderate challenge. The residents classified as having at least one severely challenging behaviour had, on average, 4.4 severely or moderately challenging behaviours each (range, 2–7).

### Change in challenging behaviour over time

Data on change in levels of challenging behaviour are only available for the NIMROD group. Data were collected on the Andover sample using the ABS Part Two but low reliability of assessment rendered them uninterpretable. Readers are referred to Felce and Toogood (1988) for anecdotal accounts of development for nine of the residents. The DAS assessment was repeated for each of the NIMROD residents at approximately six-monthly intervals over five years. At the same time, staff were asked to assess the severity of management problem reported behaviours posed.

Challenging behaviours were not found to diminish. If anything, quite the reverse occurred. Significantly more challenging behaviours were reported for the NIMROD accommodation group following admission and the passage of time (de Paiva and Lowe, 1990). Moreover, there was a shift in how these behaviours were viewed by staff, with more being seen as presenting a severe or moderate management problem by the end of the evaluation period. Table 5.4 shows the proportions of the NIMROD group who were assessed at the beginning and the end of the study as having the various severely or moderately challenging behaviours considered above.

## Change in skills and quality of life

Nonetheless, a significant increase in overall scores on the Adaptive Behavior Scale Part One (Nihira *et al.*, 1974) occurred for the NIMROD group over the same time period. On average, a score gain of 3.6 points per person per year was attained. Significant increases in the ABS domains of responsibility, domestic activity and economic activity were evident. Similar results were obtained on the Pathways to Independence Checklist (Jeffree and Cheseldine, 1982) following transition, with significant increases

**Table 5.4** Proportion of NIMROD accommodation residents with severely and moderately challenging behaviours at T1 and T8

|  | T1 | | T8 | |
|---|---|---|---|---|
|  | *n* | *(%)* | *n* | *(%)* |
| *Severely challenging behaviours* | | | | |
| Physical aggression | 8 | (36) | 11 | (50) |
| Destructiveness | 5 | (23) | 9 | (41) |
| Self-injury | 8 | (36) | 9 | (41) |
| Temper tantrums | 3 | (14) | 13 | (59) |
| Wandering off | 3 | (14) | 1 | (5) |
| Anti-social | 3 | (14) | 5 | (23) |
| Inappropriate sexual | 0 | (0) | 3 | (14) |
| *Moderately challenging behaviours* | | | | |
| Overactivity | 1 | (5) | 5 | (23) |
| Attention seeking | 3 | (14) | 4 | (18) |
| Disturbing noises | 1 | (5) | 12 | (55) |
| Objectionable personal habits | 5 | (23) | 16 | (73) |
| Stereotypies | 6 | (27) | 2 | (9) |

in overall mean scores and on each of the two domains, domestic and community skills (Lowe and de Paiva, 1990).

Further indications of improvements in residents' lifestyles were evidenced by significant increases in their contact with community amenities, both in terms of the range used and in the frequency of usage (Lowe and de Paiva, 1991). The amenities used most were shops, parks, cafes, pubs, public transport, hairdressers and learning disability clubs. Increased use over time was particularly noted in relation to pubs and learning disability clubs. Although, overall, low proportions were said to have contact with friends, there was evidence to suggest that this group increased their contact with friends to the level of people already living in the community within their family homes. The majority had contact with their relatives throughout the five years, and there was evidence that the frequency of regular contact increased, from fortnightly to weekly, after transfer.

Improvements in quality of life and skill acquisition were also found for the residents of the Andover houses (Felce, 1989). Several studies compared their opportunities for activity and their levels of participation with (a) those that they had previously in institutional settings, (b) those of similar residents in institutions and (c) those of similar residents in larger community units (Felce *et al.*, 1985; 1986a; Thomas *et al.*, 1986). Significantly greater levels of opportunity and participation were found in the small houses. The house residents each spent about half of their time meaningfully occupied in a domestic, leisure, personal care or social pursuit. The comparison with institutional or large community unit care revealed that people with similar handicaps living in other settings spent about three-quarters, nine-tenths and even nineteen-twentieths of their time either doing nothing or behaving maladaptively. In all studies, the improved levels of opportunity and participation were related to greater interaction between staff and residents in the houses.

Similarly to the NIMROD results, the Andover group experienced more frequent contact with family and friends following transfer to the houses than when they were in their previous residential settings. The small-house residents maintained an average of 70 family or friendship contacts per year compared with a level of 12 before returning to live locally. In addition, their participation in the community increased dramatically (on average, 36-fold from an institutional level of seven events per year each to a new level of 254 events per year each). This level of community involvement was also significantly higher than that of similar residents in larger community units (de Kock *et al.*, 1988).

Using the ABS Part One, skill acquisition was measured for the residents of the first small house across two 18-month periods; for the residents of the second small house across one 18-month period before transfer and a second after; for the eligible clients who remained in institutional care across two 18-month periods and for those remaining in their parental homes across two 18-month periods. Progress (i.e. change in total score) was significantly greater in the small houses than in the institutional or parental home groups (Felce *et al.*, 1986b). Changes in total score mainly reflected differences on the domestic, self-direction and independent functioning domains of the scale: a not too unexpected result when one considers the nature of the service and the level of handicap of the client group.

## Conclusions and discussion

The questions concerning ordinary housing services and people with severe learning disabilities and challenging behaviours seem to fall into two groups. The first concern is whether it is feasible to provide residential services to this group using ordinary community housing: can such behaviour be contained in such settings, can staff cope, will the community be sufficiently receptive? The second concern is whether individuals benefit from such a service: do they experience an enhanced quality of life, does their behaviour change (do they gain skills, does their challenging behaviour decrease)? The evidence from the two service schemes described here shows grounds for qualified optimism on both counts.

Regarding the feasibility issue first, both service developments unquestionably admitted people with multiple severe challenging behaviours. Both offered a service to a comprehensive, demographically-defined group of substantially handicapped people. For a variety of reasons, not all those eligible were admitted, although coverage was almost total in the more restricted Andover sample. However, no decisions were made to exclude individuals on the basis of their challenging behaviour and the groups served were representative of the total samples in critical

respects. Both groups had a higher representation of people classified according to the Kushlick *et al.* (1973) method as having
Severe Behaviour Disorder (27% and 50% for NIMROD and
Andover respectively) than the average nationally in the hospital
census (17%: Department of Health and Social Security, 1972).

The first houses in both developments were opened in 1981. In
the nine years since that time, one person has moved from
NIMROD accommodation to the locked ward of the local learning
disability hospital because of an inability to cope with his challenging behaviour. This person, who is not included in the 22
people described in Table 5.2, was living in his family home at
baseline. He had a long history of challenging behaviour and
moved into a NIMROD house in October 1982. Progress was good
for about a year but then his challenging behaviour became more
serious, apparently linked to the failing of his already poor sight.
Since he was already deaf, his loss of vision left him more cut off
from the external world. Following several attempts to change
medication and the way staff interacted with him to lessen the
level of behavioural difficulty, he was finally admitted to hospital
in October 1984. Recent follow-up visits show that he remains
behaviourally challenging and is frequently given p.r.n. medication in the stretched circumstances that pertain on the ward. All of
the people admitted to the two Andover houses have remained in
the community since.

With one exception, therefore, all people with challenging
behaviours admitted to ordinary housing services in two parts of
the country have been maintained in the community. In many
ways, this achievement is equal to what is known about the 'specialist' hospitals. Evidence is rarely presented that clients improve
in or benefit from hospital care. The case for their continuation
mainly rests on the fact that many people with the most severely
challenging behaviours currently reside in hospital and that the
feasibility of alternative service models is yet to be demonstrated.
Using a criterion of ability to cope, then, the NIMROD and
Andover housing developments have demonstrated over a period of nearly a decade that ordinary housing services can cater
for the great majority of individuals with severe learning disabilities and challenging behaviours and, in this respect, are equivalent to existing hospitals. Given the demographic basis for client
selection, we can generalize from this experience to conclude that
services of similar ethos would be capable of achieving similar

results. One can envisage only a handful of individuals in any district or region posing a level of problem which might call for a particularly different solution. Even here, such solutions may involve the provision of ordinary community housing (Emerson, 1990; see also Chapter 6).

Addressing the benefits to client welfare, it is clear, when considering the NIMROD and Andover research as a whole, that individuals living in the houses had a greater level of participation in activities typical of daily living, enjoyed a better social life and more frequent family contact and gained skills at a faster rate than would have been the case had they received a hospital or larger community unit service. Living in ordinary community housing, then, is not just an issue of principle but one which can be demonstrated to be in the person's better interests. However, the hope that these improvements would also be reflected in a lessening of behavioural challenge was not borne out. For those who moved from hospital to NIMROD accommodation, the data suggested a tendency for challenging behaviours to be reported at a higher level at the first data collection point after the move and to continue at that level subsequently. Moreover, across research subjects living in NIMROD accommodation, their family homes and hospital, there was a trend over time in the reporting of the severity of the management problem such behaviours constituted. In all settings, they were more likely to be reported as causing a greater management problem towards the end of the research period than at the beginning.

It is difficult to interpret the evidence on challenging behaviour with precision. One possibility is that they reflect an actual increase in difficult behaviour of residents as some response to the characteristics of the community settings. Alternatively, the difference may lie in the reporting of behaviour, either in the operation of different standards of what constitutes a problem or in different capabilities to observe and encapsulate behaviour. It is interesting that a similar change in the reporting of the degree of challenge of individual behaviour was found across a variety of settings over time. This may reflect changing expectations generally of what should be achieved. No data are formally reported on the change in challenging behaviour of the Andover subjects due to the lack of reliability in the administration of the ABS Part Two. However, if the uncertainties caused to interpretation by this fact are overlooked, then a similar picture to the NIMROD results would be portrayed: one of challenging behaviour continuing and becoming more diverse in the post-transfer community settings. Yet anecdotal accounts of individual development (Felce and Toogood, 1988) largely describe successful resolution of the most conspicuous behavioural problems present on admission and a broadening of activity and skills over time.

The evidence on challenging behaviour in different environments is unsatisfactory. Certainly, we cannot conclude that improvements naturally occur in ordinary housing, as this has not been demonstrated. However, neither can we accept unequivocally the opposite view that they will continue to occur at similar or higher levels. Definitive research remains to be done. Direct systematic observation of behaviour is required to overcome the difficulties of interpretation inherent in measures which rely on reports of behaviour, particularly where a change in respondent is inevitable when clients change their place of residence.

However, despite these reservations, it is clear that some level of challenging behaviour continued within the ordinary housing models or else staff would not have reported it. This is consistent with evidence on the chronicity of challenging behaviour in institutional and community environments (Eyman *et al.*, 1981; Hill and Bruininks, 1984). It is also consistent with the diversity in possible causation of challenging behaviours (Chapter 3). One would not expect change in behaviours which were a manifestation of an underlying organic state or developmental problem. Nor, if it is correct to characterize community environments as having a greater ethos to involve clients in ordinary living, would one necessarily expect a reduction in behaviours which were environmentally determined if the causation was via negative reinforcement. Individuals who exhibit challenging behaviours to avoid demands, bring activities to an end, be removed to a quiet place or from the company of others may well continue to behave similarly in community settings. Stereotypic behaviours, possibly maintained by the sensory consequences that they produce (Lovaas *et al.*, 1987), would also be likely to continue, as would any related challenging behaviours which preserved the individual's access to stereotypy. Hence, we can be fairly certain in concluding that the problem of challenging behaviour will not be solved by a move to ordinary living *per se*. Challenging behaviour is not a product of institutional environments, cured by transfer to the community, and this conclusion is supported by some of the direct observational studies of these housing services (e.g., Felce *et al.*, 1986a; Saxby *et al.*, 1988).

If challenging behaviour is not going to decrease as a natural result of the provision of better community housing in the place of our inadequate existing institutions, then it must be addressed directly. Both of the services described here maintained an emphasis on individualized planning and a structured approach, although the latter may have been seen as more important in the Andover development than in NIMROD (see discussion in de Paiva and Lowe, 1990). Skills of behavioural analysis and programme design need to be represented at some level within the service system. Moreover, Felce (1989) has argued that these will only have a sustained beneficial effect if environments have the structure to offer people with severe handicaps the routine support they need to participate appropriately in everyday activity. The orientation and competencies of staff in this respect are vital and data from research in the South East Thames Region discriminating those services which are coping well with individuals with severely challenging behaviour confirms this view (Mansell and Beasley, 1990; see also Chapter 6).

## References

Caddell, J. and Woods, P. (1984) The Bryn y neuadd degree of dependency rating scale: An extension of the Wessex mental handicap register. *Mental Handicap*, **4**, 142–5.

Campbell, V., Smith, R. and Wool, R. (1982) Adaptive Behavior Scale differences in scores of mentally retarded individuals referred for institutionalization and those never referred. *American Journal of Mental Deficiency*, **86**, 425–8.

de Kock, U., Saxby, H., Thomas, M. and Felce, D. (1988) Community and family contact: An evaluation of small community homes for adults. *Mental Handicap Research*, **1**, 127–40.

de Paiva, S. and Lowe, K. (1990) *A Longitudinal Study of Maladaptive Behaviours Among People with Mental Handicaps in Different Residential Settings*. Cardiff: Mental Handicap in Wales Applied Research Unit.

Department of Health (1989) *Needs and Responses: Services for Adults with Mental Handicap who are Mentally Ill, who have Behaviour Problems or who Offend*. London: HMSO.

Department of Health and Social Security (1972) *Census of Mentally Handicapped Patients in Hospital in England and Wales at the end of 1970*. London: HMSO.

Department of Health and Social Security and Welsh Office (1971) *Better Services for the Mentally Handicapped*. London: HMSO.

Emerson, E. (1990) Designing individualised community-based place-ments as an alternative to institutions for people with a severe mental handicap and severe behaviour problem, in *Key Issues in Mental Retar-dation Research* (ed. W. Fraser). London: Routledge, pp. 395–404.

Eyman, R.K., Borthwick, S.A. and Miller, C. (1981) Trends in maladaptive behavior of mentally retarded persons placed in community and insti-tutional settings. *American Journal of Mental Deficiency*, **85**, 473–7.

Felce, D. (1989) *Staffed Housing for Adults with Severe or Profound Mental Handicaps: The Andover Project.* Kidderminster: BIMH Publications.

Felce, D. (1991) Using behavioural principles in the development of effective housing services for adults with severe or profound mental handicaps, in *The Challenge of Severe Mental Handicap: A Behaviour Ana-lytic Approach* (ed. B. Remington). Chichester: John Wiley and Sons, pp. 285–316.

Felce, D. and Toogood, S. (1988) *Close to Home.* Kidderminster: BIMH Publications.

Felce, D., Thomas, M., de Kock, U. Saxby, H. and Repp, A. (1985) An ecological comparison of small community-based houses and tradi-tional institutions for severely and profoundly mentally handicapped adults: II. Physical settings and the use of opportunities. *Behaviour Research and Therapy*, **23**, 337–48.

Felce, D., de Kock, U. and Repp, A.C. (1986a) An eco-behavioral compari-son of small home and institutional settings for severely and pro-foundly mentally handicapped adults. *Applied Research in Mental Retardation*, **7**, 393–408.

Felce, D., de Kock, U., Thomas, M. and Saxby, H. (1986b) Change in adaptive behaviour of severely and profoundly mentally handicapped adults in different residential settings. *British Journal of Psychology*, **77**, 489–501.

Harris, P. and Russell, O. (1989) *The Prevalence of Aggressive Behaviour among People with Learning Difficulties (Mental Handicap) in a Single Health District: Interim Report.* Bristol: Norah Fry Research Centre, Uni-versity of Bristol.

Hemming, H. (1982) Mentally handicapped adults returned to large in-stitutions after transfers to new small units. *British Journal of Mental Subnormality*, **28**, 13–28.

Hill, B.K. and Bruininks, R.H. (1984) Maladaptive behavior of mentally retarded individuals in residential facilities. *American Journal of Mental Deficiency*, **88**, 380–7.

Holmes, N., Shah, A. and Wing, L. (1982) The Disability Assessment Schedule: A brief screening device for use with the mentally retarded. *Psychological Medicine*, **12**, 879–90.

Jeffree, D. and Cheseldine, S. (1982) *Pathways to Independence.* Sevenoaks: Hodder and Stoughton Educational.

King's Fund (1980) *An Ordinary Life: Comprehensive Locally-based Re-sidential Services for Mentally Handicapped People.* London: King's Fund Centre.

Kushlick, A. and Cox, G.R. (1973) The epidemiology of mental handicap. *Developmental Medicine and Child Neurology*, **15**, 748–59.

Kushlick, A., Blunden, R. and Cox, G. (1973) A method of rating behaviour characteristics for use in large scale surveys of mental handicap. *Psychological Medicine*, **3**, 466–78.

Lovaas, I., Newsom, C. and Hickman, C. (1987) Self-stimulatory behavior and perceptual reinforcement. *Journal of Applied Behavior Analysis*, **20**, 45–68.

Lowe, K. and de Paiva, S. (1989) *The Evaluation of NIMROD, a Community Based Service for People with Mental Handicap: The Service, Staff and Clients*. Cardiff: Mental Handicap in Wales Applied Research Unit.

Lowe, K. and de Paiva, S. (1990) *Effects of a Community-Based Service on the Adaptive Behaviour of People with Mental Handicaps: A Longitudinal Study*. Cardiff: Mental Handicap in Wales Applied Research Unit.

Lowe, K. and de Paiva, S. (1991) Clients' community and social contacts: Results of a five year longitudinal study. *Journal of Mental Deficiency Research*, **35**, 308–23.

MacDonald, L. and Barton, L.E. (1986) Measuring severity of behavior: A revision of Part II of the Adaptive Behavior Scale. *American Journal of Mental Deficiency*, **90**, 418–24.

Mansell, J. and Beasley, F. (1990) Severe mental handicap and problem behaviour: Evaluating transfer from institutions to community care, in *Key Issues in Mental Retardation Research* (ed. W. Fraser). London: Routledge, pp. 405–414.

Mansell, J., Felce, D., Jenkins, J., de Kock, U. and Toogood, A. (1987) *Developing Staffed Housing for People with Mental Handicaps*. Tunbridge Wells: Costello.

National Development Team for Mentally Handicapped People (1985) *Fourth Report 1981–1984*. London: HMSO.

Nihira, K., Foster, R., Shellhaas, M. and Leland, H. (1974) *AAMD Adaptive Behaviour Scale*. Washington, DC: American Association on Mental Deficiency

Oliver, C., Murphy, G.H. and Corbett, J.A. (1987) Self-injurious behaviour in people with mental handicap: A total population study. *Journal of Mental Deficiency Research*, **31**, 147–62.

Pagel, S.E. and Whitling, C.A. (1978) Readmissions to a state hospital for mentally retarded persons: Reasons for community placement failure. *Mental Retardation*, **16**, 164–6.

Saxby, H., Felce, D., Harman, M. and Repp, A. (1988) The maintenance of client activity and staff–client interaction in small community houses for severely and profoundly mentally handicapped adults: A two-year follow-up. *Behavioural Psychotherapy*, **16**, 189–206.

Sherman, B.R. (1988) Predictors of the decision to place developmentally disabled family members in residential care. *American Journal on Mental Retardation*, **92**, 344–51.

Sternlicht, M. and Deutsch, M.R. (1972) *Personality Development And Social Behavior In The Mentally Retarded*. Lexington, MA: D.C. Heath.

Sutter, P., Mayeda, T., Call, T., Yanagi, G. and Yee, S. (1980) Comparison of successful and unsuccessful community-placed mentally retarded persons. *American Journal of Mental Deficiency*, **85**, 262–7.

Thomas, M., Felce, D., de Kock, U. and Saxby, H. (1986) The activity of staff and of severely and profoundly mentally handicapped adults in residential settings of different sizes. *British Journal of Mental Subnormality*, **32**, 82–92.

Welsh Office (1978) *NIMROD: Report of a Joint Working Party on the Provision of a Community Based Mental Handicap Service in South Glamorgan.* Cardiff: Welsh Office.

Wing, L. and Gould, J. (1979) Severe impairments of social interaction and associated abnormalities in children: Epidemiology and classification. *Journal of Autism and Developmental Disorders*, **9**, 11–29.

# 6

# Individually designed residential provision for people with seriously challenging behaviours

*Peter McGill, Eric Emerson and Jim Mansell*

This chapter will describe and evaluate community-based residential services set up for people with severe learning disabilities and the most severely challenging behaviour in the South East Thames Region of England. The services considered are those set up with the assistance of the Special Development Team (Emerson and McGill, in press) but this chapter will focus on the services themselves rather than the work of the SDT.

Following a brief discussion of the background, the chapter will describe the factors which led to the services developing, the processes by which the services were set up, the clients served and other 'structural' aspects of the services, and their operational characteristics. The success of the services will be considered both from the viewpoint of a formal evaluation study (Mansell and Beasley, in press) and through a number of individual case descriptions. Finally, the common characteristics of such services will be discussed and the lessons for those involved in developing, operating and supporting them considered.

## Background

Residential services for people with challenging behaviour have traditionally been more likely to be provided in institutional settings (Chapter 2). Challenging behaviour is one of the factors most likely to lead to institutional placement (Chapter 5) and to reinstitutionalization following community placement (Chapter 11). Within institutions people with the most severe challenging behaviour have often been congregated together on one ward or unit, either with a treatment rationale or with the intention of managing the problems with less disruption to other clients and units (Newman and Emerson, 1991).

In recent years, as hospitals have begun to reduce in size and close, the phenomenon of transinstitutionalization has developed where individuals with challenging behaviour are amongst the most likely to be resettled in another institution to allow their original institution to close. There has been a growth in the provision of residential care by private psychiatric hospitals and other commercial providers, and one of their best groups of customers has been people with severe learning disabilities and challenging behaviour. This growth has paralleled the growth in community care so that the same agencies who are extensively developing housing-based services for the majority of people with severe learning disabilities are sometimes placing quite large numbers of people 'out of district' because of difficulties coping with their challenging behaviour (Hughes and Mansell, 1990; see also Chapter 11).

As the history of community residential provision is one of exclusion and breakdown it might be asked why anyone should want to develop such services for people with (the most serious) challenging behaviour and why it should be thought that such an enterprise might succeed. The services described in this chapter had four grounds for optimism. Firstly, most previous attempts have been based only to a very limited extent, if at all, on individual planning and design. Such a lack of individualization has been widely seen (e.g., King's Fund, 1980) as the source of the frequent failure to meet individual client needs and, from a different perspective, as leading to the inefficient and ineffective deployment of resources (Departments of Health and Social Security, Welsh Office, Scottish Office, 1989). By starting from the individual and tailoring the service to a comprehensive assessment of their needs, it was hoped that the resulting provision would be more responsive and successful.

Secondly, the last 15 years have seen a considerable increase in understanding of the causes of, and influences on, challenging

behaviour (Chapter 3). If this understanding could be implemented in the analysis of the problems presented by a particular
individual and in the provision of management and intervention
plans there was a better chance of containing the person's
behaviour within safe boundaries and possibly ameliorating it
over time.

Thirdly, understanding of the organization of residential placements has also greatly improved in recent years (Felce, 1989;
Mansell *et al.*, 1987; see also Chapter 10). In the light of this and the
former development the frequent failure of previous attempts
could be seen as reflecting their lack of clinical and organizational
sophistication.

Fourthly, the services to be described were all, at least initially,
operating in a relatively resource-rich environment. Thus extra
money was available to pump-prime the revenue costs of each
placement, capital was available to many of them to offset the
initial property purchasing and development costs, and 'free'
technical support was to be provided by the Regional Health
Authority through the SDT.

Despite the adverse history, therefore, there were sufficient
rational grounds for optimism to persuade many people that it
was worth having a try.

## The services

### Policy context

The South East Thames Regional Health Authority (SETRHA) is
responsible for the co-ordination of health care provided by 15
District Health Authorities and the Special Health Authority
(Maudsley and Bethlem Royal Hospitals) to 3 600 000 people
in the south east of England. During the 1980s SETRHA embarked upon an ambitious plan of institutional reprovision
centring upon the phasing out and eventual closure of Darenth
Park Hospital (Korman and Glennerster, 1985; 1990). Within this
process, the role of the RHA was perceived to be facilitation of
change through the co-ordination of planning and the establishment of financial mechanisms to enable the redistribution of the
resources currently tied up in institutions. As a result of the success of these measures, several smaller institutions within the

Region closed and the pace of the phasing out of Darenth Park Hospital increased in the mid-1980s until its eventual closure in 1988.

During the early stages of this programme, however, it was recognized that the resettlement of a number of individuals, those with special needs, would present such a challenge to receiving services that additional RHA-led initiatives were considered appropriate. Such concerns were confirmed by the experience of the hospital closure programme which demonstrated the all too familiar pattern of receiving agencies reproviding services for the most able/least needy, leaving institutional services coping, with depleted resources, with an increasingly disabled population.

Existing policy options for those with special needs involved the development of subregional treatment and residential units for those clients whose needs were considered too complex or challenging for local services (South East Thames Regional Health Authority, 1979). Increasingly, however, such plans were seen as out of step with some of the more innovative developments occurring in leading Districts within the Region which had adopted an 'ordinary life' model (King's Fund, 1980) as a foundation for service development.

These developments were reflected in the appointment of a Regional Coordinator of Staff Training in 1983 and the subsequent organization of training courses for professionals and managers on staffed domestic housing for the residential care of people with serious disabilities (Mansell, 1988; 1989). The time was right, therefore, for the development of relatively radical proposals for those groups of clients who had until then, to all intents and purposes, been 'left out' of local service developments. Indeed, a subsequent review of the RHA's Special Needs Policy (South East Thames Regional Health Authority, 1985) proposed that, instead of subregional units, services for people with severe learning disabilities and severely challenging behaviour should be set up by District Health Authorities and other local agencies with the expert assistance of a regionally funded Special Development Team.

This proposal was accepted by Regional and District officers, the support of the Regional Nursing Officer being particularly crucial to its success, as it was for much of the hospital closure and reprovision process (Korman and Glennerster, 1990). The Special Development Team was established as a five-year project in 1985 and was later funded (with a changed remit) for an additional five years (Emerson and McGill, in press).

## Clients

While it has been suggested that over 50% of people with severe learning disabilities are likely to display behaviour problems at some time or other (Chapter 2), it should be stressed at the outset that the clients considered here are those with the most extreme and durable challenging behaviour. Indeed the project was initially conceptualized as focusing on the 38 'most challenging' individuals within the Region.

Potential clients were identified in each District through a meeting between the SDT and senior managers and professional staff of local agencies (health, social services and, occasionally, education). Typically a 'short-list' of eight to ten potential clients was identified who were screened by the SDT and final decisions were then made in conjunction with local staff. The main criteria for acceptance on to the team's caseload were their level of ability (having a severe learning disability) and the severity of the challenge presented by their behaviour. Some clients were judged to be too able and the referring agency was directed on to the regionally supported initiative for clients with mild learning disabilities – the Mental Impairment Evaluation and Treatment Service (Murphy and Clare, 1991; Murphy *et al.*, 1991). Some referrals were judged to not display severely challenging behaviour. In such cases regional policy was that local agencies needed to make their own arrangements to cope with such individuals without external assistance. Services developed for these individuals are not considered here.

This process resulted in the identification of 35 clients in 14 separate District Health Authorities. To date services have been developed for 22 of these clients in nine separate Districts. Information about these 22 clients is given in Table 6.1. A number of general points can be made.

1. All clients had spent considerable periods of their lives in institutional settings.
2. Many had lived in several different placements, not counting different wards within institutions.
3. All displayed severe learning disabilities in terms of their level of adaptive behaviour.

**Table 6.1** Services set up with the support of the Special Development Team

| Client characteristics[1] | Original living arrangements | Staffing establishment | Date opened | Current status | Overall revenue costs[2] (£) |
|---|---|---|---|---|---|
| 44-year-old man, severe self-injury and destructive behaviour | Four-bedroomed house shared with three others with mild/moderate learning disability and without seriously challenging behaviour | 9 wte | 21.6.88 | Service relocated to a detached house after one year because of the amount of noise. Other arrangements still stand | 140 000 |
| 36-year-old woman, aggressive and destructive behaviour, extremely socially withdrawn | Four-bedroomed detached house in residential area shared with three others with mild/moderate learning disability and without seriously challenging behaviour | 9 wte | 25.6.90 | Original arrangements still stand | 130 000 |
| 18-year-old man, aggressive and destructive behaviour, severe non-compliance | Three-bedroomed detached house, shared with one other with severe learning disabilities and seriously challenging behaviour | 8.25 wte | 29.4.91 | Original arrangements still stand | 120 000 |
| 17-year-old man, aggressive and destructive behaviour | Three-bedroomed terraced house, shared with live-in member of staff and non-handicapped co-tenant | 4.5 wte | 23.10.88 | In April 1991 client moved to the service immediately above, partly because of the isolation arising in a single-client service, | 60 000 |

| Client | Accommodation | Staff | Date | partly because of a belief that now in a position to benefit from sharing, partly for logistic and financial reasons | Cost |
|---|---|---|---|---|---|
| 30-year-old man, aggressive and destructive behaviour | Five-bedroomed bungalow in residential area, shared with two others with severe learning disabilities without seriously challenging behaviour | 14.5 wte | 1.7.91 | Client died of natural causes in April 1992 | 210 000 |
| 39-year-old woman, aggressive and obsessional behaviour | Five-bedroomed detached house in residential area, shared with three others with severe learning disabilities without seriously challenging behaviour | 10 wte | 6.3.89 | Client died of natural causes in January 1990 | 110 000 |
| 18-year-old woman, self-injurious behaviour | Four-bedroomed detached house in residential area, shared with three others with severe learning disabilities without seriously challenging behaviour | 13 wte | 15.9.87 | Original arrangements still stand although some of the co-tenants have changed | 160 000 |
| 29-year-old man, destructive and obsessional behaviour | Five-bedroomed detached house in residential area, shared with four others with severe learning disabilities three of whom display challenging behaviour | 14.6 wte | 22.4.91 | Original arrangements still stand | 180 000 |

**Table 6.1** (Continued)

| Client characteristics[1] | Original living arrangements | Staffing establishment | Date opened | Current status | Overall revenue costs[2] (£) |
|---|---|---|---|---|---|
| 22-year-old man, aggressive and anti-social behaviour | Three-bedroomed house, shared with one other with severe learning disabilities and seriously challenging behaviour (also an SDT client) | 10 wte | 9.6.88 | In April 1991 the placement was closed and the clients resettled to another, larger service in the District to save money | 120000 |
| 28-year-old-man, aggressive and destructive behaviour | Three-bedroomed house, shared with one other with severe learning disabilities and seriously challenging behaviour (also an SDT client) | 10 wte | 9.6.88 | In April 1991 the placement was closed and the clients resettled to another, larger service in the District to save money | 120000 |
| 31-year-old man, aggressive and self-injurious behaviour | Three-bedroomed house (a 'staff' house on a campus development for 72 people – originally intended as an interim placement but the DHA was unable to obtain capital to go ahead with property purchase), shared with two others with severe learning disabilities, one of whom displays seriously challenging behaviour (also an SDT client) | 10.5 wte | 20.3.89 | Original arrangements still stand | 110000 |

| Client | Housing | Staff | Date | Notes | Cost |
|---|---|---|---|---|---|
| 41-year-old man, aggressive and destructive behaviour | Three-bedroomed detached bungalow in residential area, shared with two others with severe learning disabilities, one of whom displays seriously challenging behaviour | 10.5 wte | 20.3.89 | Original arrangements still stand | 110000 |
| 24-year-old man, self-injurious behaviour | Three-bedroomed house (a 'staff' house on a campus development for 72 people – originally intended as an interim placement but the DHA was unable to obtain capital to go ahead with property purchase), shared with two others with severe learning disabilities, one of whom displays seriously challenging behaviour (also an SDT client) | 10.5 wte | 20.3.89 | Original arrangements still stand | 110000 |
| 33-year-old woman, aggressive behaviour | One-bedroomed flat in a residential building containing a second flat occupied by four others with severe learning disabilities without seriously challenging behaviour | 14 wte (supporting both flats) | 5.10.88 | In April 1990 the client was moved within the district and, subsequently, out of the district because of difficulty in managing aggressive behaviour. With the support of the SDT a placement was reestablished in March | 70000[3] |

**Table 6.1** (*Continued*)

| Client characteristics[1] | Original living arrangements | Staffing establishment | Date opened | Current status | Overall revenue costs[2] (£) |
|---|---|---|---|---|---|
| | | | | 1991 in a single-person flat on a campus development for 48 people within the District | |
| 22-year-old man, aggressive and destructive behaviour | Five-bedroomed terraced house in residential area, shared with two others with mild learning disabilities without seriously challenging behaviour | 10 wte | 22.8.88 | On 13.9.88, as a result of difficulty in managing aggressive behaviour, the client was moved to a large mental handicap hospital in another district where he remains to date | 160 000 |
| 22-year-old woman, aggressive behaviour | Three-bedroomed semi-detached house in residential area, shared with one other with severe learning disabilities | 9 wte | 27.11.89 | Original arrangements still stand | 140 000 |
| 33-year-old woman, destructive and non-compliant behaviour | Four-bedroomed terraced house in residential area, shared with two others with severe learning disabilities without seriously challenging behaviours | 10 wte | 30.6.88 | Original arrangements still stand | 140 000 |

| Client | Accommodation | Staffing | Date | Outcome | Cost (£) |
| --- | --- | --- | --- | --- | --- |
| 29-year-old man, aggressive, destructive and sexually inappropriate behaviour | Two-bedroomed flat in residential area, living alone | 7 wte | 5.8.88 | In September 1990 the client was moved to a staff flat in a local, small mental handicap hospital because of difficulty in managing his behaviour and threat of eviction | 100 000 |
| 32-year-old man, self-injurious and destructive behaviour | Three-bedroomed semi-detached house in residential area, shared with one other with severe learning disabilities without seriously challenging behaviours | 10.5 wte | 2.5.88 | In October 1989 the client was moved to a similar but more accessible placement within the district because of a deterioration in mobility | 150 000 |
| 30-year-old man, aggression, inappropriate sexual behaviour | Three-bedroomed flat in residential area on the same site as a hostel for people with learning disabilities, shared with one other with mild learning disabilities and seriously challenging behaviour | 12 wte | 26.1.90 | Original arrangements still stand, although consideration is being given to the introduction of a third client | 160 000 |
| 28-year-old man, aggressive and destructive behaviour | Five-bedroomed detached bungalow in residential area, shared with four others with severe learning disabilities and challenging or seriously challenging behaviour (one of whom is an SDT client) | 15 wte | 2.9.91 | Original arrangements still stand | 200 000 |

**Table 6.1** (*Continued*)

| Client characteristics[1] | Original living arrangements | Staffing establishment | Date opened | Current status | Overall revenue costs[2] (£) |
|---|---|---|---|---|---|
| 33-year-old woman, aggressive and destructive behaviour | Five-bedroomed detached bungalow in residential area, shared with four others with severe learning disabilities and challenging or seriously challenging behaviour (one of whom is an SDT client) | 15 wte | 2.9.91 | Original arrangements still stand | 200 000 |

1. All client ages as of date of opening of service
2. Unless otherwise indicated revenue costs refer to the annual costs of providing the entire service i.e. including co-tenants (where applicable) as well as the SDT client. To provide some measure of comparability costs are all at 1991/92 levels. Where current costs are not available the original cost of the service has been inflated at 8% per annum to produce an approximation to the current figure. All costs should be treated as approximate
3. This refers to the cost of the single-person flat only

4. All displayed more than one seriously challenging behaviour and many displayed several. In addition to those mentioned in the table all clients displayed stereotyped behaviour of various forms. The most frequently occurring behaviours were aggression, destructiveness and self injury.
5. In all cases clients' challenging behaviour had a long history and, in a number of cases, had proved resistant to treatment at specialist units.
6. In some cases analogue assessment procedures (Iwata *et al.*, 1982) were used to assess the function of clients' challenging behaviours. These procedures suggested that demand avoidance was the most frequent function (Emerson *et al.*, 1988).

A more qualitative description of one of the clients may serve to emphasize the severity of the problems presented. An assessment report based on her institutional placement prior to resettlement included the following:

these [behaviours] include assault of others (pulling hair, pinching, scratching), manual evacuation and smearing of faeces, removing and tearing her clothes, eating inappropriate objects (e.g., torn clothing), throwing objects and stealing food. These behaviours occur on at least a daily basis if she has the opportunity. Aggression occurs regularly and persistently whenever she is approached. She currently spends the majority of her day sitting or lying under a blanket in the corner of the ward. The combination of faecal smearing and aggression on others approaching has led to her being avoided by staff unless it is absolutely necessary to approach her . . . in general she is a very challenging young woman who will respond with unpleasant aggression (faeces smeared hand in the victim's hair) if approached.

### Planning

Almost all services were based on a written individual service plan developed as a collaborative venture between the SDT, managers and professional staff in the receiving and sending services, and relatives, friends or advocates of the client. Leadership in this enterprise was usually, but not always, provided by the SDT (Toogood *et al.*, 1988). The serious disabilities of the clients precluded their effective contribution to such an abstract process, although on many occasions they were present at meetings convened to develop the plan.

Each ISP contained a detailed specification, including estimates of revenue and capital costs, of the support required to provide a high-quality community-based service for the client. The processes involved in this task drew heavily upon the types of ethnographic group work advocated by Brost *et al.* (1982) and O'Brien (1987). As a result both the process and the final product were characterized by a strong emphasis upon normalization-related values and the use of mechanisms for providing support which appeared to combine effectiveness (in achieving the desired outcomes) with conformity to local social and cultural values. Thus, for example, all completed individual service plans advocated that the client should live in ordinary domestic housing centrally located within the community so as to give ready access to as wide a range as possible of local facilities.

While District Health Authorities were inevitably involved in the planning process they did not always act as lead agency or 'provider' of the placement. Of the 22 placements developed, the Health Authority was the initial provider of 15, the local authority of three, a voluntary organization of two and a private organization of two. In a few cases there were subsequent changes or planned transfers of provision, reflecting the increasing role of private, voluntary and non-profit-making agencies in the provision of residential care.

### Client groupings

As part of the individual service planning process, consideration was usually given to a number of options involving different client groupings and the degree to which the options were likely to meet the focal client's needs. Thus, typically, living alone, living in a small group, living with a family, and a 'lifeshare' arrangement with non-handicapped co-tenants were considered and evaluated.

In retrospect, it is interesting to consider the criteria used to generate and evaluate these options, the manner in which decisions were reached about the most satisfactory option, and their actual implementation (or otherwise). The main criteria used can be categorized as ideological, pragmatic and behavioural. Ideological criteria included considering with whom the client might like to live, notions of avoiding the congregation of people with challenging behaviour, and providing the client with co-tenants who could function as positive role models. Behavioural criteria included the dangerousness of the client's behaviour to other tenants and other factors (e.g., noise) which might make it difficult for other people to live with the client. Pragmatic factors included cost, property availability, the staffing implications of single person placements, the acceptability of the option to local service mangers (e.g., its perceived 'fairness' given the resources available to other clients), and the urgency with which the placement had to be developed (e.g., because of hospital closure deadlines).

Perusal of individual service plans suggests that, while the behavioural factors undoubtedly excluded certain sorts of client groupings (e.g., highly dependent, immobile co-tenants) they had little other influence on the option selected. Ideological criteria appear to have had some influence in that practically all individual service plans proposed that the person should live in a small group with more able clients without challenging behaviour. Within these ideological boundaries, pragmatic considerations, however, were very important. Such considerations usually ruled out the most expensive options, excluded single person placements on the grounds of both cost and difficulty of organizing staff support, and generated recommendations which were relatively easy to implement and helped the agency to speedily resettle the client and others for whom they were responsible. Such pragmatic factors sometimes overruled ideological considerations, so that one shared placement was planned for two clients, both of whom had seriously challenging behaviour but had no 'special relationship', and another shared placement had places 'reserved' for people with a lesser degree of challenging behaviour.

It is clear, then, that the development of the planned client grouping reflected a process of negotiation in which some of the parties (including, but not only, the SDT) were able to force consideration of more radical options and raise the profile of ideological and behavioural criteria, while other parties (e.g., senior managers of the providing agencies) were attempting to reach decisions primarily informed by pragmatic considerations. The result of this process, the agreed client grouping, was often subject to further informal negotiation as the service was commissioned so that relatively radical plans were sometimes watered down as they were implemented. This resulted in most clients living in small groups where their co-tenants sometimes displayed challenging behaviour (18 out of 42 co-tenants did so) and usually had severe learning disabilities (33 out of 42). Three clients initially lived on their own but it seems likely that even these options were adopted at least partly on pragmatic grounds. For example, the decision making process was described in one of these clients' plans as follows: 'As ––––– has demonstrated that he can occasionally find it difficult to live with his peer group, it was decided to be in his best interests to share his home with people who would act as positive role models (non-handicapped co-tenants)'. As this statement was true of almost all the clients it seems unlikely to have been the key factor in the decision that this person should live apart from other handicapped people. Information about the client grouping in each of the placements is given in Table 6.1.

## Buildings

All properties were domestic houses or flats and were in close or reasonable proximity to generic community facilities. They were usually bought on the open market. While many properties required substantial modifications these were dictated more by the needs of the property than by the needs of the client. The modifications made to take account of the challenging behaviours presented by clients have included strengthened glass, soundproofing and electrical circuit breakers. These modifications were made selectively rather than routinely. Furniture, fixtures and fittings were selected to be as aesthetically pleasing as possible but also to minimize unnecessary risks and to withstand heavy prolonged use. These criteria sometimes resulted in more expensive, higher-quality furniture being provided.

## Staffing

The majority of the clients showed intense aggressive behaviours which would, at times, require the immediate intervention of two or more members of staff to ensure the safety of the person and of others in the vicinity. This, in effect, dictated the staffing requirements of the proposed services, i.e., two or three staff on duty at any one time. It was clear, however, that such staffing ratios would be unnecessary for the vast majority of the time because of the infrequent occurrence of such episodes. As a result, rather than develop an inefficient service in which the majority of staff were underemployed at any one time, group living options (as described earlier) were usually developed so that the 'redundant' staff time could be spent supporting other people with learning disabilities in the same residential setting. The size of staff groups in each placement is given in Table 6.1.

Staff teams invariably had a home leader, and usually had one or more deputy/assistant home leaders, with the rest of the posts being support workers/care assistants. In some cases the recruitment and appointment policies of the provider agencies meant that senior placement staff had to have nursing qualifications. In others it was possible to appoint staff with any relevant qualification or experience. Detailed job descriptions (Special Development Team, 1988) were developed to complement agencies' existing materials. Recruitment (especially to home leader and deputy home leader positions) often proved difficult (Cummings *et al.*, 1989) with few candidates having all of the desired attributes. Normal recruitment policies were used though it often proved necessary to readvertise and/or to advertise nationally as well as locally. Even following this, it was in many cases necessary to appoint individuals with limited qualifications/experience and much to learn about working with people with challenging behaviour in community settings.

Some home leaders and deputy home leaders participated in an induction training programme provided by the SDT. This programme (Special Development Team, 1988) included coverage of the organizing and setting up of services, the practical aspects of managing staff and resources in a small home, and approaches to managing and changing behaviour. In all services an induction programme of one to two weeks was provided for the whole staff group prior to the service opening. This programme was usually jointly planned and provided by the managing agency and the SDT and included coverage of the nature and causes of challenging behaviour, ways of recording behaviour, supporting client participation in activity, assessment and teaching, as well as the more routine aspects of working in a small community-based home (Cummings *et al.*, 1989).

*Costs*

The costs of the services were as shown in Table 6.1. These do not include the costs of management and professional support and the use of other generic or specialist services. The main source of variation in unit costs is the number of clients living together. Thus the single-person services are inevitably the most expensive per head.

Provider agencies were able to access RHA pump-priming monies set aside to support the development of community services for this client group. A lump sum equivalent to £45 000 per client (1990 prices) was available (usually spread over three years), in addition to any existing dowry, to help with the initial revenue costs of services established by local agencies in collaboration with the SDT. From 1986 onwards the RHA also made some capital monies available to help this process further and many of the projects which later developed used this capital to help purchase property. The possible use of these monies was usually identified within the individual service plan.

*Local professional and managerial support*

The general importance of the professional and managerial infrastructure cannot be stressed enough (Chapter 4). This was recognized in the development of these services in a number of ways. Local managers and professionals (including senior staff not likely to be involved directly in the service) were involved in the planning process in an effort to generate local ownership and commitment. The plans themselves usually contained recommendations about the need for local support and this was sometimes quantified in terms of the proportion of a local manager's or professional's time. In a number of services, at the initiative of the SDT, 'contracts' were developed which explicitly defined the kind and amount of management and professional support required by the placement (Special Development Team, 1989). In a few services (in areas characterized by an almost complete absence of local support) the obtaining of defined supports was made a condition of the provision of RHA pump-priming monies.

Despite such efforts, once placements were set up, they were frequently characterized by insufficient local support. Home leaders often voiced concern about the lack of support from their middle managers and about the shortage of specialist skills, especially in the areas of behaviour management and communication.

The lack of middle management support (for whatever reason – lack of commitment, time, or competition from other demands) resulted in many services in a failure to provide placement staff with clear expectations about what the placement should be achieving and how, a failure to monitor progress towards such achievements, and a failure to intervene at an early stage to resolve developing problems. Consequently, in some services, excessive autonomy was given to the home leader and staff group to determine working practices. While this was sometimes effective in the short term it laid the basis for problems when the home leader left. It also meant that, in some cases, the service's policy was essentially determined by the home leader, a responsibility not befitting the post and reflecting the vacuum of leadership and responsibility in the agency as a whole.

Local professional support was also very variable. While some services were able to make extensive use of clinical psychology, speech therapy, community nursing and other such resources, these were much less available to others and completely absent in some.

In some services manager–professional disputes occurred. The professional's role was primarily to provide advice in his/her area of technical expertise. (S)he had a right, however, to expect that this advice would be acted upon. Where there was weak middle management this was problematic as the home leader could, in effect, decide which advice to follow and which to ignore. In the services with the best arrangements this was handled by senior management treating professional advice (within its realm of competence) as to be followed unless there were very strong grounds for doing otherwise – which would, of course, be discussed with the professional in question. In other words, professional advice would usually be followed, would certainly not be ignored and would be contested openly if necessary.

### External support

Once placements were established, the SDT provided additional professional support during the first one to two years (and sometimes longer). While the supporting role played by the SDT varied across services, the types of activity undertaken included advising upon the implementation of agreed policies and procedures, providing specialist advice concerning the analysis and treatment of the client's seriously challenging behaviours, staff training, progress chasing within the local agency and providing practical, informational and emotional support to local staff.

The support provided to the agency by the SDT was initially often very intensive. In the months before and immediately after the setting up of the service, one member of the team often worked on an almost full-time basis with the service's staff, being involved in commissioning and staff training activities and then, perhaps most crucially, in working out 'on the ground' how to provide a good service to the individual client and how to overcome the many difficulties which inevitably arose. This period of work usually culminated with a report to the agency on the service at the end of the first six months. As well as being a description of what had happened the report sought to evaluate the success of the development to date and make recommendations to the agency concerning improvements.

As time went on the support provided by the SDT gradually reduced and become less direct, with advice and consultation being offered through local management and support structures. While the amount of support provided to individual projects varied considerably, the aim was to reduce involvement to the point where complete withdrawal could occur after 18 months to two years.

*Support structures*

In many placements, their vulnerability was recognized by the establishment of additional structures to protect them from threat. This usually involved setting up a Project Coordinating/Support Group (Special Development Team, 1988) chaired by someone other than the home leader's line manager (e.g., the principal psychologist), and recruiting as group members senior managers, client/family and SDT members as well as the staff and managers involved in delivering the service. This group usually met on a monthly basis, perhaps reducing to quarterly as time went on.

While in some placements this structure has decayed with time, in others its importance has been considerable and long-lasting, providing as it does an alternative avenue for the recognition and resolution of problems, and providing placement staff with direct access to senior managers. In the face of staff and manager turnover such a structure has also sometimes provided the key means of ensuring continuity in service provision.

### Service operation

Most services had detailed operational policies based on a skeleton developed by the SDT (Special Development Team, 1988). Typical policies stressed, explicitly or implicitly, a number of themes which can be considered to be the defining features of the way in which the placement was intended to operate.

1. **Normalization**
   Service operation was based explicitly on normalization, with the aims of the service being expressed in terms of the five accomplishments (O'Brien, 1987) and considerable attention being given to the image created and maintained of clients, e.g., through the maintenance of the physical environment, the advertisements used to recruit staff, the involvement of clients in decision making and so on.

2. **Individualization**
   It was intended that the operation as well as the planning of the placement be based on the continued use of an individual planning process to select activities and achieve goals appropriate to individual needs.

3. **Integration**
   Clients were to 'not only be physically present in their local community . . . but also actively take part in community life, regularly coming into contact with ordinary, non-handicapped people'. While technically subsumed in normalization, integration was emphasized as a theme in its own right especially in terms of the use of the community and of generic services.

4. **Structured involvement of clients in activities**
   All policies stressed the importance of engaging clients in a wide range of appropriate housework, occupational and recreational activities through a structured process of planning and staff deployment.

5.  **Staff development**
    Considerable stress was laid on the promotion of staff knowl-
    edge and skill through their experience in the service and
    additional training, and on the constructive deployment and
    use of this resource by the provider agency.

Basic service operation, therefore, was intended to involve the
structured enrichment of the client's social and physical environment in a manner similar to that implemented in the Andover
Project (Felce, 1989; Mansell *et al.*, 1987; see also Chapter 5). Primary attention was to be given to the modification of the assumed
challenging environment (Chapter 10) and the construction of
adaptive behaviour which could theoretically replace client challenging behaviour (Goldiamond, 1974). In most cases more specific procedures were also developed before the services opened
around the management and recording of client behaviour, the
promotion and recording of client activities, and the deployment
of staff.

As might be expected there was considerable variation between
services in the degree to which they successfully implemented the
kind of 'programme' outlined above. There was also variation
across time with some evidence of decay of implementation in the
face of the waning of early enthusiasm, and staff turnover. Most
failures of implementation were accidental rather than deliberate
although, in a few placements, there was more active rejection of
aspects of the policy and, if accompanied by the absence of a clear
local management lead, this sometimes resulted in the imposition
of ways of working preferred by the home leader and the staff.

## Case studies

The kind of variation that occurred in establishment and operation is perhaps best indicated by telling the stories of three services. While these cannot be properly representative they do
provide some indication of the way in which services operated in
practice, of the difficulties they faced, and the variation in outcomes that were produced. Accordingly, three stories are briefly
told below: an example of a service which was successfully set up
but did not perform well; an example of a service which broke
down shortly after its establishment; and an example of a highly
successful service. Names and other details have been changed so

that it will not be possible to match these accounts with the details of individual services provided in Table 6.1.

## Frances

Frances had lived in a learning disability hospital for over 20 years. Planning of her new service proceeded fairly smoothly against a background of increasing pressure on the District Health Authority to resettle its 'own' residents from the soon-to-close hospital. The District was in the throes of developing new community services for over 60 people and, while fairly well resourced professionally was finding its management capability stretched. Frances was found a three-bedroomed house to share with one other lady with severe learning disabilities but without challenging behaviour. The District was able to appoint relatively experienced senior staff with a strong commitment to community living and a desire to work in partnership with Frances to improve her lifestyle.

From the outset, however, problems arose. Despite the local and external professional support that was available the placement's senior staff preferred to take their own counsel. As a result there was considerable conflict between placement staff and professional workers, with the latter believing that the placement was taking too *laissez-faire* an approach and being particularly concerned abut the placement's rejection of well established approaches to the management of challenging behaviour. Attempts to resolve these conflicts were initially unsuccessful as the agency's senior managers were not able to provide placement staff with clear expectations or monitor their achievement. It eventually proved possible to establish a working support structure which brought together local professionals and managers, placement staff and the SDT and which provided some degree of accountability for the placement's operation.

While Frances's lifestyle has clearly improved the change has been far less than was hoped for and there is evidence of decay in service performance over time. Staff turnover has been high and, with the departure of the placement's senior staff, it became clear that local management commitment to the placement was limited, so that its future, as it stands now, is uncertain. The key issue in this service has undoubtedly been its lack of clear accountability to local managers. Faced with the pressure of extensive provision of new services, management time was at a

premium and the resulting vacuum allowed questionable practices to develop.

### Anne

Anne was in her late 20s when referred to the SDT. She had spent
over half her life in a variety of institutional placements. While the
plans to resettle her, with two others without severe challenging
behaviour, went relatively smoothly there was, as with Frances,
considerable pressure arising from the general resettlement and
hospital closure process. This resulted in the service being opened
without a full staff team, a decision which was later regretted. As
predicted, Anne's behaviour became more aggressive and disruptive in the early days of her new placement. Considerable support
from local managers and the SDT helped to contain the situation
though it was most unfortunate that a crucial middle manager
who had been heavily involved in the planning of the service was
on leave during the opening weeks.

Over the course of three weeks the service produced considerable improvements in most aspects of Anne's behaviour but incidents of aggression, while fewer than in the first few days,
continued at a higher rate than in her previous placement. The
improvements were obtained at a high cost to the service. Some
staff refused to work with Anne and the absence of the middle
manager meant that crucial guidelines for the management of
her behaviour were not always followed. A number of minor
injuries were incurred by staff and, as senior management became
involved, the 'story' developed that Anne's behaviour was un-
manageable in a community setting. She was returned to an institutional placement where she remains two years later.

The key issue in this placement breakdown was the inability of
the agency to mobilize the resources necessary to manage a service in crisis. This was undoubtedly partly a function of the pressure the agency was under to develop services for a large number
of clients and the lack of development, at this stage in the agency's
life, of procedures to properly support staff. The crisis also called
into question the agency's commitment, at its most senior levels,
to the task which it had taken on since, at the time when Anne was
moved, many aspects of the situation were actually improving.

### John

John was a man in his 30s who had lived in a learning disability
hospital since early childhood. The planning of his new service

was considerably delayed because of difficulties in allocating him to a District Health Authority. He had originated outside the hospital's catchment area and it took some time to establish that his local DHA would take responsibility for his future care. Most of the planning was actually carried out in collaboration with a voluntary organization which had been contracted to provide the service. This organization had previously been involved in providing another such service and had a high degree of commitment and considerable understanding of the issues.

John was found an ordinary detached house in a residential area to share with three other more able men, none of whom presented challenging behaviour. The staff team took up post some months before the service opened and, while their experience was limited, they were able to spend a considerable amount of time getting to know John and the other residents with support from the SDT and their own manager. Two weeks' induction training was provided and time was spent in planning how the service would operate.

When the service opened John's behaviour (mainly aggression and destruction) presented staff with a major challenge. After a few weeks it was clear that the support available locally and externally should be provided rather more directively and staff were helped to develop appropriate procedures and structures to promote John's adaptive behaviour and manage his difficult behaviour. The service took these on board very quickly and soon began to achieve excellent outcomes with John. Evaluation over the three years of the service shows considerable increases in the amount of contact and assistance that John receives from staff coupled with a fourfold increase in his participation in purposeful activities. Key factors have undoubtedly been a relatively stable staff team, directed and encouraged appropriately by informed local management.

## Outcomes

### *Survival and attrition*

Of the 22 projects established 15 have been maintained, 11 in the original community setting, four in new community settings resulting from planned within-District relocations. As of June 1992, these 15 services have been maintained for periods of between nine months and four and three-quarters years, an average of two years eight months. Seven have closed for a variety of reasons:

1. In two cases (two clients sharing a house) lead agency responsibility changed hands from the District Health Authority to a non-profit-making organization funded jointly by the DHA and the Local Authority. In the face of operational and financial difficulties this organization subsequently relocated the individuals to a local service for six people, most of whom presented some degree of challenging behaviour.

2. In three cases the project closed because the lead agency (two different DHAs) felt that the client's behaviour could not continue to be managed within a community-based setting. In one case the client was moved to a 'crisis intervention' placement on the periphery of a large hospital, where he remains after three and a half years. In one case the client was relocated within the District to a small learning disability hospital, where he remains after one and a half years. In the third case the client was relocated to a private psychiatric hospital, and subsequently to a private placement but, with support from the SDT, returned to a newly developed placement in her home district which is still operating a year later.

3. In one case the client died of a heart attack nine months after the placement was established; in a second case the client died as a result of status epilepticus nine months after the placement was established.

### Quality of client lifestyle

In addition to funding the establishment of the SDT, the South East Thames Regional Health Authority commissioned a formal evaluation of the services set up in pursuit of its strategy. This evaluation focused upon the lifestyle and challenging behaviours of people moving out of long-stay hospital. The study, which is still ongoing, has monitored patterns of client and staff activity to provide indicators of client lifestyle, the quality of support provided within services and changes in challenging behaviours. Eleven of the 22 placements were included in this study.

While the full results of this study are forthcoming, preliminary analyses (Mansell and Beasley, 1989; 1990; in press) indicate that, as clients moved into newly established services they:

1.  moved from large, barren environments, from parts of which they were excluded, to domestic-scale surroundings in which no rooms were 'out of bounds' and which were decorated and equipped with the wide range of furniture and domestic items found in the average household;
2.  received much higher staff ratios (1:0.9 versus 1:3.5) and were in the same room as a member of staff more of the time (90% of the time versus 74%);
3.  spent more time in small rather than large groups of clients (only client in room 63% of the time versus 33%);
4.  were interacted with much more by staff and received more staff assistance to engage in constructive activities (interaction: 22% of the time versus 7%; assistance: 9% of the time versus 2%);
5.  markedly increased their amount of time spent in participation in ordinary meaningful activity (28% versus 16%), especially practical housework tasks;
6.  experienced no overall change in the minimal amount of time spent in formal educational or vocational activities.

This overall pattern of results was also observed when the performance of the newly created services was compared against two major policy alternatives: the use of the traditional range of services typically available to a District Health Authority, including placement in the private sector (Mansell and Beasley, 1991); and the establishment of specialized staffed houses within which people with seriously challenging behaviours were congregated together (Emerson *et al.*, 1992).

As would be expected the overall pattern of results as described above masks a considerable diversity of outcomes across individual services and service users. Thus while some of the new services achieved only modest increases in quality when compared against previous institutional placements, other services demonstrated substantial gains. Key variables which appeared to discriminate between successful and unsuccessful placements will be discussed below. There was also a tendency for outcomes to be better in the early days of the new services, though later outcomes were still significantly better than obtained in the clients' previous institutional settings.

In addition to the formal evaluation of user outcomes, a number of approaches have been taken to internal monitoring of the projects. These have included:

1.  the use of management information systems for the regular collection and review of data indicating service quality (e.g., participation in community activities);
2.  reviews by the SDT of overall service quality;
3.  the establishment of local quality assurance processes, including Quality Action Groups, around some of the projects.

In general these less formal approaches to evaluation have reinforced the findings described above. Clients are reported to be participating in a larger and more varied range of personal, domestic and community activities. Doubts have been expressed, however, about the quality and sustainability of these changes. In addition, considerable scope has been found for promoting more individual and active participation. The general picture is undoubtedly one of much higher quality than represented by most clients' previous experiences, but with many of the potential benefits of community living still to be tapped.

It appears from the above that, despite the problems of implementation described earlier, the services have been relatively successful in delivering an enriched social and physical environment

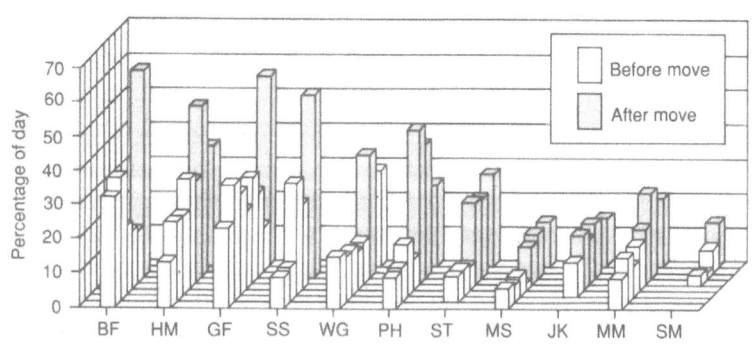

**Figure 6.1**  Engagement in constructive activity before and after transfer to community-based residential services.

which has promoted increased adaptive behaviour on the part of clients (see Figure 6.1).

## Challenging behaviour

The evaluation study also allowed comparison of level of challenging behaviour in new and old services for the 11 clients who were part of the study. Levels of minor problem behaviour (principally stereotyped behaviour) are shown in Figure 6.2. Levels of major problem behaviour (principally aggressive, destructive and self-injurious behaviour) are shown in Figure 6.3. Interpretation

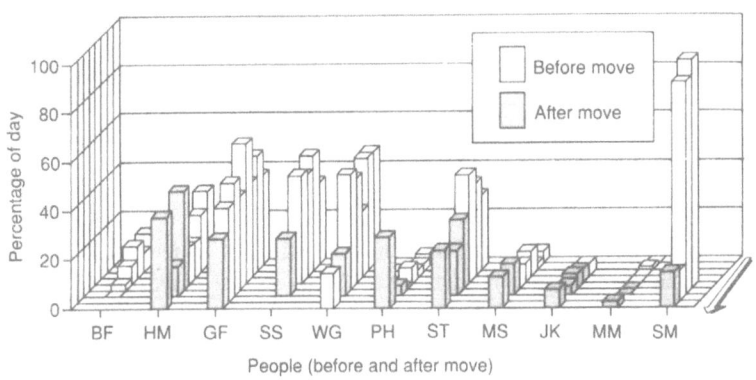

**Figure 6.2** Minor problem behaviour before and after transfer to community-based residential services.

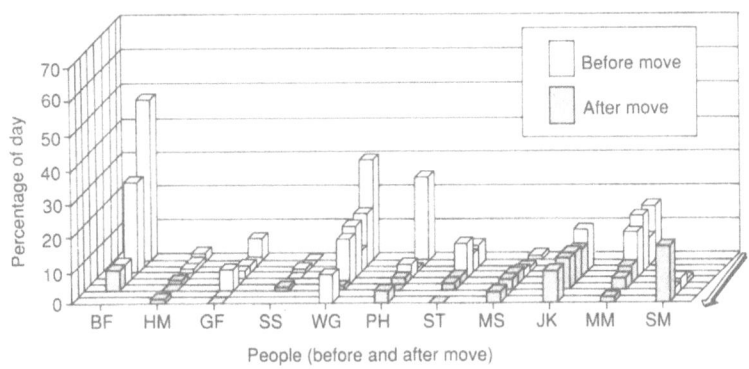

**Figure 6.3** Major problem behaviour before and after transfer to community-based residential services.

of these comparisons is complicated by the wide variability across individuals and by the presence, in some individuals, of increasing or reducing trends in challenging behaviour prior to resettlement. For minor problem behaviour following resettlement there appears to have been:

1. no change in two clients (JK, MM);
2. an increase in two clients (HM, PH);
3. an increase throughout data collection in one client which stabilized following resettlement (MS);
4. a reduction in three clients (SS, WG, ST);
5. a reduction throughout data collection in three clients which was maintained or furthered following resettlement (BF, GF, SM).

For major problem behaviour following resettlement there appears to have been:

1. no change in two clients (HM, SS);
2. an increase in two clients (MS, SM);
3. a reduction in three clients (ST, JK, MM);
4. a reduction throughout data collection in four clients which was maintained or furthered following resettlement (BF, GF, WG, PH).

Taken together these findings suggest that for nine out of 11 clients minor problem behaviour reduced or remained the same as its previous institutional level. Similarly, for nine out of 11 clients major problem behaviour reduced or remained the same. The 'increasers' were different clients so that there was no client whose minor **and** major problem behaviour increased.

While the data on challenging behaviours are encouraging they need to be interpreted carefully for a number of reasons (see Emerson and McGill, in press, for more detail):

1. Most of the seriously challenging behaviours displayed by clients were of low frequency and short duration. This explains the low levels of challenging behaviour observed in some clients and makes comparisons problematic.
2. Secondly, the coding strategy employed does not distinguish between different levels of intensity of similar behaviours (Beasley *et al.*, 1989). The data considered, therefore, provide an estimate of occurrence but not of intensity of challenging behaviour observed.

3.  Thirdly, marked improvements in staffing levels and aspects of the physical environments provided considerably greater opportunities for clients to exhibit challenging behaviours in the newly established services. Thus, for example, at a simple level there were more objects around to throw and more staff to hit.

4.  Finally, comparison of overall levels or rates of challenging behaviours across settings need to be evaluated in light of differences between settings in the rates of occurrence of events known to precipitate challenging behaviour (Carr *et al.*, 1990). For many clients, challenging behaviour was precipitated by 'demands' to participate in activities or social interaction. It is noteworthy, therefore, that such challenging behaviour generally appears not to have increased **despite** the considerable increase in such demands in newly established services (see discussion above of service operation).

Informal accounts have generally reported levels of challenging behaviour to be manageable, though, as time goes on and personnel change, even a continuing low level of serious disturbance can be difficult for services to tolerate and can lead to intermittent crises.

### Effects on co-tenants

One particular aspect of the service model described in this chapter frequently raises concern – the impact of sharing a service with someone with seriously challenging behaviours upon the quality of life of co-tenants. As noted above, the majority of services involved small group living arrangements for one person with severe learning disabilities and seriously challenging behaviours and one or more others who had a learning disability but did not, in the majority of instances, have any seriously challenging behaviours.

While no information on this aspect of user outcomes was collected as part of the formal evaluation study, some informal observations may be made as a result of information collected from internal monitoring systems. In general, the possible picture of co-tenants living a vulnerable, frightened existence has not been found. There have been very few reports of co-tenants being attacked or otherwise threatened. Undoubtedly, there have been times when they have been living in a fairly disturbed and disturbing environment but their sometimes higher levels of ability, or prior planning, have often allowed them to escape from such situations to conditions of greater privacy within or outside the house. Indeed, there is anecdotal evidence to suggest that co-tenants have benefited from the higher staffing levels, structured programming and external professional involvement associated with the projects.

It is interesting to note that concerns are rarely raised regarding services which congregate people with seriously challenging behaviours together in one setting. If people with learning disabilities have the right not to live with others who show challenging behaviour then this right must be extended to all people with learning disabilities **including people with challenging behaviours themselves**. Thus, the ethical issue is one of whether it is appropriate for **anyone** to live/work in close proximity to someone with seriously challenging behaviours. Congregating together people with challenging behaviour does not provide a solution to this problem.

### Lessons

Some people with challenging behaviour have always lived in community settings, principally with their families. As discussed earlier, however, there is evidence that challenging behaviour has been an important factor in institutional admission and the most significant contributor to reinstitutionalization after community placement. Institutional admission, reinstitutionalization and transinstitutionalization remain common outcomes for people with challenging behaviour in South East Thames. There is now, however, as the foregoing has shown, a body of experience of relatively successful development and maintenance of community-based services which suggests that institutional living is not a necessary consequence of even seriously challenging behaviour. The first, and most important, lesson from the South East Thames experience is that such services are feasible – of the 22 services set up 16 are currently maintained in some form and these placements have been maintained for an average of over two and a half years.

Such services are feasible, however, only if their common characteristics are understood and properly responded to.

## They are expensive

The average per capita revenue cost of the services described in this chapter was £53 000 at 1991/92 prices. This is the average cost for all clients, not just those with seriously challenging behaviour. These figures do not take into account the extra costs associated with managerial and professional support, day placement and so on. While there is sometimes scope for reducing these costs over time this cannot be done arbitrarily. The costs are high principally because of the number of staff required to be on duty at any one time to guarantee the safety of clients and staff with minimum recourse to restrictive methods of managing challenging behaviour such as seclusion. While the consequence of a 10% cut in staffing in an ordinary staffed house may be a reduction in out-of-house activities for clients, the consequence in a service for someone with significant challenging behaviour may be serious injury to the client, other clients, staff or members of the public. Unfortunately such services are vulnerable not just to the kind of across the board cuts likely in the current climate but, because they are often the most highly staffed and most expensive services in the locality, to being asked to take a greater share of the financial cuts which are seen as necessary. It is therefore very important if these services are to survive that there is understanding and commitment at the highest levels of provider and commissioner agencies.

## They are difficult to manage and support

While most staffed houses will survive, even if they do not prosper, with limited managerial and professional input, this is not the case with services for people with challenging behaviour. They are likely to continually raise problems for and make demands on managers. These may be directly to do with the individual's challenging behaviour, e.g. frequent incidents involving injury or damage to the environment, complaints from neighbours about noise. They may be to do with the needs of staff, e.g., to manage high levels of stress, to recruit regularly and promptly in response to higher levels of staff turnover, to have more frequent meetings and so on. Managers need to have the time to respond to such issues and also the understanding to see them as partly inevitable characteristics of the service rather than as reflecting the incompetence or lack of commitment of staff. Similarly these services are likely to make greater demands on local professional resources, especially psychology and speech therapy. Such technical expertise may well be crucial to the survival and success of the service and is likely to be needed on an ongoing basis.

### They are vulnerable to crisis and breakdown

Of the group of services considered here three have broken down at least temporarily, with the client being returned to an institutional setting, while six have had a change of service location and/or organization. The crucial tasks of early detection and crisis management (Chapter 4) are of enormous importance in the management of these services. Managers need to know enough about what is going on in the service to detect problems early and to take proactive action. When a placement is threatened, managers need to be able to devote the resources necessary to ride out the crisis or to make local rearrangements.

### They are prone to isolation

Partly because of their expense and the extra resources devoted to them, these services are often viewed with jealousy and antipathy by other parts of the service system. The potential for using the placement's experience and competence in the management of challenging behaviour is sometimes lost through the isolation that results. This isolation needs to be tackled both within the local service system and beyond it. Thus, exchange of staff between local placements and involvement of placement staff in local training can help to overcome the barriers to local integration. Bringing together staff and managers working in, and supporting, such services can help to establish other networks to which these people can relate and from which they can obtain understanding and support.

### They require highly structured approaches to the organization of staff and the provision of care

Traditionally, in institutional settings, challenging behaviour has been handled proactively by avoiding engaging with the person and avoiding situations likely to set off such behaviour, and, reactively, by restraint, seclusion and p.r.n. medication. The goals of community services are rather different and, while some of these responses may sometimes be needed, the overall frame-work needs to be one that encourages the development of an active, varied and valued lifestyle despite the person's challeng-ing behaviour. The services which have done best in South East Thames have used the sort of organizational technology de-scribed elsewhere in this book (Chapter 10). This has involved the careful short-term and long-term planning of activities, the struc-tured deployment of staff, the implementation of agreed and detailed plans for the promotion of activity and the management of challenging behaviour, and the keeping of careful records about the success of the strategies being used.

As such systems are not frequently used in mainstream com-munity services they are often opposed by staff and managers who, initially, do not understand how to use them, and may feel they are turning what should be a 'home' into a 'classroom'. While the increases in staff–client contact and client participation in activity found in the services described here are to be wel-comed, they represent relatively limited improvements given the high staff:client ratios. More rather than less attention needs to be given to these issues in the future.

## Concluding comments

It is essential that the developers and operators of community services for people with challenging behaviour understand the common characteristics of such services and provide the neces-sary supports. When this is done the potential for highly success-ful outcomes can begin to be realized. The service can deliver the kind of active, varied and valued lifestyle that is its goal. The evaluation suggests that many of the services have succeeded in doing this, at least to some extent. The service can also begin to increase its understanding of the causes of the client's challenging behaviour and begin to reduce its occurrence.

Residential services in the community for people with challeng-ing behaviour are clearly feasible. If service agencies believe in what they are doing, understand the task, are well organized, and allocate the necessary resources, then the initial successes de-scribed in this chapter can be repeated and sustained. Meeting such a challenge is crucial to both the comprehensiveness of community care and the lifestyles of the people concerned.

## References

Beasley, F., Hewson, S. and Mansell, J. (1989) *MTS: Handbook for Observers*. Canterbury: Centre for the Applied Psychology of Social Care, University of Kent.

Brost, M., Johnson, T.Z., Wagner, L. and Deprey, R.K. (1982) *Getting to Know You: One Approach to Service Assessment and Planning for Individuals with Disabilities*. Madison, WI: Wisconsin Coalition for Advocacy.

Carr, E.G., Robinson, S., Taylor, J.C. and Carlson, J.I. (1990) *Positive Approaches to the Treatment of Severe Behavior Problems in Persons with Developmental Disabilities: A Review and Analysis of Reinforcement and Stimulus-based Procedures*. Seattle, WA: Association for Persons with Severe Handicaps.

Cummings, R., Emerson, E., Barrett, S., McCool, C., Toogood, A. and Hughes, H. (1989) Challenging behaviour and community services: 4. Establishing services. *Mental Handicap*, **17**, 13–7.

Departments of Health and Social Security, Welsh Office, Scottish Office (1989) *Caring for People: Community Care in the Next Decade and Beyond*, Cm 849. London: HMSO.

Emerson, E. and McGill, P. (in press) Developing services for people with severe learning disabilities and seriously challenging behaviours: South East Thames Regional Health Authority, 1985–1991, in *People with Severe Learning Difficulties who also Display Challenging Behaviour* (eds I. Fleming and B. Stenfert Kroese). Manchester: Manchester University Press.

Emerson, E., Cummings, R., Barrett, S., Hughes, H., McCool, C. and Toogood, A. (1988) Challenging behaviour and community services: 2. Who are the people who challenge services? *Mental Handicap*, **16**, 16–9.

Emerson, E., Beasley, F., Offord, G. and Mansell, J. (1992) An evaluation of hospital-based specialized staffed housing for people with seriously challenging behaviours. *Journal of Intellectual Disability Research*, **36**, 291–307.

Felce, D. (1989) *Staffed Housing for Adults with Severe and Profound Mental Handicaps: The Andover Project*. Kidderminster: BIMH Publications.

Goldiamond, I. (1974) Towards a constructional approach to social problems. *Behaviorism*, **2**, 1–84.

Hughes, H. and Mansell, J. (1990) *Consultation to Camberwell Health Authority Learning Difficulties Care Group: Evaluation Report*. Canterbury: Centre for the Applied Psychology of Social Care, University of Kent.

Iwata, B.A., Dorsey, M.F., Slifer, K.J., Bauman, K.E. and Richman, G.S. (1982) Toward a functional analysis of self-injury. *Analysis and Intervention in Developmental Disabilities*, **2**, 3–20.

King's Fund (1980) *An Ordinary Life: Comprehensive Locally-based Residential Services for Mentally Handicapped People*. London: King's Fund Centre.

Korman, N. and Glennerster, H. (1985) *Closing a Hospital: The Darenth Park Project*. London: Bedford Square Press.

Korman, N. and Glennerster, H. (1990) *Hospital Closure*. Milton Keynes: Open University Press.

Mansell, J. (1988) *Staffed Housing for People with Mental Handicaps: Achieving Widespread Dissemination*. Bexhill/Bristol: South East Thames Regional Health Authority/National Health Service Training Authority.

Mansell, J. (1989) Evaluation of training in the development of staffed housing for people with mental handicaps. *Mental Handicap Research*, **2**, 137–51.

Mansell, J. and Beasley, F. (1989) Small staffed homes for the severely mentally handicapped: Strengths and weaknesses, in *Current Approaches: Mental Retardation* (eds V. Cowie and V.J. Harten-Ash). Southampton: Duphar Laboratories Limited, pp. 26–34.

Mansell, J. and Beasley, F. (1990) Severe mental handicap and problem behaviour: Evaluating transfers from institutions to community care, in *Key Issues in Mental Retardation Research* (ed. W. Fraser). London: Routledge, pp. 405–14.

Mansell, J. and Beasley, F. (1991) Staffed housing for people with seriously challenging behaviours. Paper presented at the Experimental Analysis of Behaviour Group Annual Conference, London.

Mansell, J. and Beasley, F. (in press) Small staffed houses for people with a severe mental handicap and challenging behaviour. *British Journal of Social Work*.

Mansell, J., Felce, D., Jenkins, J., de Kock, U. and Toogood, S. (1987) *Developing Staffed Housing for People with Mental Handicaps*. Tunbridge Wells: Costello.

Murphy, G. and Clare, I. (1991) MIETS: A service option for people with mild mental handicaps and challenging behaviour or psychiatric problems – 2. Assessment, treatment and outcome for service users and service effectiveness. *Mental Handicap Research*, **4**, 180–206.

Murphy, G., Holland, A., Fowler, P. and Reep, J. (1991) MIETS: A service option for people with mild handicaps and challenging behaviour or psychiatric problems. 1.Philosophy, service, and service users. *Mental Handicap Research*, **4**, 41–66.

Newman, I. and Emerson, E. (1991) Specialised treatment units for people with challenging behaviours. *Mental Handicap*, **19**, 113–9.

O'Brien, J. (1987) A guide to life-style planning: Using The Activities Catalog to integrate services and natural support systems, in *A Comprehensive Guide to the Activities Catalog: An Alternative Curriculum for Youths and Adults with Severe Disabilities* (eds B.Wilcox and G.T. Bellamy). Baltimore, MD: Paul H. Brookes, pp. 175–89.

South East Thames Regional Health Authority (1979) *Strategies and Guidelines for the Development of Services for Mentally Handicapped People*. Bexhill-on-Sea: South East Thames Regional Health Authority.

South East Thames Regional Health Authority (1985) *Mental Handicap Special Services*. Bexhill-on-Sea: South East Thames Regional Health Authority.

Special Development Team (1988) *Annual Report 1987*. Canterbury:

Centre for the Applied Psychology of Social Care, University of Kent.

Special Development Team (1989) *Annual Report 1988*. Canterbury: Centre for the Applied Psychology of Social Care, University of Kent.

Toogood, A., Emerson, E., Hughes, H., Barrett, S., Cummings, R. and McCool, C. (1988) Challenging behaviour and community services: 3. Planning individualised services. *Mental Handicap*, **17**, 70–4.

# 7

# Towards meaningful daytime activity

*David Allen*

## Introduction

*Policy background*

The last two decades have witnessed changes in both the availability and orientation of day service provision for people with severe learning disabilities. The industrial training focus predominant in most day centres fell increasingly into disrepute during the 1970s. Concerns were expressed over the apparent exploitation inherent in subcontract work, the reduced availability of such work, and its generally unstimulating nature. The 'readiness' model, in which users theoretically passed through progressively higher levels of day activity culminating eventually in competitive employment, was also shown to be a fallacy by studies revealing the low rates of progression that occurred and the consequent 'silting up' that resulted (Whelan and Speake, 1977; Bellamy *et al.*, 1986).

The need for day services to consider the wider developmental needs of people with learning disabilities was central to the 1977 report of the National Development Group (National Development Group for the Mentally Handicapped, 1977). The report suggested an expanded role for day centres in which training programmes relating to the development of daily living, social, leisure and educational skills would be provided in addition to preparation for employment. The continuum model still featured strongly, the revitalized 'social education' centres being seen as offering four distinct processes: admission and assessment, development and activities, special care, and advanced work.

Targets for increasing the number of day service places had been set in *Better Services for the Mentally Handicapped* (Department of Health and Social Security and Welsh Office, 1971). The White Paper had suggested that the 26 400 day care places in existence in 1970 would need to be increased to around 75 000 over a 20-year period as community services developed and hospital beds (and their associated day provision) reduced. Available places had almost doubled by 1985 but, towards the end of the decade, the average number of new centre places provided per year had fallen from 2500 to 1300 (National Audit Office, 1987). If progress continues at this rate the White Paper targets will not be achieved until the end of the century, a factor of particular concern given the recent acceleration in hospital closure programmes.

In some areas of the UK, substantial attempts have been made to relocate some of the traditional functions of day services into integrated community settings. Because of this shift, the value of 'building-based' services has been increasingly questioned. In general, though, it is apparent that the developments seen in residential care (as described, for example, in Chapter 5) have not been matched in day services (Wertheimer, 1987). The National Development Group's 15-year-old guidance, while far from comprehensively implemented, now appears outmoded to many. A recent review (Social Services Inspectorate, 1990) concluded that many local authorities have no clear policy on day services, and that accepted philosophical principles had not generally been translated into clear operational statements. While some progress has been made, the provision of occupation in segregated settings remains the prevailing model in many places.

### Day services for people with challenging behaviours

People with challenging behaviours have historically been included in the heterogeneous grouping of people with learning disabilities regarded as requiring 'special care'. The 1971 White Paper endorsed the concept of special care units attached to adult training centres, an idea further developed in the National Development Group's 1977 report. The latter regarded the presence of severe behaviour disorder as a clear qualification for admission to special care, and foresaw the use of such facilities as a potential means of overcoming the otherwise likely exclusion of this group.

In 1974, 600 special care places were in existence. By 1985, this number had risen to 2800 (Social Services Committee, 1985).

Only limited data are available on the proportion of day service places available to people with challenging behaviour. Whelan and Speake's (1977) survey of 305 adult training centres in England and Wales found that the presence of behavioural difficulties was likely to be the most common reason for refusing applicants a place (cited by 41.3% of participating centres). Harris and Russell (1990), in a study of the prevalence of aggressive behaviour in a single health district, found that the lowest rate of such behaviour (9.7%) was reported in day services (versus 38.2% in hospitals). Qureshi *et al.*'s 1990 survey of behaviour problems sufficiently severe to require special provision in seven Health Districts in the north-west of England found a similar prevalence rate of 9% in day care settings. Twenty-five per cent of subjects in a total population study of individuals displaying severe self-injury were found to have no programmed day activity (Oliver *et al.*, 1987), while McBrien (1990) reported that 54% of clients served by Plymouth Health Authority's Behavioural Services Team received no day care. Taken together, these findings suggest that people with challenging behaviour are frequently likely to be excluded from or denied places in existing day provision.

Exclusion will, however, vary as a function of local facilities and attitudes. Nineteen adult training centres in West Midlands surveyed by Crawford *et al.* (1984) reported serving 'special care' users, 20% of whom were described as having severe behaviour problems. In Qureshi's (1990) study of parents caring for young adults with learning disabilities and challenging behaviour, only just over 5% of the people concerned had been excluded from regular day services. The amount of day care received varied between five and 56 hours.

Where special care provision is not available, day care in a hospital setting may constitute the only alternative (Ward, 1982). While advocating a community-based model of care, *Better Services* had also allowed for a continuing role for hospitals. Day care for individuals with challenging behaviour was considered as one possible area for continuing hospital provision. Qureshi (1990) found that social services departments provided 86.5% of the day care received by her study participants, with 9.5% being provided by NHS services. While the evidence is limited (Department of Health and Social Security, 1984), it seems likely that individuals with challenging behaviours run the same risk of being excluded from most hospital-based day programmes as they would from their community-based counterparts. Most individuals without day care found by Oliver *et al.* (1987) were living in hospital, and Qureshi *et al.* (1990) found lower prevalence rates for challenging behaviour within day services, irrespective of whether these were located within hospital or community settings.

## The significance of day activity

What we do during the day is a major determinant of our social and financial status. It provides opportunities for the development and refinement of vocational and social skills. The availability and range of opportunities for daytime activity is therefore a significant influence on the image and competence of people who have been labelled as 'challenging'.

Day activity also serves the important role of providing respite to carers (Seed, 1988). Qureshi (1990) found that the more day care received by users with challenging behaviour the better the psychological and physical health of their mothers. Use of day care was also found to be related to attitudes towards the future. Parents who rejected any prospect of future residential care for their relative received the lowest average levels of day care. However, those who were requesting immediate alternative residential care also received low levels. It is suggested that, while the amount of day-time support received by the former group was partly self-determined, for the latter it constituted an unmet service need which placed considerable stress on the families concerned.

Absence of provision may also affect formal care systems. Failure to provide day activities may result in excessive demands being placed upon residential services (Special Development Team, 1987). The basic costs of such services will also be increased due to the need to staff daytime hours fully. The lives of users may suffer from a lack of contrast, the same carers being responsible for both daytime and domestic support.

## New patterns of service delivery

As documented elsewhere in this volume, most recent service developments for people with challenging behaviour have focused on the creation of residential facilities and peripatetic support teams. It is self-evident that equal attention must be paid to the establishment of appropriate daytime activities if comprehensive community care programmes are to be developed (Social Services Committee, 1985).

Deficiencies exist in both the quantity and quality of day service provision available for this group. Recent years have, however, seen the development of some more innovative schemes, and these appear to be of three main types:

1. specialist facilities within sheltered settings;
2. increased support within normal day service systems; and
3. integrated services.

Examples will be provided from each of these three areas in turn.

### Specialist facilities

One original rationale for locating people with challenging behaviours within special care facilities was to avoid the possible impact that their presence would have on other users and staff within the main body of the service (National Development Group for the Mentally Handicapped, 1977). The initiatives described within this section have similarly felt that the behaviours displayed by such people require separate service provision. Each project has, however, attempted to meet the needs of its users in significantly more creative ways than can be found within most traditional day service settings.

McBrien (1987) described the establishment of a specialist day unit for adults with severe learning disabilities who presented with challenging behaviour (see Figure 7.1). People using the Haytor Unit had severe learning disabilities. Their self-help skills were minimal and they were mostly non-verbal. Using the Adaptive Behaviour Scale, their behaviour was shown to be as challenging as that of adults on a locked hospital ward, and more challenging than the 'most difficult' clients attending a local training centre. Indeed, their behaviour was rated as more violent and destructive than either of the other groups. Except for one anecdotal case study, no outcome data on user progress are presented. It is stated that several people were kept out of hospital because of their attendance at the Unit. High staff morale, low staff turnover

This service was set up as an alternative to the only other available provision which was within a local hospital in a neighbouring health district. The aim of the service was not to provide permanent places but, via the use of specialized training techniques, to produce sufficient improvements in the behaviour of service users to enable them to move on to less structured settings. Users attended the unit on four and a half days per week, one of which was spent in community settings. The days at the unit were divided into 30-minute sessions, each of which was occupied by a different training activity. A structured, behavioural approach was utilized, employing techniques such as differential reinforcement of other behaviour, time-out from positive reinforcement and over-correction. Other key features of the service were hypothesized to be a 1:1 staffing ratio, weekly progress reviews, competence in applying behavioural methods and staff training. The unit was staffed by nurses.

**Figure 7.1**   The Haytor Unit, Plymouth.

and high levels of staff training were reported over the first 18 months of operation. In the next six months, turnover became much more of a problem, with only one original staff member remaining when the report was written.

While the service was felt to have been an effective model for the user group described, it proved less successful for more able people with additional psychiatric or personality disorders. Referrals of people with more moderate behavioural difficulties also had to be resisted. McBrien concludes by stating that the functional components of the service were to be replicated within local adult training centres, allowing for greater integration with more able individuals. This subsequent work is described later in the chapter.

A second example of a sheltered service is the Rivermead Employment Project (Feinmann, 1988) which was based on Bellamy's earlier work on sheltered training programmes (Bellamy *et al.*, 1981) (see Figure 7.2).

The Rivermead Project was subject to an independent evaluation conducted by the Special Development Team (1986). Their

This scheme involved people with learning disabilities being taught to assemble marketable goods in a small factory unit within the grounds of a hospital. Ten 'more difficult' hospital residents were provided with a service five days a week between the hours of 9.00 am and 3.30 pm. The people concerned had been excluded from other day services because of the challenges which they presented. The project was based on the premise that these behaviours had been generated to some extent by the inactivity and lack of purposeful tasks within the environments concerned. Meeting the needs of the identified individuals was therefore felt to depend on providing personally meaningful activities within a supportive environment. Four staff were trained in precision teaching techniques (after Bellamy *et al.*, 1981) and some 'high-status' assembly work was found. Job trainers provided users with approximately two hours' individual training and support each day within the context of a room management approach. (Coles and Blunden, 1979)

**Figure 7.2**   The Rivermead Project, Sheffield.

report concluded that the quality of life experienced by users of the service was a significant improvement on their previous experience of day care. Project workers had developed complex assembly skills and, as the availability of suitable materials allowed, were engaged in age-appropriate activities. Support staff had developed a range of sophisticated teaching skills and there had been marked decreases in the frequency of dangerous and destructive behaviour within the work setting.

Some difficulties were also apparent. The location of the service resulted in the congregation of people with learning disabilities and challenging behaviour on one site, thereby acting as a major obstacle to integration. It also deprived users of an opportunity to develop other work-related behaviours (such as travelling to and from the workplace) and adopting normal working hours. The skills that staff had developed were only used in the teaching of assembly work and not extended to the development of other vocationally related social skills. Such skills are important determinants of success in supported employment placements (Hill *et al.*, 1986; Schafer, 1987). Despite the aim of participation in high-status work activities, a significant amount of time was spent in non-functional activities common to other traditional day care settings. Finally, the financial status of users was not enhanced by their attendance at the unit.

Feinmann (1988) mentions two other important problems encountered by the scheme. First, some users did not respond to the highly structured environment, and this resulted in an increasing tendency towards the use of punitive management strategies. Second, the lack of progress of some of the people attending produced a drop in the morale of project staff.

The formal evaluation (Special Development Team, 1986) made several recommendations for the further development of the project. Among the most important were suggestions that the segregation of the service could be overcome by relocating it as an enclave within open industry (Mank *et al.*, 1986) and that high priority be given to the development of a viable range of products. While the Rivermead project has continued on the same site, lessons learnt were harnessed in the development of a second employment project described later in the chapter.

### Increased support within existing day service systems

The assumption underlying the services described in this section is that standard day service models have the essential ingredients to enable them to meet the needs of users with challenging behaviour. The people concerned simply need greater staff support to allow them to access these services.

McBrien (1990) described packages of support provided to two centres in the south-west of England that enabled them to serve users with challenging behaviour (Figure 7.3). Providing a service in this fashion resulted in local Social Services day centre places being made available to people with severely aggressive and self-injurious behaviours for the first time. No client was excluded because of their challenging behaviour and a significant growth in the expertise of staff and their line managers is reported. However, the recruitment and retention of staff were problematic and the 1:1 staff support levels were only achieved at the cost of reducing the full-time placements available to other users.

Hill-Tout (1988) describes an individualized day service (Figure 7.4) in which the aim was to establish a pattern of day

The centres concerned offered four places with 1:1 staffing ratios for users with challenging behaviour. They operated on a behavioural model, and users were provided with a structured time-table which included a mixture of community opportunities and skill training programmes. All challenging behaviours were functionally assessed and written management guidelines were produced. Weekly consultancy visits were provided by a member of the Behavioural Services Team (Chapter 8) employed by Plymouth Health Authority, during which individual user programmes were reviewed. The BST was also involved in the selection of clients and in the selection and induction of staff.

**Figure 7.3**   Centre-based services, Plymouth and West Devon.

activity for a young man whose day centre placement was felt to be inappropriate to his needs. The person concerned frequently and unpredictably threw chairs and other everyday objects, was generally difficult to engage and displayed self-stimulatory and self-injurious behaviour. His behaviour within his home environment had resulted in considerable damage to property and had required the installation of polycarbonate windows. His parents

A new day service package was put together initially involving daily 1:1 activity sessions within the centre. These were of one hour duration and focused on providing high-frequency opportunities for participation in potentially rewarding activities. No attempts were made to enforce compliance with these activities, the user concerned being able to choose when to participate. A video record of these sessions was kept as a means of monitoring progress. Within three months, full participation for the duration of the sessions was reported. Building on the success of this intervention, a range of activities was gradually developed within ordinary community settings.

**Figure 7.4**   Centre-based service, Mid Glamorgan.

were unable to keep ornaments and furniture as and where they wished, and their lives were governed by their son's behaviour. As a coping strategy in the evenings and at weekends they frequently took him out for car rides (Hill-Tout, 1990).

Reported outcomes included higher rates of participation in individual and group activities and increasing use of community facilities. Flexible funding (allowing for the provision of support staff as and when required, the purchase of equipment and materials, etc.) and a base from which to work were seen as key elements in the further development of services of this type.

Accessing existing day services has been made possible in other areas by similar financial arrangements. In South Glamorgan, for example, the Flexicare system (Newman and Cox, 1987) has been used to provide 1:1 or 2:1 staff support to enable people with challenging behaviours to attend local adult training and social education centres. The county's service for people with challenging behaviours also has the capacity to fund short- or long-term day service developments for its clients (Hill-Tout *et al.*, 1991) with ring-fenced budgets.

Where developments of this type are established, it seems essential that they form part of a well planned service package of the type described above. If this is not so, there is a substantial risk of users and their identified staff becoming encapsulated within their 'mini-service'. Locational integration, being physically located within another service, may be all that is achieved. The generation of a commitment to serve users with challenging behaviour within day services generally available to people with learning disabilities is one key factor in helping to avoid such isolation.

### Integrated services

A small number of services have adopted more integrated models that have aimed for community presence and participation from the outset. Allen *et al.* (1989) have described the development of a community-based day service for people with profound learning disabilities and additional needs (Figure 7.5). The Flexicare system mentioned earlier had enabled some individual pilot day services for challenging individuals to be established. Continuing day service deficiencies and the initial success of these pilot initiatives led to the formation of a steering group charged with the

The aim of the service was to provide a variety of reliable and appropriate daytime activities for an identified group of individuals who had been unable to access or been excluded from existing services. The service was built around two staff teams of three workers operating from different geographical patches. Each team had access to additional resources which enabled them to vary the support available to each user as required. This was at minimum 1:1, but would be increased for high-risk or demand situations. One staff team worked from a base which also served as a venue for a limited number of sessional activities. The second team worked on a totally peripatetic basis, making use solely of facilities available to the general public; this team shared an office base with their local CMHT. Users spent varying amounts of time with the service ranging from three half days to five full days each week. Professional advice was available from clinical psychologists and other therapists attached to the local CMHTs.

**Figure 7.5**   Community day service, South Glamorgan.

responsibility of planning a more substantive service. The group provided a forum for the development of a strong partnership between professional workers and some of the carers of people with severe learning disabilities seeking day support. The strength of this partnership was felt to be a key variable in securing funding for the scheme.

Eleven people used the service initially. Using categories derived from the Degree of Dependency Scale (Caddell and Woods, 1984), six users were rated as Highly Dependent, two as Highly Dependent with Severe Behaviour Problems, two as Medium Dependent with Severe Behaviour Problems, and one as Severe Behaviour Problems Only. Some 45% therefore displayed challenging behaviour, the most common forms of which were, in rank order, self-injury, damage to the environment, overactivity and physical aggression. No single management approach was employed by the service, but a key feature was detailed planning in which new opportunities and activities were provided at a rate and in a style tailored to the needs of each individual.

The scheme was subject to a formal evaluation in which the

support received by users of the new service was compared with that received by an approximately matched group attending a special care unit in the area (Allen, 1990). Based on diary data collected over two weeks on each person at two-month intervals, 72.5% of activities of users of the new service were conducted in integrated settings, versus only 6.5% of those provided in the special care unit. Substantial and significant differences were also evident in both the number and range of activities undertaken, each being superior in the new service. The types of activities provided were also significantly more desirable and age-appropriate as rated by neutral judges on five-point scales. Use of local leisure centres for activities and classes featured highly in the service's programme. Engagement levels, assessed at six-month intervals, were significantly and consistently higher than in special care.

Key factors contributing to these results were felt to be the staffing levels that permitted high levels of individual attention and the ordinary community settings that provided the venues for most activities undertaken. It is concluded that, while higher engagement levels may have been produced by increasing staffing levels within a unit-based service, this could not be taken for granted in view of research conducted within residential settings (Felce, 1988). It is suggested that the qualitative changes in the activities undertaken would certainly not have been achieved in this fashion. The cost of a full-time placement in the new service was approximately three times that of one in the special care unit.

The service was not without its problems. Activities were entirely leisure based, and there was some uncertainty about whether or not the service should be provided for life (Allen and Williams, 1991). It was also inherently fragile, the impact of staff sickness, for example, being far greater than in a building-based service. Staff sickness could cause sessions to be cancelled if appropriate relief workers could not be found, thus making the service potentially unreliable. As Qureshi (1990) observes, it is clearly a disadvantage to carers if a 'flexible' service means less reliability for them, although this does not have to be a necessary consequence.

Dispersed service models have their predictable difficulties. In particular, isolation from other services is possible. As might be expected, this was felt to be more of a problem for the service team that had its own premises than for the one based with the CMHT; far more opportunities were available to members of the latter service for informal contacts with other workers and much support was derived from this. Monitoring of individual services was also sometimes difficult, and was generally done by the team leaders working regular supervisory sessions alongside team members and their clients.

A final issue related to the service's initial 'demonstration project' status. It had deliberately been kept separate from traditional mainstream day services during its development phase to protect both its principles and resources. In one area it was suggested that this had led to unhealthy attitudes of superiority/inferiority between the two (cf. Chapter 4). Once the service had become established, formal management links with other day services in the areas concerned were agreed and this competitive element was reduced.

Despite these concerns, this service was adjudged to have been sufficiently successful for many of its essential features to be replicated within a second service established to meet the needs of more able individuals with challenging behaviour.

A similar service model has been established in Sunderland as part of the Special Projects Team (Johnson and Cooper, 1991) (Figure 7.6).

Johnson (1991) states that a key factor in shaping the development of the project has been the problem of finding open employ-

---

Since 1987, Sunderland Health Authority has run a small alternative day service for people who were felt to challenge normal day service provision. The project is jointly funded and serves 12 users. Individual weekly timetables offer a mixture of activities including work, college sessions (woodwork, dance, use of computers etc.), outdoor sessions (including skiing and abseiling), and personal development. Service users either walk or use public transport or private cars for travelling between locations. The two-room service base provides a venue for specific activities or short breaks only.

---

**Figure 7.6** Special Projects Team, Sunderland.

ment in the Sunderland area (the local male unemployment rate in 1991 being 29%). Ironically, this was seen to have brought some advantages to service users. First, full-time paid employment was by no means the only model of valued activity – service users were therefore not set apart from the local population because of being unable to obtain this. The part-time work undertaken by some users was seen as a significant achievement. Second, local conditions had led to the development of a thriving co-operative movement. Service users and their supporters have been able to establish two businesses (a sandwich bar and a craft workshop) under the umbrella of a Community Business Venture that supported co-operatives in the locality. It is now planned that these ventures should become employers for non-disabled people in the open market, while retaining an option in each business for up to two users at a time to work with support. Finally, unemployment had created the need for the development of low-cost sport, education, and leisure opportunities. Service users were therefore able to participate regularly in activities (such as the skiing and abseiling) that might have been prohibitively expensive in other parts of the country.

User progress within the service is recorded by completing Adaptive Behaviour Scales (Nihira *et al.*, 1975) every six months and by separate records of individual behaviours. An example of these data for one user is shown in Figure 7.7. The service has also developed its own quality monitoring system (Johnson, 1990) that aims to ensure that a range of appropriate social and other opportunities are regularly available to users.

While both the above projects have shown the validity of a 'meaningful life without work' (Heron and Myers, 1983), employment remains the most valued daytime activity for many people. Persons with severe disabilities are generally absent from the competitive workforce. This is especially true of individuals with severe learning disabilities and challenging behaviour.

The major UK project to tackle the area of supported employment for people with challenging behaviour so far is Intowork (see Figure 7.8).

Intowork's staffing included an Employment Development Officer to find appropriate jobs, and three Job Trainers, trained in systematic instruction, to prepare and support users. On registering with the service, Job Trainers conduct a vocational profile with the user concerned. This involves getting to know the person

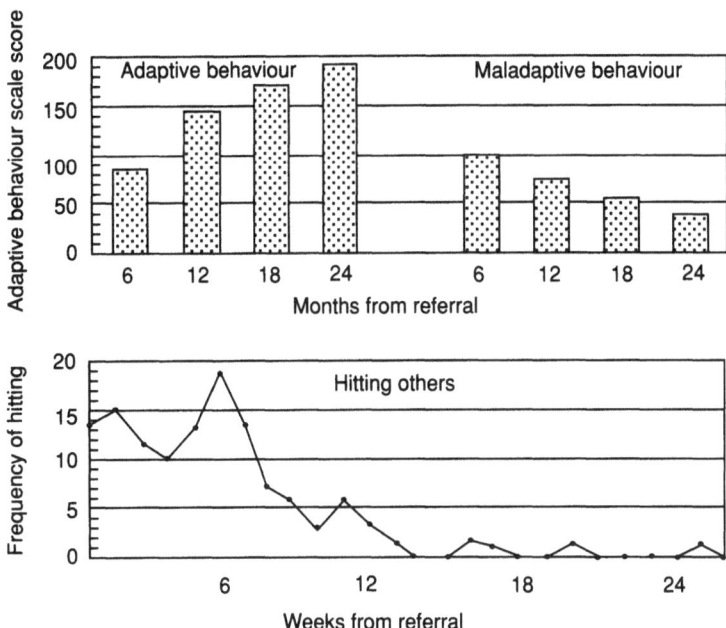

**Figure 7.7**  Illustrative changes in one person's behaviour following the involvement of the Special Projects Team.

Sheffield's Intowork service grew out of the pilot work undertaken in the Rivermead Employment Project. It was influenced substantially by systematic instruction (Gold, 1980). As with Bellamy's approach (Bellamy *et al.*, 1981), systematic instruction is based on the use of behavioural teaching strategies. In contrast with Bellamy, however, Gold stressed their use in natural work settings. The focus of the Intowork project was therefore on taking people with severe learning disabilities and challenging behaviour directly into employment settings.

**Figure 7.8**  Intowork, Sheffield.

and his/her work preferences and requirements. Once an appropriate job is found, both the vocational and social aspects of the work setting are analysed. Initial training strategies are also identified at this point. The Job Trainer then accompanies the employee to the work site and starts to train him/her in all aspects of the job. As well as skills directly related to the job, this is likely to include travelling to and from work, clocking on and using the canteen. Dependence on the Job Trainer is reduced over time as the user becomes more competent at the work involved. This may take anything between a few days and several months or years. Ongoing support is then provided to both employer and employee as required. During the training period, government subsidies mean that the employer incurs no costs. The training is also provided free. Rates of pay, following training, are negotiated individually.

Initially the three Job Trainers were involved with two people each for two days a week. Since commencing operations, Intowork has offered 75 job opportunities to 35 job seekers. Jobs have included assembly work, packing, sorting, kitchen work, cleaning, pot-washing, gardening, warehousing, food production, delivery, labouring, laundry work, garage work, care services and animal welfare.

Feinmann (1991) states that there were two main components that were central to Intowork's approach to challenging behaviour – a careful analysis of antecedents known to trigger challenging behaviours of individual workers and positive programming involving the teaching of behaviours that were functionally related or functionally equivalent to the challenging behaviours (LaVigna *et al.*, 1989). The antecedent analysis helped plan work placements that avoided known triggers but included those setting conditions likely to promote prosocial behaviours, while the work activities themselves were often a major element in the positive programming.

Market forces have now led Intowork into catering for people with severe learning disabilities as a whole. The only people excluded from the service are those individuals in their 50s or 60s suffering from degenerative disorders. Approximately 60% of the people in contact with the service so far have been labelled as challenging (Leach, 1991). Intowork staff have often had cause to question the validity of this label once the people have been found meaningful employment opportunities.

Unlike the Rivermead scheme, Intowork has yet to be subjected to a formal evaluation. Feinmann (1991) reports some anecdotal conclusions. With hindsight, it was felt that it would have been more appropriate from the outset to establish a general employment service that catered for challenging individuals as only part of its brief. The dual challenge of developing an innovative employment service and restricting its users to individuals with behavioural difficulties placed considerable pressure on the service. The right job placements were often difficult to find and, over time, the loss of key staff had an impact on the success of individual placements.

## Conclusions

Direct comparison of the various service models presented here is difficult given the likely variation in their definitions of 'challenging behaviour'. Services also vary in the degree to which they focus on 'treatment' of challenging behaviour. In the Haytor unit, for example, day service and treatment roles seem to be combined. Reductions in levels of challenging behaviour are a main effect of the service. In other projects, like Intowork and the Sunderland scheme, treatment is de-emphasized. Reductions in challenging behaviour, while clearly important, are almost seen as side effects of engaging people in meaningful activities.

Some of the key ingredients of the schemes described would appear to be as follows:

1. opportunities for participation in **valued** day activities, including both leisure (e.g., Sunderland, South Glamorgan) and employment (e.g., Intowork, Rivermead, Sunderland);
2. an increasing use of integrated settings (e.g., South Glamorgan, Sunderland, Intowork) from the outset, thus avoiding the problem of the 'continuum trap' (Taylor, 1987);
3. an ecobehavioural framework that focuses on the inter-relationships between people, their behaviour and their physical settings (e.g., Mid Glamorgan, Rivermead, South Glamorgan, Intowork) (Chadsey-Rusch and Rusch, 1986; Schutz, 1988);
4. high levels of support that allow users to access a wide range of opportunities (e.g., South Glamorgan, Sunderland, Intowork);
5. a recognition that specialist skills reside in staff, not buildings (e.g., Sunderland, South Glamorgan, Intowork);

6.  the use of effective strategies for the development of skilled behaviour (e.g., Rivermead, Intowork) and the amelioration of challenging behaviours (e.g., Haytor, Devon).

It seems likely that each of these ingredients is sometimes necessary, and no one entirely sufficient, for the establishment of meaningful day activities for people with severe learning disabilities and challenging behaviours.

Several problems are also apparent in the schemes described.

1.  Most of the schemes are fairly small scale. While this may have been a key factor in their establishment (Patton, 1986), it may also make them inherently fragile. Small scale 'pilot' schemes are often under more pressure to prove themselves within a short time, and therefore struggle to secure long-term funding (Emerson *et al.*, 1991).
2.  A combination of small staff teams and an absence of recognized bases from which to work may affect the reliability of a service.
3.  Sheltered day services established exclusively for users with challenging behaviour run the risk of encountering some of the same problems as their residential counterparts.
4.  There is comparatively limited development of vocational opportunities and some supported employment models, such as enclaves and work crews (Mank *et al.*, 1986), have apparently yet to be tried with this group of service users in the UK.
5.  Several schemes mention problems of staff retention. While this is a general problem in services for persons with severe learning disabilities it is unclear if turnover rates are any greater in services catering for individuals with challenging behaviours.

There can be little doubt that substantial developments in day service provision need to take place if sufficient high-quality community services are to be established for people with severe learning disabilities and challenging behaviour. Progress continues to lag behind that associated with residential services.

The comparative absence of meaningful activities for this group means that services have to be developed almost from first principles. While this is a daunting task, it also provides an opportunity to avoid replicating some of the pitfalls of traditional day service systems. Schemes aiming to integrate users with challenging behaviour into existing day services available to people with severe learning disabilities automatically encounter the well recognized problems of these services (such as segregated activities, low status occupation and low rates of engagement). The community-based schemes detailed in this chapter provide some early evidence to indicate that these difficulties can be avoided. The main challenges seem to lie in replicating the findings of the innovative projects described on a larger scale and in demonstrating their durability over time.

## References

Allen, D. (1990) Evaluation of a community based day service for people with profound mental handicaps and additional special needs. *Mental Handicap Research*, **3**, 179–95.

Allen, D. and Williams, M. (1991) Community based day services, in *Meeting the Challenge: Some UK Perspectives on Services for People with Learning Difficulties and Challenging Behaviour* (eds D. Allen, R. Banks and S. Staite). London: King's Fund, pp. 27–31.

Allen, D., Gillard, N., Watkins, P. and Norman, G. (1989) New directions in day activities for people with multiple handicaps and challenging behaviour. *Mental Handicap*, **17**, 101–3.

Bellamy, T., Horner, R. and Inmam, D.P. (1981) *Vocational Habilitation of Severely Retarded Adults*. Baltimore, MD: University Park Press.

Bellamy, T., Rhodes, L.E., Bourbeau, P.E. and Mank, D.M. (1986) Mental retardation services in sheltered workshops and day activity programs: Consumer benefits and policy alternatives, in *Competitive Employment Issues and Strategies* (ed. F. Rusch). Baltimore, MD: Paul H. Brookes, pp. 257–71.

Caddell, J. and Woods, P. (1984) The Bryn-y-Neuadd degree of dependency rating scale. *Mental Handicap*, **12**, 142–5.

Chadsey-Rusch, J. and Rusch, F.R. (1986) Habilitation programs, in *Severe Behaviour Disorders in the Mentally Retarded: Nondrug Approaches to Treatment* (ed. R.P. Barrett). New York: Plenum Press, pp. 99–122.

Coles, E. and Blunden, R. (1979) *The Establishment and Maintenance of a Ward-based Activity Period within a Mental Handicap Hospital*. Cardiff: Mental Handicap in Wales Applied Research Unit.

Crawford, N., Taylor, P. and Throboe, E. (1984) 'Special care' in 19 adult training centres. *Mental Handicap*, **12**, 54–6.

Department of Health and Social Security (1984) *Helping Mentally Handicapped People with Special Problems*. London: HMSO.

Department of Health and Social Security and Welsh Office (1971) *Better Services for the Mentally Handicapped*, Cmnd 4683. London: HMSO.

Emerson, E., Cambridge, P. and Harris, P. (1991) *Evaluating the Challenge: A Guide to Evaluating Services for People with Learning Difficulties and Challenging Behaviour*. London: King's Fund.

Feinmann, M. (1988) Project Intowork – how Sheffield achieved the impossible. *Community Living*, 5, 12–13.

Feinmann, M. (1991) Project Intowork, in *Meeting the Challenge: Some UK Perspectives on Services for People with Learning Difficulties and Challenging Behaviour* (eds D. Allen, R. Banks and S. Staite). London: King's Fund, pp. 31–4.

Felce, D. (1988) Behavioural and social climate in community group residences, in *Community Residences for Persons with Developmental Disabilities* (eds M.P. Janicki, M.W. Krauss and M.M. Seltzer). Baltimore, MD: Paul H. Brookes, pp. 133–47.

Harris, P. and Russell, O. (1990) Aggressive behaviour among people with learning difficulties – the nature of the problem, in *Treatment of Mental Illness and Behavioural Disorder in the Mentally Retarded* (eds A. Dosen, A. Van Gennep and G.J. Zwanikken). Leiden: Logon Publications, pp. 367–74.

Heron, A. and Myers, M. (1983) *Intellectual Impairment: The Battle Against Handicap.* London: Academic Press.

Hill, J.W., Wehman, P., Hill, M. and Goodall, P. (1986) Differential reasons for job separation of previously employed persons with mental retardation. *Mental Retardation*, 24, 347–51.

Hill-Tout, J. (1988) Personal services. *Community Care*, 4 February, 22–4.

Hill-Tout, J. (1990) Individual services to people with profound mental handicaps and challenging behaviour, in *Community Care: People Leaving Long-stay Hospitals* (eds S. Sharkey and S. Barna). London: Routledge, pp. 125–35.

Hill-Tout, J., Doyle, A. and Allen, D. (1991) The Challenging Behaviour Service, in *Meeting the Challenge: Some UK Perspectives on Services for People with Learning Difficulties and Challenging Behaviour* (eds D. Allen, R. Banks and S. Staite). London: King's Fund, pp. 40–4.

Johnson, D. (1990) Steps to a better service. *Health Service Journal*, 7 June, 844–5.

Johnson, D. (1991) Personal communication.

Johnson, D. and Cooper, B. (1991) The Special Projects Team, in *Meeting the Challenge: Some UK Perspectives on Services for People with Learning Difficulties and Challenging Behaviour* (eds D. Allen, R. Banks and S. Staite). London: King's Fund, pp. 36–40.

LaVigna, G.W., Willis, T.J. and Donnellan, A.M. (1989) The role of positive programming in behavioural treatment, in *The Treatment of Severe Behaviour Disorders* (ed. E. Cipani). Washington, DC: American Association on Mental Retardation, pp. 59–83.

Leach, J. (1991) Personal Communication.

Mank, D.M., Rhodes, L.E. and Bellamy, G.T. (1986) Four supported employment alternatives, in *Pathways to Employment for Adults with Developmental Disabilities* (eds W.E. Kiernan, and J.A. Stark). Baltimore, MD: Paul H. Brookes, pp. 139–53.

McBrien, J. (1987) The Haytor Unit: Specialised day care for adults with severe mental handicaps and behaviour problems. *Mental Handicap*, 15, 77–80.

McBrien, J. (1990) *Challenging Behaviour in Adults with Learning Difficulties:*

*Services in Plymouth and West Devon.* Paper presented at British Institute of Mental Handicap Seminar on Community Services, Bristol, 10 October.

National Audit Office (1987) *Community Care Developments.* London: HMSO.

National Development Group for the Mentally Handicapped (1977) *Day Services for Mentally Handicapped Adults.* London: Department of Health and Social Security.

Newman, T. and Cox, S. (1987) Your flexible friend . . . South Glamorgan's Flexicare Service. *Social Work Today,* **2 March,** 10–1.

Nihira, K., Foster, R., Shellhaas, M. and Leland, H. (1975) *Adaptive Behaviour Scale.* Washington, DC: American Association on Mental Retardation.

Oliver, C., Murphy, G. and Corbett, J.A. (1987) Self-injurious behaviour in people with mental handicap: A total population study. *Journal of Mental Deficiency Research,* **31,** 147–62.

Patton, M.Q. (1986) *Utilization-focused Evaluation.* Newbury Park, CA: Sage Publications.

Qureshi, H. (1990) *Parents Caring for Young Adults with Mental Handicap and Behaviour Problems.* Manchester: Hester Adrian Research Centre.

Qureshi, H., Alborz, A. and Kiernan, C. (1990) *Prevalence of Individuals with Mental Handicap who Show Problem Behaviour: Update of Preliminary Results.* Manchester: Hester Adrian Research Centre.

Schafer, M.S. (1987) Competitive employment for workers with mental retardation, in *Progress in Behaviour Modification,* vol. 21 (eds M. Hersen, R.M. Eisler, and P.M. Miller). Newbury Park, CA: Sage Publications, pp. 86–103.

Schutz, R.P. (1988) New directions and strategies in habilitation services: Toward meaningful employment, in *Integration of Developmentally Disabled Individuals into the Community* (eds L.W. Heal, J.I. Haney and A.R. Amado). Baltimore, MD: Paul H. Brookes, pp. 193–209.

Seed, P. (1988) *Day Care at the Crossroads: An Evaluation of the Local Authority Contribution to Day Care Services for Adults in Scotland.* Tunbridge Wells: Costello.

Social Services Committee (1985) *Community Care with Special Reference to Adult Mentally Ill and Mentally Handicapped People,* vol. 1. London: HMSO.

Social Services Inspectorate (1990) *Inspection of Day Services for People with a Mental Handicap: Individuals, Programmes and Plans.* London: Department of Health.

Special Development Team (1986) *A Report by the Special Development Team in Mental Handicap on the Quality of Services Provided by the Rivermead Employment Project.* Canterbury: Institute of Social and Applied Psychology, University of Kent.

Special Development Team (1987) *Annual Report 1986.* Canterbury: Institute of Social and Applied Psychology, University of Kent.

Taylor, S.J. (1987) Continuum traps, in *Community Integration for People with Severe Disabilities* (eds S.J. Taylor, D. Biklen and J. Knoll). New

York: Teachers College Press, pp. 25–35.

Ward, L. (1982) *People First – Developing Services in the Community for People with Mental Handicap: A Review of the Literature*. London: King's Fund.

Wertheimer, A. (1987) Towards a normal working life. *Community Living*, **1**, 8–9.

Whelan, E. and Speake, B. (1977) *Adult Training Centres in England and Wales: Report of the First National Survey*. Manchester: Hester Adrian Research Centre.

# 8

# The Behavioural Services Team for people with learning disabilities

*Judith McBrien*

## Introduction

Challenging behaviour teams have been established by many health and social services departments in order to provide well organized, highly skilled, peripatetic support and intervention in the community for people with learning disability whose behaviour is difficult to manage. Some of these teams are truly peripatetic, others form the outreach component of a unit-based service. This chapter describes the experience of setting up and operating, since January 1989, a specialist peripatetic team – the Behavioural Services Team (BST).

### Background

Plymouth Health Authority and West Devon Social Services have coterminous boundaries and since 1984 have been pursuing a joint strategic plan for services to adults with learning disabilities. The main purpose of this plan was to accomplish the resettlement from long-stay institutions of all those people of local origin who have learning disabilities. By early 1991, all 176 people due to be resettled had returned to the area, including those with challenging behaviour.

Some 1200 adults with learning disabilities live in the locality (general population c. 320 000). The service is widely dispersed in community settings. Approximately 60% of service users live at home with their families and residential care is provided for the remainder within voluntary and private sector homes. Day services, respite care and field social work are provided by social services, while specialist health input is provided by the usual range of health professionals with the addition of the BST. There also exists a small psychiatric in-patient facility for adults with learning disability and psychiatric disorder.

This pattern of service provision was planned and monitored by a Joint Planning Group which has met monthly since 1984. When the joint strategic plan was into its third year, it was realized that, in the main, the resettlement programme had selected those who could be easily resettled into fairly minimally staffed group homes (typically ten residents to two or three staff on duty). As a result, those hospital residents whose behaviour was challenging, some of whom were residing on locked wards, had yet to be considered seriously for resettlement. There was not, at that time, agreement that all of these people would or could be resettled. In addition, there was also a recognition that people with challenging behaviour who had always lived locally were not having their needs met in a coordinated way.

As a result, a small multi-agency group was set up during 1986 to produce a strategy for adults with learning disability and challenging behaviour. The resulting strategy made explicit a commitment to resettle all those of local origin regardless of level of disability or degree of challenging behaviour. The strategy itself consisted of four main strands: that those with challenging behaviour should be placed in existing homes with a comprehensive back-up service and additional staffing; that, in addition, a number of small and well staffed houses should be established via a new charitable body which would be able to take some people with challenging behaviour; that a specialist Behavioural Services Team of people with skills in behavioural techniques should be appointed to provide peripatetic support specifically for these users; and that a steering group be created to guide the implementation of this new service.

The basic contention was that a high-quality service would be achieved primarily by the provision of well trained and well motivated staff. Special buildings, the congregation of difficult people or the use of remote settings did not form any part of the recommendations. The policy drew heavily on work by the South East Thames Regional Health Authority's Special Development Team (Chapter 6).

The proposed service was to be seen as a 'layer of expertise' within the existing framework of services. Therefore the proposed service was designed to provide the additional expertise and staffing to enable users to access and benefit from existing services without exception.

Unfortunately, however, the planned service failed to take account of the respite needs of those living with or caring for people with challenging behaviour. It was erroneously assumed that the respite service already in existence, two 12-bed units, could cope with any additional demands, especially since it was envisaged that, as people with challenging behaviour would commonly be living in staffed housing, they would not therefore need respite care. In practice, it has emerged that 30% of those with challenging behaviour live with their parents. These families do need respite but the nature of the existing service means that someone with difficult behaviour has often to be turned away because of the possible danger they pose to other, frailer users. Plans are now under way to rectify this.

## The Behavioural Services Team

### The service model

The model underlying the BST is one of taking expertise and resources to the client and his/her carers. As an example of the delivery of appropriate health care in community settings, the model has implications beyond the client group and can be used to illustrate the role of health care staff in fostering the aims of the recent NHS and Community Care Acts. In particular, the model lends itself to fulfilling the aims of promoting practical support in the home, the development of proper assessment and case work, the fostering of skills in the independent sector and the building in of quality standards. Service provision is highly complex for this group and the notion of a specialist team is a relatively new concept. Above all, clarity of input and close partnership between agencies are required if such an approach is to be effective.

### Definitions

The BST provides a specialized service to adults and school leavers with moderate to severe learning disabilities and challenging behaviour. 'Learning disabilities' are defined as an impairment of learning that has resulted in moderate to severe deficits in the acquisition of adaptive behaviours, a disability that would first become apparent in childhood. The original brief was to work only with adults with severe learning disabilities (as opposed to mild or moderate). This has been found impossible to hold to in practice. The brief was therefore extended to embrace people with a range of learning disabilities. In practice this generally means anyone already in 'the system', i.e. attending a day centre and/or living in a residential home for people with learning disabilities. Priority nevertheless goes to those with more severe handicaps. The team does not accept people who appear to have no, or only mild, learning disabilities. Such people are referred to more appropriate sources of help.

'Challenging behaviour' refers to behaviour of such an intensity, frequency or duration that the physical safety of the person or others is placed in serious jeopardy, or behaviour which is likely seriously to limit or deny access to and use of ordinary community facilities. This definition and much of the operational policy are borrowed from or based on the work of the South East Thames Regional Health Authority's Special Development Team (Emerson *et al.*, 1987). Practice has shown that challenging behaviour (to some extent) lies in the eye (or rather the mind) of the beholder. Some staff and parents are prepared to tolerate and work with some very difficult behaviours without feeling the need to call in extra help – merely taking it in their stride. In other settings, what would appear to be minor problems are seen as major challenges (see also Chapter 2). Day-to-day practice has been dictated by the view that, whatever the apparent problem or degree of seriousness, if placement breakdown is threatened or the well-being of clients or carers is in jeopardy, then the behaviour is challenging and help is required. Where it can be identified that the problem is not in itself serious, the emphasis shifts from treating the individual to helping carers gain a more balanced view or acquire the skills and confidence to cope more effectively.

### Objective and philosophy

The objective of the BST is to reduce challenging behaviour and increase skills and quality of life for people referred, through the provision of advice and technical support based upon an explicitly behavioural approach. The behavioural approach is adopted on the basis that the available evidence suggests that interventions informed by applied behaviour analysis are effective in reducing unwanted behaviour and building up appropriate alternatives (see for example Donnellan *et al.*, 1988; Durand, 1990; Meyer and Evans, 1989). The service is available for any adult fulfilling the criteria stated above who lives in, or is due to return to live in, the catchment area. This entails working in facilities run by any agency and includes working with school leavers. The service is peripatetic and not bed-based. The team is an additional layer of expert advice and practical help for these clients and not a substitute for the range of specialist and generic services available to adults with learning disabilities. Thus, the team works in close conjunction with staff of these other services.

The team adheres to the principles of providing a high-quality service via the least restrictive environment, using the least restrictive treatment methods compatible with reducing the challenging behaviour and increasing quality of life. The values subscribed to are those embodied in 'the five accomplishments' (O'Brien, 1987) and adopted by the local service in general.

## Staffing and organization

The BST is employed by Plymouth Community Services NHS Trust (formerly Plymouth Health Authority) and forms a part of the Department of Clinical Psychology. It has its own budget and is directly managed from within the learning disability specialty of the psychology department. It has a two-tier staffing structure of advisers and technicians. Funding allows for a team leader, who is a clinical psycholigist, and gives 50% of his/her time to being the team leader and 50% to clinical psychology in learning disabilities. There are a further two full-time behavioural advisers. The advisers must have a relevant professional qualification (e.g., clinical or educational psychology, nursing, social work, teaching, occupational therapy). In addition they must have expertise in applied behaviour analysis and have experience of working with people with challenging behaviour. Five posts exist for behavioural technicians who form a pool of staff who can be deployed flexibly by the advisers. Technicians generally have experience of the client group but need not have formal qualifications. They undertake a competency-based induction training on taking up their posts.

In establishing the BST it was firmly felt that a behavioural approach was not the prerogative of any particular professional group and that a key to success would be the appointment of staff who brought with them a knowledge of applied behaviour analysis as well as their own professional skills. This, of course, produced an immediate problem of how to grade the team members since, as all advisors had identical roles, it would be unacceptable to grade and pay each member differently. The final solution was to place all team members on the Administrative and Clerical pay scale and to tie the salaries of advisers as closely as possible to nurse behaviour therapists and those of technicians to salaries of day-centre staff. In practice it has been difficult to maintain parity over time, large pay awards having been made to both nurses and day-centre staff.

The advisers began work in January 1989 and the five behavioural technicians were appointed subsequently, with full strength being reached in May 1990. It was necessary to hold two rounds of interviews to appoint two advisers and three rounds of interviews to appoint five technicians. All BST staff are accountable to the team leader no matter what their professional background. This was felt to be essential and has worked well in practice. Staff turnover was low in the first two years with only one person leaving (one of the technicians). Turnover of technicians is expected as most of these staff intend to undertake professional training in due course. The first adviser to leave spent two and a half years with the team before taking promotion to a similar team. The first Team Leader (the author) left after 3 years; recruitment of Team Leaders and advisers has proved extremely difficult.

The role of the behavioural adviser is to take on individual referrals for assessment, analysis and intervention; to plan and conduct staff training courses and workshops; to offer consultancy on challenging behaviour to other staff; to plan and conduct relevant service evaluation studies and contribute to service planning. The role of the behavioural technician is to act as hands-on staff with clients referred to the team. This entails assessment, direct observation, functional analysis and implementing intervention programmes with clients. They also play an important role in contributing to evaluation studies and staff training. The technicians are supervised by the behavioural advisers.

## Activities of the BST

These will be described under separate headings. An approximate breakdown of time spent under each heading taken from the annual statistics shows that case work occupies 45% of advisers' time, staff training 20%, consultancy and service planning 20%, service evaluation 15%. For technician staff, most time is spent on case work (approximately 60%), with the rest of the time divided between service evaluation and staff training.

### *Case work methods*

There are three broad types of case work undertaken by the team, described below. Referrals may come from any source and must be in writing unless urgent. Each referral is allocated to one of the behavioural advisers who will then initiate the case work according to the agreed format.

### Therapeutic work

Therapeutic work consists of three stages, input ceasing at any stage according to need and the co-operation received from carers. These stages are: (1) initial screening by an adviser to assess suitability of the referral and feasibility of effecting change; (2) detailed assessment and analysis of the problem, of the client's skills and of his/her quality of life and general circumstances; (3) intervention to reduce the problem/s and improve quality of life and/or skills. At the end of the second stage, a report is presented to the referrer/carers and a meeting held to agree the next steps (e.g., full-scale intervention by the team, written advice only, modelling and training for carers to implement advice, refer elsewhere). The format currently followed is that of the Behavioural Intervention System (BIS) developed by McBrien and Felce (1992).

### Intensive support

In addition to the above, the team can respond quickly to bolster the staffing levels provided for a referred client. The technicians have a key role here and can go at short notice to any residential home or day centre to act as staff members for the referred client. Their role in these cases is carefully discussed with the manager of the home or centre to ensure that it is purposeful (e.g., modelling for staff, further assessments). During 1990 this kind of intensive support was provided for 12 clients in residential homes and respite units. The input has varied from three or four evenings (6 pm to midnight) to several weeks of full days, managed in rotation by all five technicians. The team has the facility of placing its members on call for a referred client through the use of a radio pager.

**Assessments for purchasers and providers**
Some referrals are made directly by purchaser or provider agencies. For example, where an agency is asked to fund a placement for a person with difficult behaviour, the BST may be asked to assess level of difficulty, appropriate staffing levels and so on. Other examples include input to decisions regarding the rationing of scarce resources such as access to a one-to-one staffed daycentre place. In these cases the BST has provided an objective assessment of all candidates which can be used by managers to compare with the recommendations of those more closely involved. Meeting such requests entails assessment and analysis, as for other cases, combined with the preparation of a useful report for the funding agency or provider. As may well be imagined, this is a sensitive task. The value of using the BST is that an objective (and hopefully expert) opinion can be given by staff who are at arm's length. This is a growing area of work as the separation of purchasers and providers become a reality for both health and social services.

*Priorities and conditions for case work*

Priorities in accepting referrals have been made explicit in the *Operational Policy* (Behavioural Services Team, 1993a) and *Guide to Referrers* (Behavioural Services Team, 1993b). These centre on giving higher priority to people whose residential placement is threatened by their behaviour, particularly those who live with their parents. A second level of priority is to those with no day activity outside the home or to those whose day placement might break down.

All professionals will be familiar with the difficulties of gaining the co-operation of staff and carers to carry out assessments and interventions. There can be much time wasting when charts are not filled in, staff do not keep appointments or fail to communicate with one another. To try to offset this, the BST brings to bear a number of factors which influence the acceptance of a referral and the continuation of case work. These include a consideration of the degree of commitment shown by the carers and clear statements of circumstances under which the BST cannot continue with a case (e.g., when action by others is required first, such as medical assessment or suspension of unsuitable management methods). In some circumstances, the living or working environment of the referred person may be so antipathetic to an improvement in behaviour that intervention would be judged to be unethical without a change of environment or drastic improvements in it. In these cases, the BST would not undertake direct work with the client but would endeavour to set in motion a change of location or the desired improvements. Such situations are brought to the attention of the appropriate service managers.

## Case work over the first two years

Initially, case work was divided into two distinct types – community referrals and pre-discharge hospital referrals. These will be described separately.

Over the first two years (1989 and 1990) 117 community referrals were accepted on to the caseload of the BST (57 in 1989, 60 in 1990). The rate of referral in year one averaged 4.2 per month (range 1–7) and in year two averaged 5 per month (range 1–13). The proportion of referrals of ex-hospital patients resettled to the area was 39% in year one, 35% in year two. Overall, there were 70 men and 46 women, the average age of referrals being 30 years with a range of 16–68 years. Analysis of the modal age for the men referred in 1990 reveals a peak at 20 years, confirming the impression that the BST is increasingly dealing with the younger, school-leaving age group. These are young people who in the past may have been admitted to long-stay institutions but who are now remaining in the community. The types of challenges cited at the time of referral are illustrated in Figure 8.1.

Over the first year the BST had an input to 53% of the existing private homes and 56% of the voluntary sector homes. All the large day centres bar one had an input as did most of the smaller

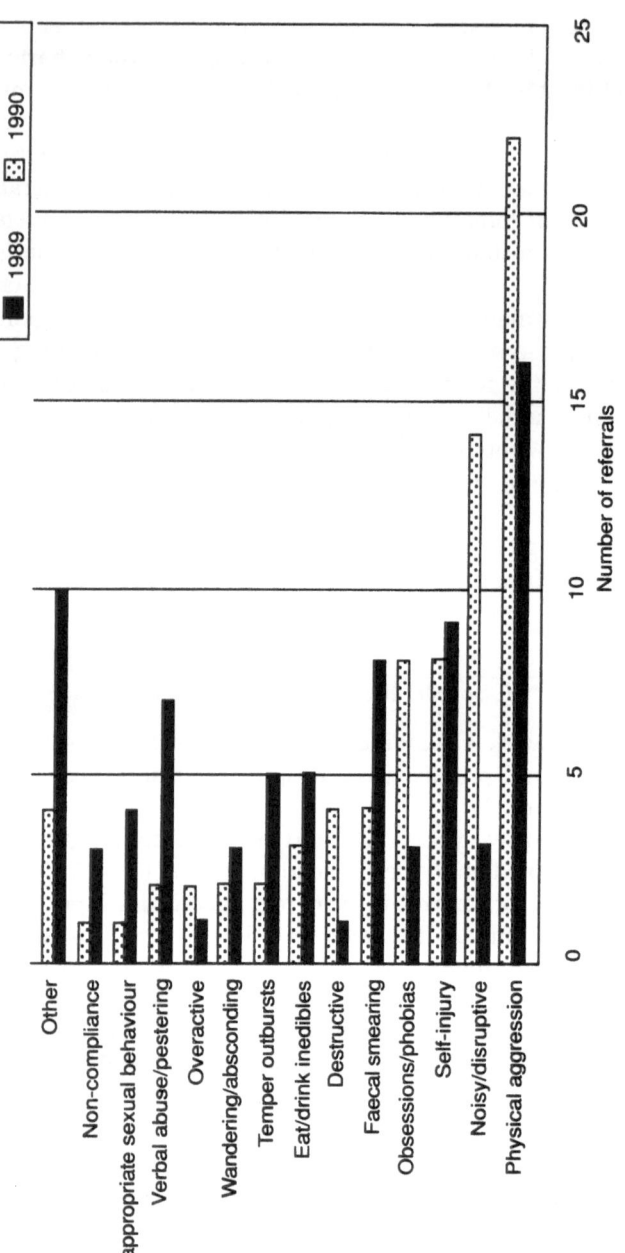

Note: more than one problem may be cited per referral.

**Figure 8.1** Problems cited at time of referral to the BST.

more specialized centres. The residential location of referrals received during 1990 is illustrated in Figure 8.2.

The source of referrals received during 1989 and 1990 is presented in Figure 8.3 and the nature of the day service they received in Table 8.1.

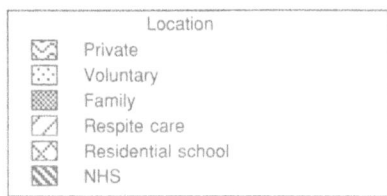

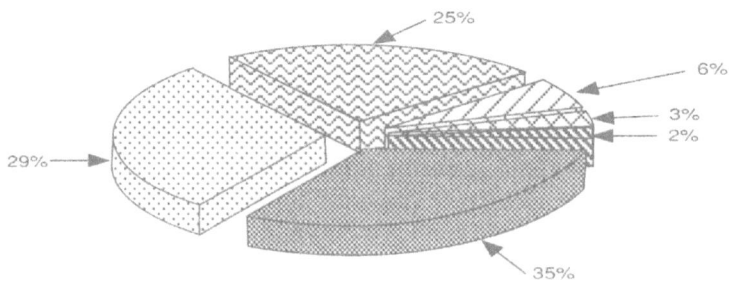

**Figure 8.2** Place of residence at time of referral to the BST.

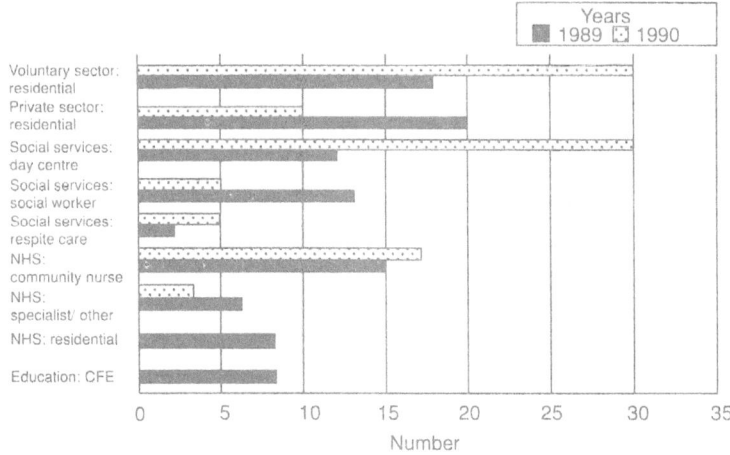

**Figure 8.3** Source of referrals to the BST.

**Table 8.1** Daytime location of clients at time of referral to the BST (1989–1990)

| Type of day care | | 1989 | | 1990 | |
|---|---|---|---|---|---|
| | | n | (%) | n | (%) |
| None | | 20 | (35) | 26 | (43) |
| Adult day services: | 1:10 | 25 | (44) | 21.5 | (36) |
| Staff ratios | 1:3 | 1 | (2) | 4 | (7) |
| | 1:1 | 4 | (7) | 2 | (3) |
| F.E. college | | 5 | (9) | 2 | (3) |
| School | | 2 | (4) | 4.5 | (8) |
| Total | | 57 | (101) | 60 | (100) |

Inspection of Table 8.1 reveals that 43% of those referred in 1990 had no day-care place, an increase over 1989 when 35% had no day care. The increase for 1990 is accounted for partly by over half of these people having been resettled to the area very recently. Within local services, day placements are not normally sought until each person has a chance to settle in their new home. However, there also exists a shortfall in day placements providing intermediate levels of staffing ratios, i.e., between 1:10 and 1:1, especially since those places staffed at a 1:3 ratio are reserved for people with profound and multiple disabilities. This has to be taken in the context, however, of the observation that many people with a challenging behaviour are catered for in larger groups with a staffing ratio of 1:10.

There are a number of reasons for higher staff ratios sometimes being required. In some cases, of course, the seriousness or frequency of the behaviour itself dictates the need for high staffing ratios. In other instances, however, the tolerance of the carers or the philosophy of the managers appears to be a more important factor, tolerance being dictated, at least to some degree, by the level of training and experience of staff. A full report was made to the management of social services concerning those people with no day activity outside the home. While providing appropriate day time activity is a priority, it would be a mistake to believe that merely providing it would serve to reduce the challenge posed. Referrals by day centres for assistance with challenging clients made up 30% of the team's referrals in the second year.

## Case work stages

As regards the use of the three stages of case work – screening, assessment and analysis, intervention – of the 60 new referrals during 1990, five turned out to be inappropriate (largely through having no challenging behaviour but requiring other services, for example psychological assessment, counselling) and the rest moved on to the second stage of detailed assessment and analysis. Of the 55 referrals passing to the second stage and for whom the assessment process has been completed, input ceased with the presentation of the assessment and analysis for 19 cases, while input continued into the intervention stage for 29 people. This distribution of activity is shown in Table 8.2.

Concerning those for whom input ceased following the assessment and analysis phase: two died; for five the advice was that a change of residence or day care should precede any further involvement of the BST; one person was referred on to the psychology service as needing long-term psychotherapy; in nine cases the initial agreement was to assess only (for advice on future placement or suitability of current situation or management); and finally, for two people long delays on the part of referrers or carers ensued following the assessment which led to termination of case work.

**Duration of case work and case workload**

Data on the number of hours spent per case are routinely collected. Time spent varies enormously. The most intensive intervention has been five six-hour days conducted in one week by two technicians, followed by daily visits during the week after and subsequent case review follow-ups. This had of course been preceded by a considerable amount of assessment and analysis. In

**Table 8.2** Case work stages for 1990 referrals at 31.12.90

| Stage of case | n (total = 60) |
| --- | --- |
| Screening only | 5 |
| Assessment only | 19 |
| Assessment ongoing | 7 |
| Intervention by BST completed | 18 |
| Intervention by BST ongoing | 11 |

terms of the number of weeks or months over which the contact is spread, this too is very varied. Looking at completed cases in 1990, the time span varies from four weeks to six months. As regards case workload, in a typical week the team worked with an average of 19 different clients, with a range of 13–25.

### Termination of case work

An analysis of all 112 referrals to date which went beyond the screening stage has been made. At the end of 1990, of the 112 people who had been taken on, 59 were no longer being seen by the team, 22 were being seen for follow-up only (individual planning meetings, case reviews), 31 were being seen regularly (i.e. once a fortnight or more often).

### Re-referrals

During 1990, nine clients were re-referred to the team after an interlude. In only two cases was re-referral for the same or similar problems again causing concern in the same setting. In three cases the same problem was occurring but in a different setting (the client having changed residence). In four cases re-referral was for a different problem (three of these occurring in the original setting and one in a changed setting).

### Admissions to the Health Services treatment clinic

The clinic provides short-term admission for the treatment of psychiatric disorders in adults with learning disability. Over the two years 1989 and 1990, of 112 referrals to the BST which went beyond screening 12 people have been admitted to the clinic following or during involvement by the BST. Seven of the 12 were admitted for problems other than those for which the team was seeing them. However, five of the 12 were admitted for the same problem. Two of these five were admitted to the clinic not only because of their behaviour and other problems but because they were homeless. These two might have had respite from social services had their behaviour not made this impossible under current respite provision.

### Types of assessment

Assessment always commences with detailed interviewing of all carers and, where possible, the client. It then always includes direct observation by BST staff using a variety of methods (e.g., time sampling, continuous coding of behaviour by hand-held computer). The direct observation would typically include coding of levels of engagement, staff contact and the challenging behaviours in question. In this way a picture of the individual's quality of life and interaction with others and his/her environment is built up. In many cases the challenging behaviour itself is too infrequent to be accessible to direct observation (e.g., occurring once or twice a week or less). In such instances, the BST will request carers to complete charts of behaviour as an essential part of the assessment process. This is most commonly done through the use of ABC charts, thus incorporating the beginnings of a functional analysis. Considerable training is given to front-line staff in the completion of such charts. Videotaping is frequently used to provide opportunities for more detailed observation of behaviour and to demonstrate to carers conflicting or inconsistent practices across groups of staff in the same or related settings.

A major aim of assessment is to attempt to analyse the function served by the person's challenging behaviour (Chapter 3). Where ABC charts do not provide sufficient information, analogue assessment methods may be employed to test hypotheses about the function of behaviour which have been generated by interviews, observations or record keeping (see Emerson *et al.*, 1990; Oliver, 1991).

The case of Tom may help to illustrate a very simple assessment process which led to a self-evident intervention. Tom lived in a group home of ten residents with a total staff group of 16 working in shifts of three to four at a time. Tom was referred for violent temper outbursts while being shaved. He would shout, scream, lash out at staff, hold on to the basin and at times go quite rigid. Following initial interviews, a member of the BST staff videotaped each member of the day staff as they shaved Tom early in the morning. The tapes showed startling differences in practice among staff – some held Tom round the neck in the crook of the arm while applying the electric shaver with the other hand; some sat beside him and gently prompted him to shave himself using hand-over-hand guidance. Some staff reacted to his tantrums by holding him tighter and reprimanding him, some paused in their demands. Some staff gave much praise and helped him to look in the mirror, others said little throughout. The videotapes were watched by the whole staff group at a staff meeting. It was then straightforward to agree on best practice and to draw up guidelines incorporating this to be used consistently by all staff. However, follow-up some months later revealed that Tom now had a beard.

A more complex example is that of Bernard, a middle-aged man with no mobility and no sight who was referred for severe self-injury to his face. Neither clinical interviews nor straightforward observation suggested any clear function for his self-injury. Consequently, a full suite of analogue assessments was carried out in collaboration with the day centre staff. These demonstrated that his self-injury was exacerbated by noise and by absence of staff attention. Interestingly, the policy of the residential staff was to respond to self-injury by placing him alone in his bedroom with *The Sound of Music* playing, as they felt that this calmed him. Despite the preparation of advice and many meetings, the residential home could not be persuaded to implement any changes in this practice. This latter point illustrates a difficulty for any team in that their role is one of providing advice without being in a line management relationship to the service provider. In a multi-agency service there will be times when advice is rejected and there may be little that can be done.

### Types of intervention
The types of intervention developed by the BST are too varied to enumerate in detail. All are informed, however, by the rationales of applied behaviour analysis, whether applied to the client's behaviour, the carers' behaviour, the organization of the environment or whatever. The focus of the intervention may be skills training for the client to teach functionally equivalent behaviour which can replace the challenging behaviour with something more acceptable but just as useful to the individual; it may entail altering the antecedents of the behaviour (e.g., filling people's time more meaningfully, altering the way in which demands are made); it may involve changing the consequences of the behaviour. Some interventions centre on teaching self-control to the individual, some on teaching self-control to staff! Very often the focus becomes one of training carers in particular skills or the passing on of explanations of behaviour. A case history is given after the next section to illustrate the kind of input the BST has provided.

### Hospital referrals
At its inception, the BST was asked to assess 25 people living in out-of-district hospitals who were thought to have challenging behaviour and who had been scheduled for resettlement. A suite

of assessments was used which included direct observation, standardized assessments of skills and problem behaviours, an intellectual assessment, a staff questionnaire on the function of behaviours, prospective logs of behaviour problems and off-ward activities and a summary of the hospital file. These assessments were labour-intensive, taking on average ten hours per person (not counting considerable travelling time) and had not been possible before the creation of the team. The information was used in three ways.

Firstly, it was used to advise those responsible for finding accommodation and deciding on groupings of people to live together. Secondly, it was used to inform the staff of the receiving homes about the needs and characteristics of the residents. Following resettlement, the usual referral service was offered. Of the 25, 13 (52%) had subsequently been taken on as individual referrals at the time of writing, with the rest having settled satisfactorily to date. Thirdly, the assessments provided an excellent set of data on each person before they left hospital. This is being used to monitor and evaluate resettlement of this group (see below).

### Case history of Hannah

Hannah had lived in a long-stay hospital for 22 years from the age of nine. Her learning disability would be described as severe, with impaired mobility, no speech and minimal communication skills. She was unable to look after her personal needs but could eat with some help. She had a history of behaviour problems including faeces-smearing, injury to staff and residents, self-injury, removing and tearing her own clothes and non-compliance. It was reported, before her resettlement, that she had rarely exhibited these behaviours in recent years. Indeed, Hannah had not been referred to the BST as one of the hospital referrals, presumably on the assumption that she would resettle easily. Hospital notes and some direct observation on the ward suggested she spent most of her time in the ward, sitting in a chair, turning the pages of a catalogue. She was often dressed in an all-in-one suit to prevent her from removing her clothes or injuring herself.

Hannah moved to a spacious, well designed bungalow with high standards of furnishings and decorations with five other ex-hospital residents as part of the resettlement programme. As noted above, difficulties were not anticipated. However, within two days Hannah was refusing to go to bed, demanding constant attention from the staff, grabbing and hurting staff and residents, smearing faeces, refusing to sit on the toilet, eating her meals separately because of aggression to other residents at the table and because of stripping off her clothes at mealtimes. The other residents were finding Hannah's behaviour unsettling. Staff were finding that Hannah's demands coupled with her aggression prevented them from involving other residents in activities.

After a week of this behaviour, the BST was asked to visit to advise on management strategies. It was agreed that the most immediate problem was Hannah's refusal to go to bed, particularly as medication had already been used to no effect. Hannah was observed by the adviser that evening and a sleeping routine was devised on the spot. Within three days Hannah was settling at night and going to sleep within an hour of staff implementing the routine. This early success raised staff morale and allowed at least a peaceful evening and night. It also increased staff confidence that following management strategies consistently could bring results.

As Hannah was constantly demanding attention during the day, it was agreed that a rota should be organized so that staff were allocated to Hannah for 30–60-minute periods at a time. Although staff were resistant to this degree of structure, it meant they knew they would only have Hannah for a set period before someone else took over. This reduced staff stress. It was then possible to analyse Hannah's behaviour and to assess her skills in more detail so that longer-term intervention could begin.

A behavioural technician from the BST was allocated to Hannah for two to three hours each afternoon, seven days a week. The technician went to the house and used the time to explore new activities for Hannah, to assess her abilities and to monitor her aggression (whilst providing regular respite for staff). Three weeks of this intensive input saw a significant reduction in staff stress and anxiety and an increase in their confidence and competence. Regular discussions took place between staff, the adviser and the technician to look at ways of reducing the inappropriate behaviours. The intensity and frequency of the various behaviours reduced rapidly over the first six weeks.

Subsequently, a technician visited Hannah twice a week for two to three hours with the aim of completing a formal skills assessment prior to devising specific skill teaching programmes for staff to carry out. The adviser visited weekly to monitor progress and discuss new strategies as Hannah's behaviour altered. Ultimately Hannah was sitting with other residents without injuring them, did not demand constant attention and was only occasionally grabbing staff. She continued to settle well at night and to sleep through until the morning.

Some months later she was re-referred by day-centre staff when she achieved a part-time day centre placement. At that stage more detailed analysis of her self-injury was undertaken, leading to further interventions.

### Staff training and dissemination

High priority is placed within the services provided by the BST on training staff to understand and deal with difficult behaviour. A number of nationally recognized courses are routinely offered to local staff and other courses are tailored to meet specific needs of staff groups. Induction training is given to staff recruited to care for clients with challenging behaviour.

The BST disseminates its work to other staff groups of local and national agencies as appropriate. This may take the form of reports, seminars, conference presentations, etc. Each year an annual report is written and circulated.

### Consultancy and service planning

The BST offers periodic and regular consultancy to other staff concerning named clients or concerning more general issues of relevance to the client group. For example, the two day centres offering one-to-one staffed places for those with challenging behaviour each receive a half day per week from a behavioural adviser. The team contributes to multi-agency planning groups concerned with clients with challenging behaviour. They initiate such planning where service deficiencies are revealed by their other activities.

### Evaluation and research

**Aims and methods**
The BST has a brief to evaluate its own activities and to research areas pertinent to clients with challenging behaviour. The South

Western Regional Health Authority group on challenging behaviour has a subgroup for evaluation studies which has provided an essential forum for discussing Region-wide evaluation plans and for exchanging expertise in research methods.

## Case evaluation

Data on the intensity of the case work and the hours spent per case are routinely recorded by all BST staff. Standard information on changes in challenging behaviour and quality of life is collected for all clients seen by the BST. To introduce the possibility of comparative data with other teams, a suite of measures has been put together (in collaboration with the RHA core group) which are designed to evaluate the impact of a service on the individual client and his/her carer. Client measures include: the nature, frequency and duration of challenging behaviour, quality of life, engagement in daily activities. For carers measures are taken of attitude to the client pre/post-intervention, satisfaction with the team's input and perceptions of improvements post-intervention. It will also include a measure of carer stress.

As an illustration of individual case evaluation, the work with Angela can be described. Angela was referred for throwing objects at the day centre (e.g., laden trays, plates of food). The instructor responsible for her collected data on an ABC chart for three months (direct observation failed to provide an example of throwing due to its relatively low frequency). The data showed nine incidents of throwing over these three months. During this time information was also gathered on how Angela spent her days at the centre and on how her instructor reacted to throwing. The instructor's response when Angela threw something was first to tell her off and then to take her to a quiet room where he spent 10 minutes sitting silently beside her and then a further 20 minutes engaging her in a one-to-one activity of her choice. On occasion, as an alternative, the instructor would telephone her mother who then had to ask her father to leave his place of work and come and collect her forthwith from the centre. Angela quite enjoyed being at home with her mother on these occasions as there was actually more to do at home.

At the start of the baseline period the instructor completed an attitude scale concerning his attitude towards Angela. This scale, devised by the BST, is a five-point Likert-type scale with nine polarized statements with dimensions such as Calm/Not calm, Irritated/Not irritated, I do know what to do/I don't know what to do, I understand her behaviour/I do not understand her behaviour.

The intervention consisted of written guidelines on providing Angela with a more meaningful timetable at the centre and a changed consequence for throwing which centred on not giving undivided positive attention but requiring her simply to pick up and clear away the thrown items. No incidents of throwing occurred in the three months following intervention. The instructor again completed the attitude scale which showed a 50% improvement in his attitude towards Angela. He also completed a Satisfaction Questionnaire which asks a series of questions about the BST's input. He rated his satisfaction as 100%. Nevertheless, in the fourth month following intervention, throwing occurred three times and on investigation it was found that the instructor had reverted to his previous responses to throwing. Input then recommenced along the same lines but including the involvement of the manager of the day centre.

**Resettlement studies**
The baseline measures collected on 25 people in hospital prior to resettlement are being repeated at intervals. A six-month follow up on the first eight is complete, as is a 12-month follow up on a further six. Presentations of the findings have been made to the provider agency, regional research meetings and the staff of the homes. The voluntary agency which provides the staffed group homes has asked for the measures to be repeated for a third time 18 months after resettlement.

## Conclusions

### *Demand for the service*

The referral rate has been fairly steady over the first two years, with large fluctuations from month to month. There has been a gradual increase in the demand for staff training. So far demand has not outstripped available staff time, although there is always a danger of decreasing the intensity of work and spreading the service too thinly. The main attraction of the team for many service providers is the level of intensity of individual case work which has been offered to date. Careful attention must be paid to maintaining staff numbers and the balance between the various activities. Some referrers request intensive case work with people who have no challenging behaviour but who would undoubtedly benefit from detailed one-to-one training. Such activity would undermine the purpose of the team.

Some challenging behaviour teams adopt a more intensive model of case work than the BST, carrying very small case loads at any one time and working virtually full time with the referred person and their carers. An example of such an approach is the Intensive Support Team in Kidderminster Health Authority (Burchess, 1990; Burchess *et al.*, 1991). This team works with as few as five referrals at one time but offers very detailed input. A 30-page assessment report is prepared on each person, following which a contract is agreed whereby the Intensive Support Team gains exclusive control over interventions (including changes in medication, introduction of changes of location and so on). They can offer 24-hour support by moving a member of the team into the client's home. While there would seem to be great advantages to such an approach in terms of maximizing the chances of success with any single individual, these must be balanced against the disadvantages inherent in a service that reaches very few people and is therefore relatively expensive and restricted in impact.

The BST has found that many referrals do not require this level of intensity but nevertheless do require some input. Where improvement can be gained by a brief input this would seem worthwhile. One advantage in taking on many referrals is that the availability of the service is more widely dispersed and more opportunities for spreading good practice occur. It is an important tenet of the BST that carers should be enabled to understand and manage behaviour themselves. Although it can take longer to produce change when working through front-line carers, it is hoped that this will increase skills in the long term and foster their application to future difficulties.

Monitoring and review, including the consumer/carer perspective, is important to ensure the right kind of service is offered by the team. To this end a 'road show' consisting of a one-hour presentation and discussion is given regularly by the team to parent groups, homes and day centres to explain the methods of working and to solicit feedback.

*Partnership with carers*

The implication for the referrer of referring someone to the team is not always apparent to them. It generally means extra time and effort required by the carers to complete assessments, keep charts and in many cases devote extra time and energy to the referred person, perhaps indefinitely. As one means of stemming referrals which are ill thought out or not serious, written referrals only are accepted. This demonstrates at least a minimal commitment on the part of the referrer. Within the BST, much debate has taken place on whether or not to introduce contracts between the team and the referrer. While a contract seems a straightforward solution, in practice it would mean introducing a foreign concept not used by any other professional group providing a service to the same users. This might result in a reluctance to refer and a tendency to use other options (e.g., exclusion or medication), options which, in many instances, tend to be preferred by some carers. Continued use of the team will only be ensured by successful case work becoming the norm.

The experience of the BST suggests that it is extremely important to bring to people's attention the details of the practical mechanics for achieving behaviour change, i.e. that it may require detailed and carefully thought-out work over a long time scale. In a widely dispersed service with high staff turnover, this means continual attention to staff induction and in-service training. In addition, attention needs to be paid to maintaining changes in staff practices which underlie successful interventions. Repeated experience has shown that in many cases a successful intervention is allowed to slip, with a consequent re-emergence of the challenging behaviour, once the team's input has ceased. The availability of the technicians has meant that this danger has lessened as they are able to spend extended periods of time in a setting ensuring an intervention is acceptable and effective. However, even where this input has been daily for three or more months and been faded out very gradually, there have still been cases where the intervention then ceases to be used. This may arise through a feeling that, since the difficult behaviour has reduced or disappeared, the intervention is no longer needed, or through a genuine lack of staff within the establishment.

## Advisers and technicians

The positive impact of having a pool of technician staff cannot be overstated. Their flexible deployment with well designed briefs makes the advice offered by the qualified team members far more effective than it would otherwise be. There are, however, attendant risks in technician use. For example, they may be seen as merely a source of extra staffing and used to bolster poor staffing levels.

The balance of employing two and a half advisers and five technician staff worked well while the advisers were in post. However, this is a delicate balance and was destroyed during the long-term absence on sick leave of one of the full-time advisers and the subsequent difficulty in appointing a Team Leader. Technician staff tend to be people preparing for admission to professional training courses (e.g., clinical psychology, social work) and the posts provide suitable experience for this. The posts do not, however, provide scope for promotion within the NHS without first gaining a professional qualification. Adviser posts can serve as excellent experience as part of a longer-term career plan within psychology, social work, etc., or for branching out into other specialist forms of work with the client group.

## A bed-free service

It was an explicit intention from the outset to provide a peripatetic service and not to have the team attached to any beds. This has worked well in practice, with the capacity to place team members on call through a radio pager strengthening the team's ability to respond in a crisis to prevent placement breakdown. Anecdotally, it appears that several teams which have been associated with a residential unit have suffered from becoming bogged down in staffing the unit itself in times of staff shortages and have, consequently, been unable to provide the peripatetic outreach service in the way envisaged.

The success of a truly peripatetic team relies, in part, on all other elements of a comprehensive service for people with challenging behaviour being in place and functioning adequately

(Chapter 4). The weaknesses in the respite service mentioned above have meant that periodically crises have occurred and users with challenging behaviour have found themselves admitted to the health service's psychiatric treatment clinic. Meanwhile, two useful indicators of the extent to which a 'bed-free' service is effective, are the number of referred cases who have been sectioned and the number who have been sent to live outside the district. Of 112 referrals taken up by the BST in the first two years, only five were admitted to the psychiatric treatment clinic for reasons solely to do with their challenging behaviour, of whom only one was placed on a section. Of these, all but two returned to their original address following the admission. Only one person taken up by the BST has been sent to live out of district and this for two years' residential schooling only.

### Partnership with other professionals

Although in theory the inter-relationships between the team, the treatment unit, the respite units and the community team staff are clear, in practice these are often blurred. The BST is the newest element in service provision and has yet to make its full impact on referral habits. Meanwhile, there are homes or centres which have developed a tradition of referring in a certain direction which is hard to alter. Greater liaison between the various elements of local services should help to overcome this difficulty. Shortages in community nurse and social work staff have meant that the team's intention of working closely with these staff has often been frustrated. Fewer referrals than expected have been made by community nurses and social workers (compared to residential homes and day centres who refer directly to the team). This has led to a situation where parents have not been as aware of the service as they might have been since the team had assumed (wrongly) that parents would access the service through their community nurse or social worker. Attempts have been made to rectify this by the team addressing parent groups directly and setting up a parent support group. The existence of professional jealousy also needs to be acknowledged. Traditionally, certain professional groups guard their territory and may act in their own interests rather than in those of the users.

Looking to the future and the likelihood of a more severely rationed service, what chance does a highly labour-intensive service such as the BST have? It may be seen as cheaper to herd difficult people together – thus requiring fewer staff, less need for staff training across the board and no need for a specialist team. Maintaining the attention of involved agencies on quality and service philosophy is crucial. If services are designed to promote quality of life and are provided in integrated settings, then peripatetic support becomes an essential part of the whole. Specialist teams must be able to demonstrate effective help delivered to those who need it. Such teams must also be able to demonstrate that they provide a service which is complementary to, and not a duplication of or substitute for, services which are, or should be, delivered by other groups.

Detailed evaluation including costings remains to be done to compare the efficacy of such specialized teams with other models of service delivery. In the meantime many such teams have been set up and some have already collapsed. It is important to gather information on their successes and failures before drawing conclusions as to their final place in the range of services offered to those few but significant people who present a major challenge to the future of care in the community.

## References

Behavioural Services Team (1993a) *Operational Policy*. Plymouth: Behavioural Services Team.

Behavioural Services Team (1993b) *Guide for Referrers*. Plymouth: Behavioural Services Team.

Burchess, I.D. (1990) *The Intensive Support Team: Discussion documents 1, 2, 3*. Kidderminster: Kidderminster Health Authority.

Burchess, I.D., Walker, J., Dearn, J. and Heath, D. (1991) The Intensive Support Team, Kidderminster, in *Meeting the Challenge: Some UK Perspectives on Community Services for People with Learning Difficulties and Challenging Behaviour* (eds D. Allen, R. Banks and S. Staite). London: King's Fund Centre.

Donnellan, A.M., LaVigna, G.W., Negri-Shoultz, N. and Fassbender, L.L. (1988) *Progress Without Punishment: Effective Approaches for Learners with Behavior Problems*. New York: Teachers College Press.

Durand, V.M. (1990) *Severe Behavior Problems: A Functional Communication Training Approach*. New York: Guilford Press.

Emerson, E., Barrett, S., Bell, C., Cummings, R., McCool, C., Toogood, A. and Mansell, J. (1987) *Developing Services for People with Severe Learning Difficulties and Challenging Behaviours*. Canterbury: Institute of Social and Applied Psychology, University of Kent.

Emerson, E., Barrett, S. and Cummings, R. (1990) *Using Analogue Assess-*

*ments.* Canterbury: Centre for the Applied Psychology of Social Care, University of Kent.

McBrien, J.A. and Felce, D. (1992) *Working with People who have Severe Learning Difficulty and Challenging Behaviour: A Practical Handbook on the Behavioural Approach.* Kidderminster: British Institute of Mental Handicap.

Meyer, L. and Evans, I.M. (1989) *Nonaversive Intervention for Behavior Problems: A Manual for Home and Community.* New York: Teachers College Press.

O'Brien, J. (1987) A guide to life style planning: Using The Activities Catalogue to integrate services and natural support systems, in *The Activities Catalogue: An Alternative Curriculum for Youth and Adults with Severe Disabilities* (eds B. Wilcox and G.T. Bellamy). Baltimore, MD: Paul H. Brookes, pp. 175–189.

Oliver, C. (1991) The application of analogue methodology to the functional analysis of challenging behaviour, in *The Challenge of Severe Mental Handicap: A Behaviour Analytic Approach* (ed. B. Remington). Chichester: John Wiley, pp. 97–118.

*Part Three*

---

# Determinants of Quality

# 9

# Values, attitudes and service ideology

*Eric Emerson, Richard Hastings and Peter McGill*

## Introduction

The role played by social values and cultural ideologies in shaping the form of services for people with disabilities has received extensive attention over the past two decades (e.g., Wolfensberger, 1972; 1975; 1980). Indeed, it nowadays appears to be accepted as something of a truism that such a 'value base' underpins the very existence of welfare services and exerts a pervasive and powerful influence upon their everyday practice.

As a result, service agencies have expended considerable effort in attempting to clarify their value base, and hence the 'theory of action' upon which they operate (Dowson, 1991; Tyne, 1987). The concepts of normalization (Nirje, 1980; Perrin and Nirje, 1985; Wolfensberger, 1972; 1980), social role valorization (Wolfensberger, 1983) and service accomplishments (O'Brien, 1987) appear to have been widely adopted by many service agencies for people with a learning disability. Indeed, agency 'mission statements' and job adverts which do **not** make specific reference to at least one of these concepts have become quite a rarity. In addition to clarifying underlying values and agency goals, services have also devoted considerable resources to orienting staff to these ideological 'foundations' of service provision.

There can be little doubt that these activities have had a profound impact upon the ways in which we describe publicly the aims of services for people with severe disabilities (e.g., Departments of Health and Social Security, Welsh Office, Scottish Office, 1989). In general, however, the assumptions that organizational values exert a powerful influence over service quality, or that organizational performance may be effectively improved through changing the attitudes of staff, have received little critical scrutiny. This may, in part, be explained by the atmosphere within which these developments have taken place. Indeed, attempts to orientate both organizations and individuals towards specific service ideologies have often taken a form akin to a religious crusade, in which challenging the orthodox teachings of 'Saint Wolfensberger' constitutes an unspeakable heresy.

In this chapter we will explore some of the ways in which values and staff attitudes may relate to the quality of services for people with severe learning disabilities and challenging behaviours. It is not our intention to provide a comprehensive analysis of all the possible relationships between societal, personal and service values and service quality. Such an aim would be far too ambitious. Rather, we aim to point to some issues of potential importance to managers and practitioners within services. In doing so we hope to provoke discussion rather than resolve it. Specifically, we will address two main questions.

1. What influence do the personal beliefs and values of staff have on the quality of services provided? What can be done to increase positive effects and reduce negative effects?
2. What influence do service beliefs and values have on the quality of services provided? What can be done to increase positive effects and reduce negative effects?

Prior to addressing these questions, however, it is important that we clarify the ways in which we intend to use the terms 'values', 'attitudes' and 'ideology', and that we make explicit our assumptions concerning the types of staff and organizational practices which we believe to be characteristic of high-quality services for members of this client group.

## What constitutes 'good practice' within services for people with severe learning disabilities and challenging behaviours?

For the purpose of the current chapter we will assume that services exemplifying 'good practice' will have two complementary aims. Firstly, they will seek to enable users to respond more constructively to the types of situations which currently elicit their challenging behaviours. Secondly, they will try to ensure that, to the greatest extent possible, users maintain and/or develop their participation in activities associated with social roles which are valued within the mainstream culture of our society.

In order to achieve these aims we believe that staff will need to develop, consistently implement, monitor and revise a logically coherent plan for providing support to service users which takes into account:

1. factors which have been shown to underlie the person's challenging behaviours;
2. pragmatic issues relating to the management of episodes of disturbed and disturbing behaviour;
3. ethical considerations regarding the user's rights to effective support and freedom from harm;
4. the known effectiveness of specific procedures for reducing challenging behaviours and building up constructive alternatives; and
5. the resources available to achieve the overall objectives of such a plan.

This may, at times, include the development, implementation and monitoring of technical interventions to reduce or replace specific challenging behaviours. In all situations, however, it will include procedures to ensure that staff consistently establish the general conditions which 'set the occasion' for appropriate or alternative behaviours to emerge (Chapter 10).

## What are values?

In the following discussion we will use the terms 'values', 'attitudes' and 'beliefs' interchangeably to refer to the set of beliefs held by an individual concerning the social worth or value of another individual or group of individuals and the meaning or interpretation of their behaviour. We will use the term 'ideology' to refer to a set of values or attitudes which is characteristic of a particular religious, social or ethnic group.

In general, attitudes, values and beliefs can be thought of as rules which enable individuals to make sense of their world by predicting the likely consequences of their actions (cf. Skinner, 1988). Thus, for example, a belief that a person's challenging behaviours result from their negative life experiences (e.g., discontinuities in social relationships and/or segregation from normative life experiences), can be thought of as a rule which suggests that replacing such negative life experiences with more positive ones should lead to an amelioration of such behaviours.

It is, of course, possible to classify the attitudes or values held by individuals in a number of ways. We will be concerned, however, to distinguish between two broad classes of values: generic values relating to appropriate conduct within society and specific values relating to the nature of learning disabilities and challenging behaviours. In addition, we may consider each of these two classes of values to be operating at three levels: within society in general, within service agencies and at the level of individuals employed by service agencies.

### Societal values

While values are, in the last analysis, held by individuals, certain values are of general importance as they either reflect the ways in which resources are allocated within a society or represent a broad consensus of opinion about the meaning or interpretation of an individual's behaviour. As we noted above, two aspects of societal values will be of importance to our discussion: general values reflected in the patterns of social organization evident in the UK, and disability-specific values.

In some ways it would appear inappropriate to try to identify general social values. Society does, after all, contain a plethora of social, cultural, ethnic and religious groups embracing a remarkable diversity of ideologies. The importance of pluralism can, however, be taken too far. Consideration of the ways in which resources are allocated within society, the values permeating the education of our young and the values expressed within popular media do reveal certain consistencies. British society does, in general, place greater value on a number of inherited or acquired characteristics. These include such factors as gender, ethnicity, wealth, power, intelligence, entrepreneurial skills, beauty, youth and fitness. While different social groupings may place different emphasis upon such characteristics, it would be inadvisable to neglect the importance of such common values. The importance of such values is reflected in the existence of formal and informal discriminatory practices (identified by their various -isms, e.g., racism, sexism, ageism, handicapism) which operate against individuals who do not belong to such valued groups.

The nature of societal values specific to people with a disability has received much attention. In general, of course, most disabilities are defined by their exclusion from generally valued social groupings, e.g., the beautiful and/or fit or the entrepreneurial and/or intelligent. Such exclusion is often associated with a range of formal and informal discriminatory practices (Bogdan and Biklen, 1977).

In addition, however, Wolfensberger (1972; 1975) has suggested that there exist a number of more specific stereotypes or 'deviancy role perceptions' which characterize a culture's interpretation of, and response to, deviancy. These stereotypes include the perceptions of the disabled person as being subhuman, a menace, sick, an object of pity, a burden on charity, an object of ridicule or an eternal child (Wolfensberger, 1975; Wolfensberger and Thomas, 1983).

## Service values

Service agencies commonly espouse a specific set of values concerning the social worth of the agency's clientele and the interpretation of, and appropriate response to, their disability. The values reflected in the manifest (if not the latent) aims of contemporary service agencies are characterized by a commitment to equality, fairness and stewardship (Bank-Mikkelsen, 1980; Departments of Health and Social Security, Welsh Office, Scottish Office, 1989; Committee of Enquiry into Mental Handicap Nursing and Care, 1979; Nirje, 1980; Perrin and Nirje, 1985; Tyne, 1987; Wolfensberger, 1972), although it should be noted this has not always been the case (Hollander, 1989; Wolfensberger, 1981).

Service agencies do differ markedly, however, in the more specific beliefs according to which they interpret, or make sense of, deviant behaviour. Thus, for example, in different agencies a person's challenging behaviour may be interpreted as being the result of such varied factors as faulty metabolism, adaptation to a dysfunctional environment, negative life experiences or diabolic possession. Such interpretations are, of course, likely to be associated with different ways of responding to the person (e.g., treatment, care, prayer).

Over recent years, Wolfensberger's conceptualization of normalization (Wolfensberger, 1972; 1980) and social role valorization (Wolfensberger, 1983) has had a powerful impact within the UK upon the ways in which services interpret and respond to challenging behaviours (e.g., Blunden and Allen, 1987). These recent developments appear to have displaced, at least in part, more specific behavioural or medical models which had previously provided the main frameworks within which challenging behaviours had been formally interpreted.

### Personal values

It would be naive to assume, of course, that either the general or disability-specific values held by individual members of staff within an organization are consistent with the agency's manifest ideology. Indeed, it is likely that the personal values held by individuals within an organization will reflect a broad mix of societal and service-related values. But in what general proportion? A number of factors may serve to determine the spread of values held by individuals within an organization and their congruence with organizational aims.

Firstly, the range and strength of societal values pertaining to a specific disability will vary over time and across cultures. Such variation is likely to be reflected in the general socialization processes to which all members of society are subjected. Thus, for example, in contemporary society the role of people with learning disabilities as objects of (mild) ridicule or pity is closely woven into the fabric of popular culture (Bogdan *et al.*, 1982). For example, incompetence often serves as the main vehicle for much TV comedy. These socializing processes, along with actual contact with members of the disabled group, may be expected to help shape both the nature and strength of disability-related values held by members of society, including potential employees of service-providing agencies.

Secondly, the extent to which agency practices embody the values reflected in the organization's manifest aims will influence this relationship between agency and personal values. Agencies with a highly explicit value-based 'mission' which is **also** reflected in day-to-day practices are unlikely to either attract, recruit or retain staff holding markedly different values. There are, for example, few Satanists in most Franciscan monasteries. Few human service agencies, however, have such explicit value-based missions or, more importantly, such a close correspondence between their mission and everyday practice. As a result the natural selection and 'weeding out' processes which operate within organizations are much less likely to be effective than those found in, for example, ecclesiastical orders. As a result there is likely to exist a much poorer fit between agency values and the personal values held by individual members of staff.

Such correspondence as does exist may be expected to decrease as we examine the relationship between personal and agency values in areas more peripheral to the agency's mission. Thus, for example, while there may be close correspondence between agency and personal values about the meaning of learning disability within an agency providing residential provision, poorer correspondence may occur with regard to the interpretation of challenging behaviours shown by residents. We will return to the relationship between agency and personal values in the sections below.

### In what ways do personal values influence staff performance (and consequently service quality)?

As we noted above, we will address two main issues in this chapter. Firstly, we will focus on the influence which the personal beliefs of staff may have on service quality. We will then attempt to draw out some suggestions for practice.

Staff performance in services for people with challenging behaviour may be most appropriately viewed as the result of complex interactions between a number of factors. These include:

1. the behaviours and characteristics of service users;
2. the formal or planned rules and contingencies operating within the setting (e.g., operational policies, shift plans);
3. the informal or unplanned rules operating within the setting (e.g., peer pressure); and
4. the resources available to staff.

The behaviours and characteristics of service users may influence staff performance in a number of ways. In general, the personal appearance and behaviours of users may set the occasion for either staff approach or avoidance (Dailey *et al.*, 1974). More specifically, the challenging behaviours shown by service users may produce a number of emotional reactions among staff including fear, irritation, anger and disgust. In general, those individuals within a setting who show the most serious challenging behaviours are also likely to receive the greatest amount of staff attention (e.g., Emerson *et al.*, 1992). Such attention, however, may be disproportionately negative in character (Grant and Moores, 1977; Moores and Grant, 1977), involve lower rates and different types of supportive contact (Carr *et al.*, 1991) and may even be abusive (Rusch *et al.*, 1986). Challenging behaviours elicited by staff contact or staff demands may deter staff approaching the person in the future (Carr *et al.*, 1991). Thus, the challenging behaviours shown by service users may have a pervasive negative influence on staff performance and hence service quality. Unfortunately, there is little corresponding evidence to suggest that positive changes in user behaviour act as effective reinforcers for staff and hence promote future contact (Woods and Cullen, 1983).

A variety of formal or planned rules and contingencies operate within any workplace (Chapter 10). These involve the explicit aims of the agency, the roles it assigns to staff and systems for ensuring that actual performance meets with the agency's expectations. They may be divided into performance expectations regarding what staff should be doing, systems for monitoring actual performance against such expectations and providing feedback to staff regarding the appropriateness (or not) of their performance. Within many human services, of course, these systems are often fragmented and ineffectual. Staff often have little specific idea of what is expected of them, are rarely monitored in any reliable way and even more rarely receive effective or constructive feedback.

In the absence of formal systems, a range of informal rules and contingencies often exert a powerful influence over staff performance. That is, peer groups define what should be done, monitor each other's performance against these (often implicit or unstated aims) and provide effective (if not always constructive) feedback. Unfortunately, however, these informal rules and contingencies may support practices at odds with the explicit aims of the service itself (Ryan and Thomas, 1987). Thus, for example, it is not uncommon in residential services for these informal rules and contingencies to constitute a powerful barrier against initiatives which involve staff assisting residents to perform activities themselves, rather than staff completing these activities (in a shorter time) for them.

These three dimensions of environmental demand interact with staff resources to produce specific patterns of staff performance. 'Staff resources' in this context refers not only to the numbers of staff available and access to material resources but also to such resources as skills, knowledge, attitudes and beliefs.

It is, of course, extremely common for problems within services to be explained in terms of resource deficiency. Increasing staff numbers or skills has come to be seen as a panacea for solving virtually all service-related difficulties. Sufficient resources, however, must be seen as a necessary but certainly not sufficient condition for ensuring quality in service provision. Indeed, the available evidence suggests that increasing staffing levels has little impact on either the extent or nature of support received by service users (Harris *et al.*, 1974; Mansell *et al.*, 1982; Seys and Duker, 1988) and that training *per se* has little lasting impact on staff performance (Reid *et al.*, 1989; Ziarnik and Bernstein, 1982).

Within this framework the personal values, attitudes and beliefs held by individual members of staff constitute some of the important resources available within the setting. Below we will examine in more detail the nature of these resources and the conditions under which they are likely to have an active influence on staff behaviour and, hence, service quality.

In general, we tend to view people as rational creatures whose behaviour is guided by the beliefs they hold about the world around them. Indeed, most of us feel rather uncomfortable if we cannot find a reason for something important that has happened in our environment. Based upon such a premise, we may, therefore, expect care staff's responses to challenging behaviours to be consistent with their beliefs about such behaviours.

This notion of 'reasoned action' has been developed into a formal theory by social psychologists who have been concerned with the relationships between attitudes and behaviour (Ajzen and Fishbein, 1980; Fishbein, 1979). At a basic level this model states that the intention to perform a particular behaviour is the best predictor of the occurrence of that behaviour. This self-reported intention to do something is, in turn, influenced by (1) the subject's attitude towards that behaviour and (2) what is termed the subjective norm. Attitudes towards a behaviour combine beliefs concerning the likely outcomes of different courses of action and the evaluation of the **value** of such outcomes. Similarly, the subjective norm combines the subject's beliefs about how others would interpret the possible courses of action open to him/herself and the subject's own motivation to comply with these normative beliefs.

Thus, for example, the model suggests that the response of a member of staff to a particular episode of challenging behaviour will be influenced by:

1.  their subjective evaluation of the likely consequences of possible courses of action (e.g., ignoring it may decrease the behaviour over time; shouting at the person may stop the behaviour);
2.  the value they place on these potential outcomes (e.g., the relative value of short- and longer-term effects);
3.  their beliefs about how others (e.g., other members of staff, managers, the public) may react to the possible courses of action open to the member of staff (e.g., open support, peer hostility, dismissal); and
4.  the extent to which the person is motivated by the reactions of others.

From this perspective, therefore, both care staff's personal beliefs about challenging behaviours and their interpretation of wider social influences (other care staff's beliefs, the service's beliefs and society's beliefs) will affect their response, different components of this equation becoming dominant for different people in different contexts.

As we have noted above, these basic processes can also be encompassed within a behavioural framework which emphasizes the role of the verbal rules which govern behaviour. Society in general, the service and colleagues provide various rules that staff may follow when dealing with people with learning disabilities and challenging behaviours (e.g., the law, service policies, behavioural programmes). Care staff also use their own personal rules to guide their behaviour, commonly called 'experience'.

We can easily find out what the services that deal with challenging behaviours believe about such behaviours and the nature of their policy on intervention. Similarly, professional staff have ideas and recommendations based on their perceptions of challenging behaviours. Finally, it is possible to identify written and unwritten beliefs in society at large relevant to the treatment of 'deviant' behaviours. However, we know very little about the beliefs of individual staff members or the extent to which these beliefs are influenced by others. This must be considered a major omission given the importance of care staff in providing ongoing daily support to people with severe learning disabilities.

A preliminary interview study designed to look at such issues (Hastings and Remington, submitted for publication) suggested that, as would be expected, care staff have divergent views on the reasons for the occurrence of challenging behaviours. These ranged from medical or biological determinants to the seeking of attention and communication difficulties. Most respondents reported that challenging behaviours are (at least to some extent) 'intentional', although this did not necessarily mean that they considered that service users were personally responsible for their behaviour.

A small number of studies have attempted to determine the typical responses of staff in residential services to episodes of challenging behaviours. Bruininks *et al.* (1988) asked care staff in community and public residential facilities how they responded to incidents of challenging behaviour. Seventy-three per cent said that they responded verbally or physically to such behaviours, rather than by encouraging other behaviours or ignoring incidents. Similarly, respondents in the Hastings and Remington (submitted for publication) study also reported this tendency to stop challenging behaviours by intervening physically or verbally. A commonly cited reason for this response was to protect people engaging in the behaviours and other people and property. Finally, Maurice and Trudel (1982) asked the staff of three large institutions how they typically responded to self-injurious behaviour. The results indicated a diversity of reactions, including verbally reprimanding users in 45% of instances, reassuring the user in 12% of instances and hitting the client in 2.5% (or one in 40) of cases. Observational studies of the behaviours to which care staff respond support the above results, showing that challenging behaviours, and not more socially acceptable behaviours, draw the attention of staff (Felce *et al.*, 1987).

Although care must be taken in making comparisons across studies conducted in differing contexts, the above results do suggest examples of conflicts between different sources of values. Care staff's reported beliefs about the reasons for challenging behaviours match closely those suggested by professionals and researchers. However, these beliefs alone do not seem to guide their actions. Rather, as predicted by the notion of 'reasoned action', individual responses to challenging behaviours reflect the interaction between personal beliefs regarding the meaning of behaviour and other beliefs, for example, the valuation of outcomes (e.g., concerns for the protection of fellow human beings overriding longer-term reductions in challenging behaviour).

Services have often emphasized the caring or protective aspects of the role of care staff. Staff, of course, often feel responsible for what happens to clients and this may lead to the emphasis on terminating episodes of challenging behaviours as soon as they occur. The choice of a method for terminating a person's challenging behaviour appears, in many instances, to be determined by personal beliefs (or experience) regarding the likely effectiveness of different strategies, e.g., verbal reprimands, punishment. They may also, however, reflect 'lay' beliefs regarding the reasons for challenging behaviour. Thus, for example, reassuring a person who is self-injuring may constitute either a pragmatic strategy for terminating the episode and/or a response based on the belief that self-injury is the external manifestation of inner torment.

Whatever the exact relationship between beliefs and staff performance their influence cannot be denied. Furthermore, in many situations this influence may serve to undermine planned responses to challenging behaviour. Thus, for example, behavioural programmes and other policies commonly describe how people **should** respond (reactively) to episodes of challenging behaviours. However, our previous discussion suggests that immediate responses to incidents of challenging behaviours may not be driven by technical beliefs about the reasons behind such behaviour. Rather, they appear to be determined by more general beliefs about what should be done when people engage in challenging behaviours (e.g., protect them from harm).

Like all resources, however, the impact of beliefs may be modified by a number of other factors. These include the emotional reaction of people to challenging behaviours and the formal and informal rules and contingencies operating within a setting.

Care staff report strong and upsetting reactions to self-injurious behaviour, including disgust, despair and sadness (Hastings and Remington, submitted for publication). Similarly, aggressive behaviour elicits fear, and stereotypy is commonly reported as being annoying. It is possible that such emotional responses 'set the occasion' for staff responses. Thus, for example, disgust may set the occasion for responses focusing on the immediate termination of the behaviour or withdrawal from the vicinity of the service user. Fear may set the occasion for avoidance. Anger or annoyance may set the occasion for abuse. Such emotional responses may, of course, either facilitate responses congruent with personal beliefs or not. Fear in response to aggression may well aid compliance with an intervention programme based upon the withdrawal of staff from the vicinity of the person, but is likely to act as an impediment to the implementation of a programme based on calmly redirecting the person back to the activity in hand.

The determining effects of beliefs may also be overridden by the formal and informal rules and contingencies operating in a setting. As we have noted above, however, the formal rules and contingencies which operate within services are often rather ineffectual in determining staff performance. Expectations may be unclear, monitoring unreliable and feedback ineffective. The informal rules and contingencies, which are usually considerably more powerful, constitute the subjective norms within settings. Again, these may or may not be consistent with the personal beliefs and attitudes of individual members of staff. However, a marked disparity between a person's beliefs and the beliefs and actions of others in the setting may lead to the person absenting him/herself from the setting, possibly by seeking alternative employment.

Given these considerations, what can be done to maximize the beneficial effects that personal beliefs may have on staff performance and minimize any untoward effects? A number of possibilities arise from consideration of the above framework.

The beneficial effects of beliefs become apparent when they are consistent with service beliefs and values. In such instances, individual members of staff may be expected to act in ways consistent with organizational aims even under conditions in which the formal rules and contingencies are ineffective or absent. Ensuring as close a match as possible between individual and service values may be approached through staff selection, training, supervision and retention.

### Staff selection

Staff selection procedures would, therefore, need to find more accurate ways of assessing applicants' beliefs concerning the 'meaning' or reasons for challenging behaviour and beliefs about what should be done when someone displays such behaviours. Traditional interview practices are, of course, rather ineffective in this area as the applicant's behaviour is likely to be primarily determined by the demands of the interview situation itself. If the selection of individuals whose personal beliefs mirror the prevailing service ideology appears impossible, then consideration should be given to the selection of staff from as broad a mix of backgrounds as possible in order to minimize the chances of a powerful informal staff counter-culture which may emerge more readily within a staff group of similar ages, backgrounds and experiences. Similarly, congruence between organizational expectations and staff behaviour may be increased by the selection of individuals with a history of rule-following, i.e. individuals whose behaviour appears to, in general, be more effectively controlled by external, rather than by internal, rules.

### Staff training

Staff training has frequently been employed in an attempt to change the beliefs upon which members of staff operate. Unfortunately, however, evidence from such diverse areas as health education and race relations suggests that information and training may be ineffectual in changing personal beliefs, attitudes or behaviour. This should not be surprising given the competing influence of education, everyday 'experience' and popular culture in shaping our beliefs. The effectiveness of training may be enhanced, however, by basing it upon an analysis of the individual's current beliefs, increasing its intensity and linking it to practical experience (e.g., through on-the-job training). Thus, for example, while the types of full-time intensive training over extended periods which are characteristic of professional training may stand some chance of changing participants' values, much in-service training is likely to represent an ineffective use of service resources, especially given the high staff turnover rates evident in many services.

Staff training or counselling may have an important role to play, however, in situations in which the emotional reactions of staff to episodes of challenging behaviour are serving to undermine planned responses or, even, more appropriate responses determined by the individual's beliefs. As noted above, for example, fear in response to an episode of aggression may set the occasion for staff withdrawal rather than any response based upon calmly redirecting the person back to the task in hand. In such instances training staff in the skills required to manage aggression in a manner consistent with service values may have a significant beneficial impact upon future staff performance.

### Staff supervision

Staff supervision and retention procedures may play an important role in maximizing the congruence between personal and service values. Staff supervision may be considered a more effective approach to attitude change since it is, by definition, individualized, occurs over extended periods and is linked to practice. Perhaps more importantly, however, effective supervisory practice should ensure that service values are reliably translated into everyday practice in terms of generating clear performance expectations, reliable monitoring and effective feedback. While such procedures should serve to override the influence of personal beliefs which are inconsistent with service aims, they are also likely to 'weed out' members of staff whose belief systems are at odds with service ideology.

There are, of course, potential drawbacks to maximizing the congruence either between individual beliefs and service values or between service expectations and individual behaviour. While such a situation may help ensure that organizational aims are achieved, it is also likely to diminish the capacity of an organization to reflect self-critically upon its own goals and procedures. There may, therefore, be a case for explicitly recruiting staff who hold a variety of personal beliefs (within certain boundaries) and to support staff who will, in a constructive way, challenge the organization's prevailing orthodoxy. Through such processes a creative tension may be established in which the chances of constructive self-scrutiny are maximized. Attaining an appropriate balance in this area does, however, represent a formidable task.

### In what ways does service ideology influence staff performance (and hence service quality)?

While the personal values of members of staff may have a direct influence upon staff performance, the impact of service ideology is more indirect. Service values may set limits of action surrounding managerial decisions concerning service organization in relation to, for example, size and groupings, the manifest (if not latent) 'mission' of services and the acceptability of procedures employed to achieve agency goals. These may all be (partially and with corruption) translated into the formal and informal expectations, monitoring and feedback operating within service settings. Below, we will explore in more detail these modes of influence, especially as they relate to the introduction of the notions of normalization and social role valorization into services.

### Service ideology and the agency 'mission'

One of the most obvious manifestations of recent developments has been the explosion in the number of agency 'mission statements' making specific reference to the value base upon which services are purported to operate. Clarification of an agency's mission may, of course, have some considerable benefits in providing a clear pointer to service aims and the types of activity which may legitimately be undertaken in pursuance of these aims. 'Mission statements' in and of themselves, however, are unlikely to have an impact upon staff performance unless they are translated into practical aspects of service organization and management. An agency's mission needs to be made manifest in **all** aspects of service activity.

There are, of course, some considerable difficulties associated with attempts to introduce new 'missions' into old services. Services serve a multiplicity of important functions, many of which may bear only a tangential relationship to the explicit aims of the service. Thus, for example, while the aims or mission of day services are commonly (and appropriately) phrased in terms of outcomes or benefits for service users, one of their most important functions lies in providing daytime respite for carers. The effective translation of an agency's mission into everyday activity will need to take into account these latent functions of services if opposition from important stakeholders is to be avoided. Somewhat unfortunately, however, the recent emphasis upon clarifying the manifest mission of services has, if anything, drawn attention away from the analysis of its latent functions. As a result the potential impact of such activity is placed in jeopardy.

### Service ideology and service organization

The values held by an organization are one source of influence which helps determine the ways in which its services are structured and employees deployed. This influence may be seen most clearly when organizations develop new types of service activity. Thus, for example, service ideology appears to have played an important role in the development of supported employment as an alternative to traditional centre-based day care. Similarly, changes in service ideology may be influential in establishing the boundaries of what is considered an acceptable form of service organization (e.g., the maximum advisable size of residential facilities). As noted above, however, service ideology is only one factor in a complex field of forces which shape service activity. As a consequence, the translation of ideology into practice needs to be approached within the context of a detailed analysis of the various forces shaping service development. Again, the recent emphasis upon 'values' may have had the effect of drawing attention away from such a pragmatic process.

Service ideology may also have a pervasive impact in determining broad aspects of employees' roles within organizations. Thus, for example, over recent years the role of care staff within community-based services has been redefined in an attempt to avoid the impersonal or paternal/maternal models typical within many institutions. Unfortunately, however, such attempts may have had a negative impact upon staff performance by reducing the clarity of **informal** performance expectations through the abandonment of more clearly understood staff roles. Many staff working with people who present major challenges now find themselves (in the absence of clear direction – or even sometimes with it) cast into the multiple conflicting roles of friend, enabler, advocate, teacher, jailor, home-maker, carer and therapist. The conflicting expectations of these amorphous roles often serve to paralyse effective action and may set the occasion for (possibly unhelpful) personal beliefs to shape actual performance.

## Service ideology and service activity

Similarly, service ideology may help define the boundaries around what should be considered legitimate activity within an organization. Normalization, for example, pays considerable attention to the means used by services as well as the ends to which these means are aimed. Thus, for example, the recent controversy surrounding the use of 'aversive' methods in the treatment or control of seriously challenging behaviours appears to be guided more by ideology than by evidence (Mulick, 1990). The risk involved, of course, is that, as service ideology is given a greater emphasis, service activity may come to be determined by moral principle rather than by evidence. Indeed, the impact of normalization as a service ideology has been criticized on the grounds of its failure to evaluate the veracity of its own propositions (Emerson, 1992).

## Service ideology and staff management

In order to have a significant impact upon staff performance, service ideology will need to be translated into routine procedures for setting performance expectations for staff activity, monitoring actual activity and using the results of this to give effective feedback to staff based on the relationship between expected and actual performance. Service ideology is likely to have an influence on both the content and style of staff management procedures. Clearly, the nature of performance expectations should reflect the aims of the service and service beliefs regarding what may be considered legitimate and effective means to achieve such aims. Service ideology may also have an impact upon the style of staff management practised within an organization (e.g., Dowson, 1991). Thus, for example, service ideology may help determine the actual procedures by which performance expectations are set, performance is monitored and feedback given. Effective management need not, of course, be associated with a hierarchical bureaucracy.

The translation of service ideology into the day-to-day practices of staff management is clearly essential if service values are to have an impact upon service activity. The influence which service ideology may have on defining service models and broad aspects of service organization provides a framework of opportunities. Taking advantage of these opportunities requires effective staff management.

Unfortunately, however, the impact of normalization as a service ideology upon staff management procedures has left much to be desired. As we noted above, in many services effective management procedures simply do not exist. Staff are unclear regarding their general roles and specific duties, are not monitored in a reliable fashion and rarely receive effective feedback which may sustain 'good practice'. Such a pattern is also evident in services driven by normalization-related values. Indeed, such values appear in some instances to be associated with a distinct lack of clarity and resistance to (at least formal) methods of staff management along with a general atmosphere of anti-professionalism. Such services commonly place a strong emphasis on selection, orientation and training methods in an attempt to ensure that staff adopt agency values at a personal level and hence act as a guide to staff action in the absence of external controls. We have argued above, however, that such an approach is unlikely to be effective when considered in the context of our limited effectiveness in changing the types of personal values and beliefs which underlie action and the ever-changing nature of the workforce in community-based services.

## Conclusions

The control of the social and physical environment provided by services constitutes the main means by which services can improve the behaviour and lifestyle of service users. The task is no less than the design of a culture which will support clients in living quality lifestyles. Much attention has been paid to the role of staff behaviour in such a culture and, similarly, though to a lesser extent, to the role of the physical and programmatic environments. Such work has often foundered on a failure to maintain appropriate staff behaviour or appropriate environments in the longer term. Short-term change, usually in the context of close supervision and leadership, is relatively straightforward but longer-term maintenance is more problematic. Services can, and have, responded to this problem in several ways. They can endeavour to provide explicit supervision and control over staff behaviour through the kind of organizational technology described elsewhere in this book (Chapter 10). Alternatively, or additionally, they can try to generate a self-sustaining culture which is mediated either by the personal values of staff or by the broader values of the organization. In the former approach, the assumption is made that by recruiting staff who care enough about the right things ('committed' staff) they will directly maintain and develop the culture experienced by service users. In the latter, the assumption is made that the organization controls staff by inculcating (or indoctrinating) them with its values. In a sense the outcomes of these two strategies are likely to be similar, though the locus of control remains different.

In this chapter we have attempted to review the value of these strategies. While this review has pointed to the limitations of such approaches it has also sought to identify how, given what we currently know, their effects can be maximized.

We have argued that service ideology and personal beliefs are important factors influencing staff performance and, consequently, service quality. Service ideology may help define the agency's 'mission', the legitimacy of different ways of approaching these aims and the day-to-day framework within which staff will operate. We have suggested, however, that within current services the ideologies made explicit in agency 'mission statements' have, to date, been ineffectively translated into service activity. In addition, the ideology of normalization or social role valorization may have had some unhelpful consequences in generating confusion concerning staff roles and devaluing the importance of effective staff management procedures.

In the absence of formal procedures for determining staff activity the personal values and emotional responses of individual members of staff may come to play an important role in shaping their actions. We have provided a framework for conceptualizing the ways in which attitudes and beliefs may be related to behaviour and made suggestions concerning strategies for ensuring consistency between service ideology and personal beliefs.

Failure to attend to these issues will mean that fertile ground will continue to exist for the growth of informal staff cultures that may either subvert or impede the attainment of service aims. The task ahead may be conceptualized as one in which both the informal staff culture operating within services and the personal beliefs of individual members of staff are either consistent with or, when in conflict with notions of good practice, overridden by service ideology.

## References

Ajzen, I. and Fishbein, M. (1980) *Understanding Attitudes and Predicting Social Behavior*. Englewood Cliffs, NJ: Prentice-Hall.

Bank-Mikkelsen, N.E. (1980) Denmark, in *Normalisation, Social Integration and Community Services* (eds R.J. Flynn and K.E. Nitsch). Austin, TX: Pro-Ed, pp. 51–70.

Blunden, R. and Allen, D. (eds) (1987) *Facing the Challenge: An Ordinary*

*Life for People with Learning Difficulties and Challenging Behaviours*. London: King's Fund.

Bogdan R. and Biklen, D. (1977) Handicapism. *Social Policy*, **7**, 14–9.

Bogdan, R., Biklen, D., Shapiro, A. and Spelkoman, D. (1982) The disabled: Media's monster. *Social Policy*, **12**, 32–5.

Bruininks, R.H., Hill, B.K. and Morreau, L.E. (1988) Prevalence and implications of maladaptive behaviours and dual diagnosis in residential and other service programs, in *Mental Retardation and Mental Health: Classification, Diagnosis, Treatment, Services* (eds J.A. Stark, F.J. Menolascino, M.H. Albarelli and V.C. Gray). New York: Springer-Verlag, pp. 3–29.

Carr, E.G., Taylor, J.C. and Robinson, S. (1991) The effects of severe behavior problems in children on the teaching behavior of adults. *Journal of Applied Behavior Analysis*, **24**, 523–35.

Committee of Enquiry into Mental Handicap Nursing and Care (1979) *Report*, Cmnd 7468. London: HMSO.

Dailey, W.F., Allen, G.J., Chinsky, J.M. and Veit, S.W. (1974) Attendant behavior and attitudes toward institutionalised retarded children. *American Journal of Mental Deficiency*, **78**, 586–91.

Departments of Health and Social Security, Welsh Office, Scottish Office (1989) *Caring for People: Community Care in the Next Decade and Beyond*, Cm 849. London: HMSO.

Dowson, S. (1991) *Moving to the Dance or Service Culture and Community Care*. London: Values Into Action.

Emerson, E. (1992) What is normalisation?, in *Normalisation: A Reader for the 1990s* (eds H. Brown and H. Smith). London: Routledge, pp. 1–18.

Emerson, E., Beasley, F., Offord, G. and Mansell, J. (1992) An evaluation of hospital-based specialized staffed housing for people with seriously challenging behaviours. *Journal of Intellectual Disability Research*, **36**, 291–307.

Felce, D., Saxby, H., de Kock, U., Repp, A., Ager, A. and Blunden, R. (1987) To what behaviors do attending adults respond? A replication. *American Journal of Mental Deficiency*, **91**, 496–504.

Fishbein, M. (1979) A theory of reasoned action: Some applications and implications. *Nebraska Symposium on Motivation*, **27**, 65–116.

Grant, G.W. and Moores, B. (1977) Resident characteristics and staff behavior in two hospitals for mentally retarded adults. *American Journal of Mental Deficiency*, **82**, 259–65.

Harris, J.M, Veit, S.W., Allen, G.J. and Chinsky, J.M. (1974) Aide:resident ratio and ward population density as mediators of social interaction. *American Journal of Mental Deficiency*, **79**, 320–6.

Hastings, R.P. and Remington, B. (submitted for publication) Implementing behavioral programmes for challenging behavior: Toward an understanding of care staff.

Hollander, R. (1989) Euthanasia and mental retardation: Suggesting the unthinkable. *Mental Retardation*, **27**, 53–61.

Mansell, J., Felce, D., Jenkins, J. and de Kock, U. (1982) Increasing staff ratios in an activity with severely mentally handicapped people. *British Journal of Mental Subnormality*, **28**, 97–9.

Maurice, P. and Trudel, G. (1982) Self-injurious behavior: Prevalence and relationships to environmental events, in *Life-Threatening Behavior: Analysis and Intervention* (eds J.H. Hollis and C.E. Meyers). Washington, DC: American Association on Mental Deficiency, pp. 81–103.

Moores, B. and Grant, G.W. (1977) The 'avoidance' syndrome in hospitals for the mentally handicapped. *International Journal of Nursing Studies*, **14**, 91–5.

Mulick, J.A. (1990) The ideology and science of punishment in mental retardation. *American Journal of Mental Retardation*, **95**, 142–56.

Nirje, B. (1980) The normalization principle, in *Normalization, Social Integration and Community Services* (eds R.J. Flynn and K.E. Nitsch). Baltimore, MD: University Park Press, pp. 31–49.

O'Brien, J. (1987) A guide to life style planning: Using The Activities Catalogue to integrate services and natural support systems, in *The Activities Catalogue: An Alternative Curriculum for Youth and Adults with Severe Disabilities* (eds B. Wilcox and G.T. Bellamy). Baltimore, MD: Paul H. Brookes, pp. 175–89.

Perrin, B. and Nirje, B. (1985) Setting the record straight: A critique of some frequent misconceptions of the normalization principle. *Australian and New Zealand Journal of Developmental Disabilities*, **11**, 69–74.

Reid, D.H., Parsons, M.B. and Green, C.W. (1989) Treating aberrant behavior through effective staff management: A developing technology, in *The Treatment of Severe Behavior Disorders: Behavior Analysis Approaches* (ed. E. Cipani). Washington, DC: American Association on Mental Retardation, pp. 175–190.

Rusch, R.G., Hall, J.C. and Griffin, H.C. (1986) Abuse-provoking characteristics of institutionalised mentally retarded individuals. *American Journal of Mental Deficiency*, **90**, 618–24.

Ryan, J. and Thomas, F. (1987) *The Politics of Mental Handicap*, 2nd edn. London: Free Association Books.

Seys, D. and Duker, P. (1988) Effects of staff management on the quality of residential care for mentally retarded individuals. *American Journal on Mental Retardation*, **93**, 290–9.

Skinner, B.F. (1988) An operant analysis of problem solving, in *The Selection of Behavior: The Operant Behaviorism of B.F. Skinner* (eds A.C. Catania and S. Harnad). Cambridge: Cambridge University Press, pp. 218–36.

Tyne, A. (1987) Shaping community services: The impact of an idea, in *Reassessing Community Care* (ed. N. Malin). Beckenham: Croom Helm, pp. 80–96.

Wolfensberger, W. (1972) *The Principle of Normalization in Human Services*. Toronto: National Institute on Mental Retardation.

Wolfensberger, W. (1975) *The Origin and Nature of Our Institutional Models*. Syracuse, NY: Human Policy Press.

Wolfensberger, W. (1980) The definition of normalisation: Update, problems, disagreements, and misunderstandings, in *Normalization, Social Integration and Community Services*. (eds R.J. Flynn and K.E. Nitsch). Austin, TX: Pro-Ed, pp. 71–115.

Wolfensberger, W. (1981) The extermination of handicapped people in

World War II Germany. *Mental Retardation*, **19**, 1–7.

Wolfensberger, W. (1983) Social role valorization: A proposed new term for the principle of normalization. *Mental Retardation*, **21**, 234–9.

Wolfensberger, W. and Thomas, S. (1983) *PASSING: Program Analysis of Service Systems Implementation of Normalization Goals*. Toronto: National Institute on Mental Retardation.

Woods, P. and Cullen, C. (1983) Determinants of staff behaviour in long-term care. *Behavioural Psychotherapy*, **11**, 4–17.

Ziarnik, J.P. and Bernstein, G.S. (1982) A critical examination of the effect of inservice training on staff performance. *Mental Retardation*, **20**, 109–14.

# 10

# Organizing community placements

*Peter McGill and Sandy Toogood*

## Introduction

This chapter will first point to the ways in which placements for people with challenging behaviour often fail to deliver a satisfactory service. It will be argued that this failure is directly related to the occurrence and exacerbation of challenging behaviour. The characteristics of a more successful service will be described. The main part of the chapter will consider the ways in which services can organize themselves to produce such characteristics. Finally the chapter will consider the arguments often used against such an organizational technology and point to some of the requirements for successful implementation.

## The environmental context of challenging behaviour

While very little is known about the factors correlated with the original onset of challenging behaviour (Chapter 2) it is becoming increasingly clear that, to explain already existing challenging behaviour, we need to look both at individuals and at the environments with which they interact (Chapter 3). Thus, there is good evidence (Duker and Remington, 1991) that poor communication skills (an individual factor) are correlated with challenging behaviour and this has led to the development of intervention strategies which stress the development of functional communication abilities (Carr and Durand, 1985). Similarly, it is clear that challenging behaviour may be correlated with an absence of social contact or materials with which to interact (Durand and Crimmins, 1987; Horner, 1980). We are concerned in this chapter particularly with these sorts of environmental factors and with the kind of intervention strategy which may redress them. There is no doubt that the kinds of strategies described here will often need to be complemented by intervention strategies which focus on changing the individual's behaviour.

Recent advances in our understanding of challenging behaviour have come primarily from a conceptualization of challenging behaviour as functional (Chapter 3). In other words, it usually can be understood as a way in which the individual succeeds in controlling his/her environment. This, of course, is in the context of individuals who often have no other effective ways of controlling their environments or communicating their needs.

Functional analysis (Chapter 3) has stressed the importance of individual assessment to determine the function or functions served by a particular behaviour of a particular individual in a particular environment. This process usually involves collecting detailed information about the person's behaviour and the circumstances in which it occurs. Such analyses, despite their individual orientation, have tended to produce explanations for particular challenging behaviours which, while differing in their detail, have focused on certain common functions (O'Neill *et al.*, 1990).

1. **Escape or avoidance of aversive situations** – for example, where the behaviour appears to produce the effect of helping the person escape from demands to do things (activities, etc) or avoid being asked to do them altogether. Loosely put, people are left to their own devices if they kick up a fuss when an attempt is made to get them to do something.

2. **Increased social contact** – where the behaviour appears to be an effective way of obtaining social contact (e.g., from staff). Unfortunately, the notion of 'attention seeking' behaviour has become just another way of dismissing an individual's behaviour as not worthy of attention.

3. **Adjustment of levels of sensory stimulation** – there are a number of variations here. Most importantly there is evidence that some challenging behaviour serves the function of increasing the general level of sensory stimulation (perhaps self-injurious behaviour in a very barren or unstimulating

| ■ Behaviour maintained by ■ | ■ Environment characterized by ■ |
|---|---|
| Escape or avoidance of aversive situations | Intermittently high levels of overt and covert social control and abuse |
| Increased social contact | Low levels of social contact |
| Adjustment of levels of sensory stimulation | Barren, unstimulating environments |
| Increased access to preferred objects and activities (tangible reinforcement) | Regimes which rigidly control access to preferred objects/activities |

**Figure 10.1** Functional characteristics of the environments in which challenging behaviours occur.

environment); there is also evidence that some challenging behaviour is maintained by specific sensory consequences, e.g., the visual stimulation that it produces (Rincover and Devany, 1982); finally there is some suggestion that challenging behaviour may serve the function of reducing the general level of sensory stimulation, when it may be equivalent to escaping from an aversive situation (Donnellan *et al.*, 1984).

4. **Increased access to preferred objects or activities (tangible reinforcement)** – for example, food, a bath, new clothes, etc.

In considering these functions it is very important to be conscious of the context in which they often arise (Figure 10.1). It does not seem coincidental that services, both institutional and community-based, for people with severe learning disabilities are frequently characterized by:

1. intermittently high levels of overt and covert social control (Koegel *et al.*, 1987) and abuse (Zirpoli *et al.*, 1987), i.e., there are plenty of aversive events to escape from, especially if clients are not very good at understanding or doing what is required;
2. low levels of social contact (Mansell and Beasley, in press);
3. barren, unstimulating environments (Horner, 1980);
4. and regimes which rigidly control access to preferred objects and activities or which have very few of either (King *et al.*, 1971).

In other words the functions which challenging behaviour appears to most commonly serve should not surprise us and perhaps tell us something about the nature of service provision as well as the nature of challenging behaviour or severe learning disabilities.

This leads to the conclusion that these environmental character-istics are, in a sense, 'challenging'. While there is no doubt that people with severe learning disabilities have challenging needs – personal characteristics that make it more likely they will display challenging behaviour – challenging behaviour does seem to be more likely in 'challenging' environments. More technically, the common characteristics of services for people with challenging behaviour can be conceptualized as 'establishing operations' (Michael, 1982; see also Chapter 3) in that they increase the rein-forcing value of certain events, e.g., a low level, or deprivation, of social contact may establish attention as an effective reinforcer for challenging behaviour.

## Providing helpful environments

One of the tasks facing services, then, is to provide a helpful or supportive environment which will reduce the likelihood of chal-lenging behaviour. This will not, of course, 'cure' challenging behaviour. Rather, it will act as a kind of prosthesis (Lindsley, 1964). In the same way that a wheelchair can promote mobility without curing paralysis or spasticity a helpful environment can encourage adaptive rather than challenging behaviour.

Helpful environments are characterized by the opposites of what are found in challenging environments:

1. support and assistance instead of demand and control;
2. high levels of social contact, mainly contingent on adaptive behaviour;
3. meaningful activities instead of a lack of stimulation;
4. materials and activities which are readily and predictably available.

Such environments are, however, very rarely found in services for people with severe learning disabilities. They appear to be unlikely to develop 'naturally', i.e., without special organization or design. Where they exist they are often very difficult to main-tain – natural contingencies seem to support a return to a less helpful environment. We need, therefore, a conscious, systematic approach to service design.

What can be done to ensure the provision of a helpful rather than a challenging environment? One answer is to develop an organizational technology which determines what will happen to whom under what conditions and to what degree of success. To take an analogy from the world of education – what would it be like if children or students turned up whenever they liked for whatever classes and were met by teachers who decided on the spot what to teach and how to teach it, and later decided spontaneously that it was now time for an examination? In fact, of course, educational services do not (usually) operate in this way. They have a set of systematic procedures for achieving their goals (an organizational technology) that include a number of components:

1. **the curriculum** – which determines what will be taught;
2. **the timetable** – which determines who will teach whom, where, and when;
3. **lesson plans** – which determine how students will be taught;
4. **an assessment system** – which determines how well students have learned.

### Determining what will happen

What sorts of activity and interaction should be going on in placements? This depends on both individual and environmental requirements. From the environment's point of view there will be certain necessary activities. If the environment is a house then clearly it will need to be cleaned, food will need to be prepared and so on. If it is a sheltered workshop there will be contracts to be fulfilled. Within these limitations there is considerable scope for individual variation. Two people living in the same house are likely to spend their time differently on the basis of how they like to spend their time and what they are good at. The person who likes cooking may spend a lot of time preparing a meal from the raw ingredients. The person who is not so good at cooking but likes gardening may heat something up in the microwave in order to spend more time weeding.

In looking at this in more detail let us take the example of a staffed house. Figure 10.2 lists the activities required by such an environment, the 'routines and rhythms' of everyday life. This is obviously a summary of the major 'survival' activities required in

| Daily | Weekly | Less frequently |
|-------|--------|-----------------|
| Preparing meals | Shopping | Celebrating special days |
| Eating | Clothes washing | Paying bills |
| Clearing up after meals | Cleaning | Going on holiday |
| Dressing | Planning | Dentist |
| Sleeping | | Optician |
| Washing/personal hygiene | | Doctor |
| Cleaning | | Cleaning |
| Planning | | Maintaining health |
| | | Planning |

**Figure 10.2**  Routine activities in a residential placement.

a residential service. Figure 10.3 lists the activities which need to be considered from the individual's point of view. Two clients living in the same staffed house might end up with quite different patterns of activities because of differing abilities and interests. In the same way a couple living together might have quite distinct, though overlapping, patterns of activity and two children attending school might study different, but overlapping, combinations of subjects.

In this context the curriculum is the pattern of activities and interactions which are supported for individuals by the service. In considering how such curricula can be developed for people with severe learning disabilities it is worth looking at the situations of

✔ Personal care (dress, appearance, personal hygiene etc)
✔ Daily living (cooking, housework, shopping, travelling etc)
✔ Maintaining health (medication, contact with doctor, diet, exercise etc)
✔ Maintaining sensory functioning (hearing, vision)
✔ Communicating (expression, understanding)
✔ Social interaction (casual contacts, neighbours, friends, family)
✔ Organizing self (time and activity planning)
✔ Expressing emotions
✔ Asserting individuality
✔ Acceptable behaviour
✔ Maintaining or obtaining work
✔ Maintaining or obtaining leisure activities
✔ Maintaining or obtaining education

**Figure 10.3**  Areas to be considered in developing an individual pattern of activities and interactions.

people without learning disabilities. Many people spend large parts of their lives in routine activities over which they may have little control. Such activities include work, childcare, maintenance of the environment (housework, gardening etc.), body maintenance (sleeping, washing, dressing etc.). There may or may not be choices about the exact kind of work, or about the quality of the product (e.g., how neat the garden is). Whatever, such activities still take up large proportions of most people's available time. More choice may be exercised or at least felt in respect of social and leisure activities. Thus, while most people spend a proportion of their time in such activities this may mean watching TV for one person and abseiling for another.

Within these confines people may have certain aims, e.g. to give up smoking, to spend more time with the children, to write a novel, and so on. Such aims are a crucial part of most people's lives in that they provide a sense of purpose and control. Their achievement may, however, involve changing the pattern of their activities in a way which turns out to be very difficult because of the constraints exercised by their more mundane but necessary routines.

It is clear from this discussion that my curriculum, your curriculum, is likely to be determined largely by our current life circumstances (which, hopefully, we will have chosen sometime in the past) with a relatively small proportion of our time being available for new activities or directions. It is interesting to compare this pattern with how people with severe learning disabilities typically spend their time. Four differences seem particularly notable.

1. Instead of having too much to do they often have too little to do.
2. Instead of being subject to the demands of their current life circumstances they are often 'protected' from these by staff or carers who deal with such things for them.
3. There may be a complete absence of certain sorts of activities, e.g., work, which normally occupy a great deal of **our** time.
4. In so far as the pattern of their activities is defined by procedures such as individual programme planning they are often expected to spend the **majority** of their time in new activities and directions, e.g., learning new skills, losing problem behaviours and so on.

If individual programme planning is to effectively function as a mechanism for defining individual curricula it perhaps needs to change its emphasis in a number of ways.

1. It should seek to develop a curriculum which is relatively full and includes the range of activities (work, leisure, maintenance etc) present in the non-disabled person's life.
2. It should emphasize the requirements of the environment in which the service is provided, e.g., if this is a house, the curriculum should typically include some housework.
3. It should allow the person (within the constraints of typicality and environmental requirements) to choose his/her own pattern of activities.

The product of such a planning process is likely to include a list of the mundane activities of everyday life, a set of relationships to be maintained and/or created, and a **small** number of goals or changes to be sought (e.g., new skills to be learned). There is growing evidence that the kind and mix of activities provided for individuals has a considerable effect on the level of challenging behaviour likely to be displayed. Challenging behaviour is less likely when clients are engaged in preferred activities (Koegel *et al.*, 1987), when they have chosen from the range of activities on offer at any particular time (Dunlap *et al.*, 1991), and when activities that require learning are mixed with ones that have already been mastered (Winterling *et al.*, 1987).

### *Determining when, where and with whom it will happen*

If, as a student, you were told that you could study Maths, Physics and Astronomy but weren't told when or where the classes were, or who were the teachers, you would be naturally aggrieved and might well display some challenging behaviour. Yet this is often what happens in services for people with severe learning disabilities. Some kind of individual plan specifies what the client will be learning or what activities they will be doing but the details of this are left up to individual staff so that, all too often, when the plan is reviewed, we find that many of the objectives have not been achieved.

A curriculum cannot be implemented without a timetable which determines when, where and with whom activities will take place. The nature of the timetable depends on the nature of the service. In a day service, for example, there may be a fairly rigid repetition of activities from week to week so that it is possible to specify that, for example, John does pottery on Wednesday afternoon. Even in residential services such a pattern is likely to apply to at least some extent. For example many people do their main shopping or clothes washing on the same day each week. Few households go to the extent of writing these patterns down since there are generally only a few people sharing resources and contributing to the completion of household activities, most contributors have the capacity to carry the information with them, and there are adequate feedback loops and correction systems operating in the natural environment when the routines are not done or not done properly ('Where's my shorts, Mum?').

Routines received bad press in the early years of community care, mainly because they were seen as one of the worst features of institutional life. But it was the **rigidity** of routine (King *et al.*, 1971) that was problematic not routine itself. Routines, are in fact, functional in a number of important ways, e.g. creating a sense of security, providing a measure of the passing of time and making time to do other, more interesting activities. The desirability of routine is attested to by the extent to which it is present, explicitly or implicitly, in the majority of our everyday lives.

But routine, especially in shared service environments, serves another important function – its capacity to liberate. Where clear routines are absent, people who rely on services usually become prompt dependent ('It's time to go to bed now'), are more likely to be corrected by staff for 'getting it right – but at the wrong time' and are less likely to be rewarded by the natural contingencies that should apply when they take the initiative. On the other hand people with learning disabilities can exercise real autonomy within the boundaries of safe and predictable routines. If sensibly handled, routines can provide a structure or plan from which deviation can safely be made **and** a structure to return to later. For example, when planning a weekend away someone who normally washes their clothes on Sunday might choose to do them on the preceding Friday or to leave it until after the trip. Thereafter they might resume washing on Sundays until the next preferred activity interrupted the pattern. If the weekend routines were consistently interrupted then they might decide to reschedule their routines to accommodate other demands. Routine in services should feature this degree of flexibility.

Such routines, while useful and necessary, are not, however, the whole story. What does it mean to say that 'John does pottery on Wednesday afternoons'? Unfortunately, when John has severe learning disabilities and challenging behaviour it often means that he sits in the pottery room doing nothing for most of the time. In this case the timetable has not succeeded in delivering the curriculum. The timetabling approach, therefore, needs to be extended to cover how staff are deployed within a shift or period of time (Felce and de Kock, 1983). Staff–client ratios are usually such that they will not always be able to work individually with every client. They need, therefore, to systematically share themselves across individuals and groups of clients.

One parallel to this in the family setting might be the discussions which take place over dinner about who is going to do what, when, and what sorts of allowances are required to make things happen. The result of this type of discussion is usually an activity plan, e.g., 'Dad will run Kate to the skating rink and drop Alex off at his friend's house after they have each done their homework. Mum will pick them up on her way back from evening class while Dad gets that long-standing job done'. In this example, people are allocated to tasks and to be with others for defined periods of time. Some activities are contingent upon the completion of others, each knows what the others are doing and where they will be, activities that do not start and end at the same time are brought together in a coherent plan for the evening. People who need help (e.g., to get from A to B) get it and time to attend to the environmental necessities is created.

In service arrangements, where people may have substantial communication and skill deficits, the need for this type of planning is even more crucial. The need is heightened further where support is provided by staff who are present for only part of each day and who may not see each other for many days at a time. An example of this kind of more detailed timetable, or 'shift plan' is given in Figure 10.4. Notice that activities do not start and stop at the same times, everyone is accounted for throughout the period, alternative strategies are planned in at some stages of the day and staff work with different clients throughout the day – which may be important when working with people who are difficult to be with. If things go wrong at some stage the entire day is not thrown into confusion as there is a plan to return to. Opportunity plans and skill teaching programmes are scheduled into the plan,

# TIME AND ACTIVITY PLANNER

| Time | Support person 1 | Support person 2 | Support person 3 |
|------|------------------|------------------|------------------|
| 2pm | John + Sam shopping and Cafe<br><br>Sam : magazines + radio whilst John does his laundry (OP) | Gardening = Peter<br>(OP= use the mower) | |
| 4pm | Prep veg = Peter<br>Peter phone Dad @ 4.30 pm<br>Peter lay up table | Peter tea break<br>Sam magazines + radio<br>Meal Prep = Sam + John | ← tablets. |
| 6pm | Evening<br>clear table + tidy up    Peter | meal<br>wash up  Sam<br>Dry      John | * if Sam is difficult switch activity with Peter |
| 7.30 pm | Peter get ready to meet Phil + Mary at 8pm<br><br>Peter out with Phil + Mary \| John assemble the wheel on his bike    watch Tv | Sam Cash point PIN number.<br><br>Sam : shower + hair Perm<br><br>Watch Tv | |

**Figure 10.4**  An example of a completed 'shift plan'.

the balance between chores and leisure activities can be checked at a glance and environmental requirements for food preparation, cleaning, etc., are fully met.

The plan is prepared at the beginning of the session and its detail and complexity depend on what is required. In working with someone whose behaviour is very challenging it may be necessary to change activities and/or staff very frequently and to have contingency plans available for those situations where the original plan cannot be followed, perhaps because the client has refused to participate in the activity. Figure 10.4 includes such an example.

## Determining how it will happen

The presentation of activities is often a trigger for challenging behaviour. It is very important, therefore, that the manner of presentation is not left to chance and individual variation. The degree of detail will depend on the activity and the individual. Preferred activities, for example, may require less preparation than non-preferred activities. The member of staff will often, however, need the following information.

### The 'way' in which the activity is to be done

If you take six people and ask them to make a bed the chances are that you will see six different ways to make a bed. If these six people then each try to help the client make a bed in their own way the client is likely to become unnecessarily reliant on prompts, risks being corrected by one person for doing the task someone else's way, and, at worst, will become confused and demotivated. All those supporting the client in an activity need to have agreed on the way in which the activity will be carried out with this client. This will mean staff relearning well-practised skills but it is easier for six able people to learn one new method than for a person with severe learning disabilities to learn six new methods.

In practice staff should identify all the major activities that will occur on a regular basis, conduct a task analysis of each, write down the one agreed way of doing each task in the form of a manual and stick to that way of doing it. The manual serves as a useful job aid for new staff teams. As staff teams become more experienced they will internalize the client's way of doing things.

As turnover occurs new staff can be asked to learn the client's way of doing tasks according to the manual.

At times task analysis has been taken to extremes, e.g., Gold (1980) includes sample task analyses of vocational tasks having up to 76 steps. A much more global approach is usually all that is required. An example is given in Figure 10.5.

### The kind of assistance required

Gaining the client's participation in the task is the first and, often the most difficult, step. As discussed above such participation will partly depend on the task having been selected appropriately. It is still often necessary to define clearly how the task will be introduced to the client as a mistake at this stage will often set up a battle of wills which will inevitably result in challenging behaviour. Useful approaches to this problem include the use of 'pretask requests' – requests to the client which are highly likely to be followed – as a way of establishing 'momentum' which can carry forward into participation in the task itself (Horner *et al.*, 1991). Similarly, where a very active client is being requested to participate in a task which requires him/her to sit still for a period of time, the task may usefully be preceded by a period of physical exercise if this reduces the subsequent likelihood of challenging behaviour (Kern *et al.*, 1984).

The client may be able to do some bits of the task entirely independently while others have to be done by the member of staff. In between, a range of assistance is likely to be required. More generally the helper needs to know the kind of assistance

---

1.  Open machine
2.  Check and fill up the water
3.  Fill empty columns with cups
4.  Fill sugar container
5.  Put everything back
6.  Close top
7.  Lock lower cupboard
8.  Wash drip tray

---

**Figure 10.5** Task analysis of filling a vending machine (after Brown *et al.*, 1988).

that is most useful to the individual and the kind that is most likely to set off difficult behaviour. It is very common, for example, to find staff using complex verbal instructions that are completely beyond the understanding of the client. In such circumstances, where the client does not understand what (s)he is being asked to do, escape-motivated challenging behaviour is very likely. An example of written guidance for staff is given in Figure 10.6.

### The kind of reinforcement required

The almost stereotypical use of praise for task completion or on task behaviour is often neither necessary nor useful. Reinforcers should, as far as possible, be natural (so that they are obtained irrespective of the presence of a member of staff), intrinsic (so that the person does not need to stop doing the task in order to consume them), chosen by the individual (Dyer *et al.*, 1990) and based on a systematic assessment of what events are reinforcing for the person (Berg and Wacker, 1991) (so that they actually do work as

---

John can perform some parts of the task independently, though they may take him a long time. He will often continue with one part of the task when it is really finished so needs encouragement to move on. With some parts of the task he will need physical assistance, particularly lining up the nails and screws in the right positions and gluing in the right places. When using the hammer he may need some physical help until the nail is sufficiently deep in the wood. Similarly with the screws, and it may be helpful to have pre-screwed the holes beforehand. When part of the task is complete remove unnecessary tools to one side so that John can focus on the next part. This is particularly important when moving from a specially favoured activity (e.g. hammering) to a less favoured activity (e.g. using the brush). Your speech should be clear and simple, stressing the key nouns and verbs. John responds well to praise, eye contact and smiles.

---

**Figure 10.6**   Helping John to make a nesting box from prepared wooden components (based on guidance originally written by John Shephard).

reinforcers). What is required will, then, depend on the individual and the activity. The activity may well have been selected because it contains intrinsic reinforcers for the individual, e.g. the completed sandwich, the TV switched on and so on. With some clients compromises may have to be made in respect of these guidelines because of the paucity of events which appear to be reinforcing for the individual. Such a situation should, however, also prompt staff to try to extend the range of events which operate as reinforcers.

**The way in which challenging behaviour is to be handled**
Much of the above is intended to prevent, as far as possible, challenging behaviour. When it does occur, however, staff need to respond in a consistent manner which takes account of what is known about the function of the behaviour. An example of written guidance for staff is given in Figure 10.7. There are two main factors which should influence the way in which staff respond to challenging behaviour. The first is the need to contain the behaviour in a way which, as far as possible, avoids injury to anyone or damage to the environment and which gets the incident over with as quickly as possible so that concentration can again be given to delivering the curriculum. This requires a 'reactive strategy' (LaVigna *et al.*, 1989) (such as ignoring the behaviour and attempting to redirect the person back to the activity) which is essentially about damage limitation.

Staff need to be careful, however, that their reaction does not inadvertently reinforce the person's challenging behaviour and that they take advantage of the behaviour's occurrence to respond in a way which will reduce its future probability. Seclusion, for example, is often used in institutional settings as a reactive strategy and may well be effective at some kinds of damage limitation. If the person's challenging behaviour is motivated by escape from demands, however, this may also reinforce the behaviour and make it more likely to occur the next time demands are placed on the individual. In such a situation it is more appropriate to try to get the person to continue participating if only for a short time or, at the very least, to ensure that the person participates in completing the task later. The repeated occurrence of challenging behaviour in response to demands should prompt staff to reconsider the support they are providing to the person and to look at

Currently, Anne finds it difficult to do things 'on other people's terms'. That is to say, when she is asked to do something, she will often refuse.

In order to increase Anne's competence, independence and respect, staff need to help her better cope with this. If she doesn't get the opportunity to participate in activities she will never become more competent and will be totally reliant on staff.

The service is currently practising the current management plan. Anne will be presented with two activities every hour. **Anne is only expected to do a small part of the activity**. So be clear about what part of the activity she is to do (e.g. to wipe the table after you have sprayed polish, dry the cup etc). If Anne shows signs of wanting to go on with the activity or do a different part, then let her.

It is more likely than not that Anne will try to hit herself or bite her hand. **YOU NEED TO BE READY TO STOP HER DOING THAT** by restraining her hand. Anne may possibly then put herself on the ground and try to bang her head off the floor, on the wall or off other objects. **It is important before you present the demand/activity to have a cushion or similar available to move about and put under her head.**

Your role here is to stop Anne hurting herself – be careful not to wind her up further by the restraint itself: sometimes you can leave her go and she will not bite herself. **Just be ready to stop her if you think she will.**

Do not talk to Anne or look at her while she is trying to injure herself. At some point you will feel her relax (you will notice that she is very tense when she is distressed). At that point give her a full physical assist to continue with the activity. Do not make her do more than a few seconds of the activity after the challenging behaviour if you know that she is quite distressed. The point of the current programme is to ensure that Anne doesn't spend lengthy periods of time doing nothing and also to help her learn that there are times that she has to do something. The activity itself is not supposed to be a punishment for her.

**Figure 10.7** Managing Anne's challenging behaviour (based on guidance originally written by Heather Hughes).

the possibilities of teaching the person a more appropriate way to escape, or take a break from, activities.

### Determining how it will be evaluated

Recording what happens serves a number of functions. It tells us what the service is 'doing' with an individual and thus enables a judgement about the match between the plan and the result. If a service says that it provides a two-hour activity session every morning for clients but the records suggest that the session only happens 50% of the time because of staff shortages we have learned something important. Such information about occurrence of activities, teaching sessions and so on can also provide an early warning about decay of quality. Figure 10.8 provides an example where records kept of participation in activities show a decline over time. The service thought it was still doing well; the records suggested otherwise.

More detailed recording can provide important information about the achievements of the service and the need to make changes to the way it is provided. This will be crucial if, for example, the client is being taught a skill and there is a need to adjust the teaching method because of lack of progress.

Recording is often seen as a chore and is done poorly. It is crucial that the service builds in procedures for quickly summarizing records so that staff can see their work being used. This will

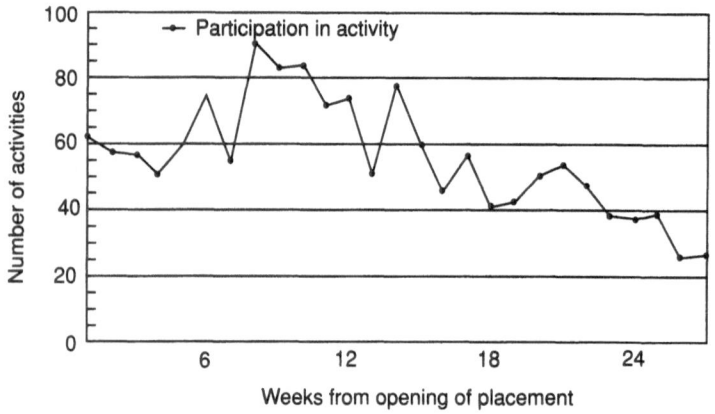

**Figure 10.8** Reduction over time in the weekly number of activities provided.

often involve certain staff taking responsibility for producing and updating graphs which can be used at the staff meeting and other such fora to evaluate progress.

### *Putting it all together*

It has been suggested above that a service needs procedures to determine what will happen (the curriculum), where, when and with whom it will happen (its timetable), how it will happen (its guide to activity and interaction), and how it will be recorded (its evaluation system). A wide variety of procedures exist for achieving such outcomes, as listed in Table 10.1.

In selecting procedures for a particular service it is important to combine them efficiently and coherently. One possible combination of procedures is shown in Figure 10.9. The system shown has a range of subsystems which are functionally separate but complementary. For example, the IPP system contributes to the development of the curriculum by identifying a range of medium-term goals for the individual client. These goals are likely to be timetabled through staff meetings and the time planning and management system. As required, more or less detailed strategies

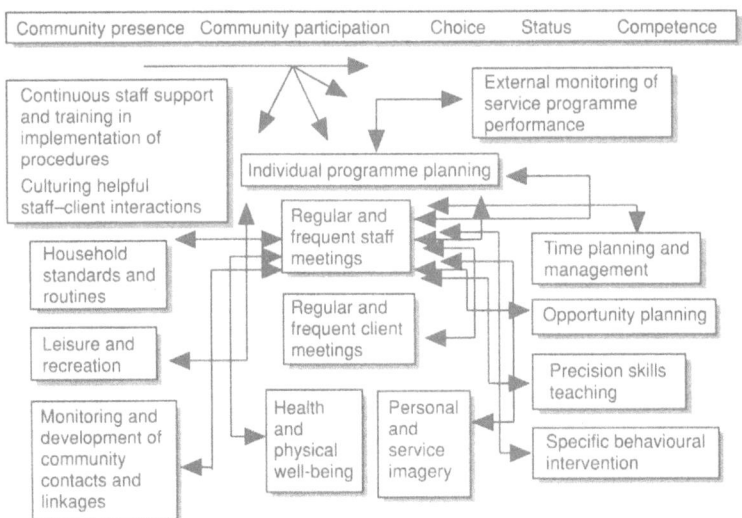

**Figure 10.9**   One possible combination of organizational procedures in a community placement.

**Table 10.1** Organization procedures for community placements

| | Procedure | Function |
|---|---|---|
| Determining what will happen | Individual programme planning | Identify a list of the mundane activities of everyday life, a set of relationships to be maintained and/or created, and a small number of goals or changes to be sought (e.g. new skills to be learned) |
| | Routines and rhythms | Establish the activities which have to be done to maintain the environment or lifestyle and specify how often they need to be done |
| | Activities catalogues | Provide a large display of possible activities from which the individual can select |
| | Activity sampling | Systematically expose the individual to a range of different activities in order to establish individual preferences and abilities |
| | Environmental audit | Identify the behaviours required to participate in a particular environment |
| Determining when, where and with whom it will happen | Duty rota | Provide supporters in the right place at the right time in the right combination |
| | Weekly schedule | Specify what routine activities have to be carried out, when, over the course of a week |
| | Diary | Specify what the person is doing, when and where |
| | Shift planning | Plan the deployment of staff to enable activities to take place |
| Determining how it will happen | Task analysis | Break down activities into their constituent steps to allow them to be presented in consistent ways to the person |
| | Support planning | Identify the kind and amount of assistance required by the person to complete the activity |

| | | |
|---|---|---|
| | Opportunity planning | Arrange regular opportunities to practise particular behaviours |
| | Precision teaching | Provide planned, systematic individual teaching of new skills |
| | Behavioural management | Respond to challenging behaviour consistently and constructively |
| | Incidental teaching | Teach new skills in the context of naturally occurring activities |
| Determining how it will be evaluated | Participation index | Record frequency and variety of participation in household activities |
| | Log of community activity | Record frequency of social contacts and presence in community settings |
| | Opportunity planning | Record rate of implementation of planned opportunity plans and rate of achievement of goals set |
| | Precision teaching | Record rate of implementation of planned teaching sessions and rate of achievement of goals set |
| | ABC charts | Record occurrence and circumstances of challenging behaviour |
| | Direct observation | Record engagement in purposeful activity, staff–client interaction and challenging behaviour |
| | Individual programme planning | Record rate of implementation and achievement of planned goals |

for how goals will be achieved will depend on the availability of planned opportunities, precision teaching strategies or specific behavioural interventions. The impact of the service on the client can be evaluated by using the information generated by the system, e.g., the number of IPP goals achieved, the level of client participation in household routines and so on. Arrows indicate the flow of such information.

Placements also need efficient ways of communicating their working practices to new or temporary staff. One way to do this is to develop one file for each client – the individual service specification – and one file for the service as a whole – the service maintenance specification. The structure of an individual service specification is based on the list of activities given in Figure 10.3. The file contains up to date accounts of how the person spends his/her time, the support s(he) needs in the whole range of activities, the way in which his/her behaviour is managed, and any special records that need to be kept. The file is a kind of a script (Saunders and Spradlin, 1991) for the service provided to the client – what is required of the service in order to meet the client's needs. An example of a partially completed specification is given in Figure 10.10.

The structure of the service maintenance specification is shown in Figure 10.11. This contains all the necessary procedures that are not specific to an individual client e.g., shift planning. An example of a partially completed specification is given in Figure 10.12.

By reviewing and practising the contents of these files new staff can be rapidly inducted into the service and all interested parties can rapidly see what it is that this service seeks to do for its clients.

What sort of impact would we expect such an approach to have on the environment experienced by clients? Properly used, these systems serve very well to modify the potentially challenging environment.

1.  They provide carefully tailored amounts of assistance to clients making it less likely that demand-avoiding challenging behaviour will occur.
2.  They increase the amount of social contact which clients get – making it less likely that social contact-seeking challenging behaviour will occur.
3.  They increase the amount and variety of activities (engage-

**Assistance needed in personal care (dress, appearance, personal hygiene etc.)**

Frank needs help to wear clothes rather than pyjamas during the day regardless of whether or not he is going outdoors. Until recently, Frank was only willing to wear clothes when going out and became very aggressive if he was not allowed out once he had dressed himself. This link seems to have been broken fairly quickly by Frank being required to wear clothes at all mealtimes and then being accompanied on a walk shortly after each meal. Frank now gets dressed for meals and for walks separately. This progress needs to be generalized by Frank being required to be dressed for other things. The support team needs to be systematic in the way it addresses this.

Frank requires some help dressing particularly in ensuring that clothes are not inside out. He needs some teaching on how to put his socks on. He cannot tie his shoe laces.

Frank is incontinent of urine after every single drink (he is obsessive about drinks and tries to drink constantly). He has been known to wet without drinks. Frank needs to be reminded to use the toilet every 15 minutes and before and after every drink. Over the past year and a half, Frank has taken to urinating on his bed and then going to the toilet. This needs to be recorded. Every aspect of this behaviour needs to be better monitored, possibly intensively for a short space of time (maybe a month) prior to any functional analysis. Working with Frank's incontinence (or excessive drinking) is likely to be a long-term goal considering the current staffing shortfall and the inconsistency between parental home and service. The short-term goal should concentrate on Frank wearing clothes.

Frank needs help to choose appropriate clothing: even in the height of summer he likes to be well covered up.

**Assistance needed in daily living (cooking, housework, shopping, traveling etc.)**

Frank can set the table with assistance and put away the dried up dishes. He can also clear away his plate with verbal prompting. Frank can help himself from a serving dish on the table but needs help to ensure that he does not spill any and does not take it all. Frank needs to be told to look at what he is doing. Frank needs assistance to move the hot iron over his trousers to avoid burning them and to replace the iron on the correct part of the ironing board when he is not actually using it. Frank will participate in polishing the coffee table if the table is close to where he is sitting. He needs to have the activity modelled for him by staff with a running commentary which invites him to join in without putting him under pressure.

**Figure 10.10** An example of part of an individual service specification (based on guidance originally written by Heather Hughes).

- Staff deployment and planning
- Staff meetings
- Staff supervision
- On the job training
- Induction training
- In-service training
- Maintenance of physical environment
- Administration
- Recording and maintaining client participation
- Recording and maintaining client development
- Recording and maintaining acceptable client behaviour
- Individual planning

**Figure 10.11**   Headings in the service maintenance specification.

**Induction training**
All staff attend five days induction training within three months of taking up post. The five days are spread over a five-week period to allow staff to do practical exercises in between training days. During their first week in post staff are regarded as supernumerary and work alongside experienced staff including at least one shift with the house manager. They are given time to complete a checklist of activities including reading individual service specifications and service policies. During this time an experienced member of staff acts as a 'mentor' to aid understanding of the requirements of the job. . . .

**Recording and maintaining client participation**
The Participation Index should be completed daily with all clients and discussed at handovers. Summary records are discussed at the fortnightly staff meeting and action agreed if there are problems around the amount or variety of participation. . . .

**Recording and maintaining acceptable client behaviour**
Agreed strategies for managing client challenging behaviour are contained in client service specifications and reviewed/updated on a three-monthly basis with the help of the clinical psychologist. All instances of aggressive, destructive and self-injurious behaviours are recorded and discussed at staff meetings. Special record forms are used for two clients as indicated in their service specifications. . . .

**Figure 10.12**   Part of a service maintenance specification.

ment opportunities) making it less likely that stimulation-seeking challenging behaviour will occur.
4.  They make materials and activities readily and predictably available making it less likely that tangible reinforcer-seeking challenging behaviour will occur.

There is good evidence that the use of such an approach is associated with reduced rates of challenging behaviour, increased rates of participation in activity and skill development in clients (Felce, 1989; see also Chapter 6).

## Successful implementation

Despite its apparent benefits it is a common experience to find resistance to the use of the above approach. The resistance seems to occur for a number of reasons.

1.  **The approach is seen as reducing the amount of choice and increasing the amount of control over clients' lives.**
    While this is an understandable objection it is usually false. Returning to the educational analogy, is it easier for students to choose and exert control in a chaotic or a structured environment? Chaotic environments are extremely difficult to control as they do not operate according to easily seen rules. Structured environments, because of their predictability, allow greater choice and control. As the student I can choose not to take the examination only if I know when it is. I can complain that the examination does not match the curriculum only if there is a well-recognized curriculum. Procedures are also increasingly being developed that allow clients more participation in the use of the organizational technology itself. For example the use of pictorial timetables (LaVigna *et al.*, 1989) potentially allows clients to participate in making up their own timetable; the use of pictorial representations of activities (Wilcox and Bellamy, 1987) potentially allows clients to participate in the development of the curriculum.
2.  **The approach is seen as reducing the amount of choice and increasing the amount of control over staff behaviour.**
    To some extent this is true but the choices which are reduced are, generally speaking, not legitimate anyway. In many services staff can choose to do nothing or do something for

themselves rather than clients. Such choices are illegitimate but in an unstructured service there is usually no way of saying what the staff should be doing instead. Helping people live 'an ordinary life' is sometimes an excuse for leaving people alone to do what they 'like', however destructive and self-destructive this is. There are some things over which staff delivering the service do not have legitimate control. To return to the educational analogy, the nature of the curriculum is not under the control of the teacher. We might disagree with the current political view on what that curriculum should be but we are unlikely to believe that what students are taught should depend on the whim of the individual teacher. Teachers do, however, have a great deal of control and choice over the manner in which the curriculum is presented. This is possible in services also, though it should be noted that the teacher is usually a 'lone wolf' while staff teams have to ensure consistency. It is the staff team that should exercise a considerable amount of control and choice not the individual staff member.

3. **The approach is imposed without consultation with users.** Just as with the implementation of other technologies this, unfortunately, is often true and such an imposition encourages staff to be similarly autocratic in their interactions with service users. The discussion in the previous section has tried to stress the functions of the various procedures (e.g., to determine the timetable) rather than the actual procedures themselves (e.g., shift planning). It is important that staff are given the opportunity to participate in the design of the system and that their ideas are used to develop better procedures rather than standard procedures being introduced without consultation. Such opportunities, however, should not constitute a *carte blanche*. It is crucial that the service organization accepts its responsibility to develop policy and monitor its implementation. This may mean that the goals of placements (the general direction of the 'curriculum') are not under the immediate control of placement staff. The organization needs to combine clear expectations regarding the kind of service which should be delivered to clients together with effective and sensitive management of the staff who will deliver such services.

The authors' experience in the face of the above resistances suggests that successful implementation is most likely when the procedures and materials used are:

1. informative and easy to use – providing clear guidance to staff and service users through their use of text and schematic representations;
2. accessible – easily available to staff as required rather than being locked in the bottom drawer of the filing cabinet;
3. kept and used discreetly – not usually being visible to a casual visitor;
4. efficient – taking the minimum of time away from direct client support;
5. designed and redesigned as far as possible in partnership with staff and service users.

## Concluding comments

Community placements for people with challenging behaviour face a difficult task. They have to deal with potentially dangerous situations in contexts of limited managerial and professional support (Chapter 6), often without being part of a comprehensive service strategy (Chapter 4), employing staff who are often young, inexperienced and likely to stay for relatively short periods of time. If such placements are to deliver a good quality of life to clients they must be organized robustly to protect good practice from decay. The kind of technology described in this chapter provides one way of doing this. Placements which lack such a technology are likely to be characterized by staff behaviour determined by uncontrolled and uncontrollable factors – such as what they usually do in their own homes, the way in which they interact with their children, and so on (Chapter 9). While such unpredictable behaviour sometimes produces apparently good results (for example, a close and facilitative relationship between a member of staff and a client) it cannot consistently produce the sorts of environment that are necessary to prevent, reduce and avoid exacerbating challenging behaviour.

## Acknowledgements

Christine McCool participated in the early discussions which led to this chapter. We are grateful for her contribution to its design.

We are also grateful to Heather Hughes and John Shephard for their permission to adapt their work for some of the examples used.

## References

Berg, W.K. and Wacker, D.P. (1991) The assessment and evaluation of reinforcers for individuals with severe mental handicap, in *The Challenge of Severe Mental Handicap: A Behaviour Analytic Approach* (ed. B. Remington). Chichester: John Wiley, pp. 25–45.

Brown, H., Bell, C. and Brown, V. (1988) *Teaching New Skills.* Bringing People Back Home Series of Video-assisted Training Packages. Bexhill-on-Sea: South East Thames Regional Health Authority (available from Outset Publications, St. Leonards).

Carr, E.G. and Durand, V.M. (1985) Reducing behavior problems through functional communication training. *Journal of Applied Behavior Analysis*, **18**, 111–26.

Donnellan, A.M., Mirenda, P.L., Mesaros, R.A. and Fassbender, L.L. (1984) Analyzing the communicative functions of abberant behavior. *Journal of the Association for Persons with Severe Handicaps*, **9**, 201–12.

Duker, P.C. and Remington, B. (1991) Manual sign-based communication for individuals with severe or profound mental handicap, in *The Challenge of Severe Mental Handicap: A Behaviour Analytic Approach* (ed. B. Remington). Chichester: John Wiley, pp. 167–87.

Dunlap, G., Kern-Dunlap, L., Clarke, S. and Robbins, F.R. (1991) Functional assessment, curricular revision, and severe behavior problems. *Journal of Applied Behavior Analysis*, **24**, 387–97.

Durand, V.M. and Crimmins, D.B. (1987) Identifying the variables maintaining self-injurious behavior. *Journal of Autism and Developmental Disorders*, **18**, 99–115.

Dyer, K., Dunlap, G. and Winterling, V. (1990) Effects of choice making on the serious problem behaviors of students with severe handicaps. *Journal of Applied Behavior Analysis*, **23**, 515–24.

Felce, D. (1989) *Staffed Housing for Adults with Severe or Profound Mental Handicaps: The Andover Project.* Kidderminster: BIMH Publications.

Felce, D. and de Kock, U. (1983) *Planning Client Activity: A Handbook.* Winchester: Health Care Evaluation Research Team.

Gold, M.W. (1980) *Try Another Way Training Manual.* Champaign, IL: Research Press.

Horner, R.D. (1980) The effects of an environmental 'enrichment' program on the behavior of institutionalized, profoundly retarded children. *Journal of Applied Behavior Analysis*, **13**, 473–91.

Horner, R.H., Day, H.M., Sprague, J.R., O'Brien, M. and Heathfield, L.T. (1991) Interspersed requests: A nonaversive procedure for reducing aggression and self-injury during instruction. *Journal of Applied Behavior Analysis*, **24**, 265–78.

Kern, L., Koegel, R.L. and Dunlap, G. (1984) The influence of vigorous versus mild exercise on autistic stereotyped behaviors. *Journal of Au-*

*tism and Developmental Disorders*, **14**, 57–67.

King, R., Raynes, N. and Tizard, J. (1971) *Patterns of Residential Care*. London: Routledge and Kegan Paul.

Koegel, R.L., Dyer, K. and Bell, L.K. (1987) The influence of child-preferred activities on autistic children's social behavior. *Journal of Applied Behavior Analysis*, **20**, 243–52.

LaVigna, G.W., Willis, T.J. and Donnellan, A.M. (1989) The role of positive programming in behavioral treatment, in *The Treatment of Severe Behavior Disorders* (ed. E. Cipani). Washington, DC: American Association on Mental Retardation, pp. 59–83.

Lindsley, O.R. (1964) Direct measurement and prosthesis of retarded behavior. *Journal of Education*, **147**, 62–81.

Mansell, J. and Beasley, F. (in press) Small staffed houses for people with a severe mental handicap and challenging behaviour. *British Journal of Social Work*, (in press).

Michael, J. (1982) Distinguishing between discriminative and motivational functions of stimuli. *Journal of the Experimental Analysis of Behavior*, **37**, 149–55.

O'Neill, R., Horner, R., Albin, R., Storey, K. and Sprague, J. (1990) *Functional Analysis: A Practical Assessment Guide*. Sycamore, IL: Sycamore Publishing Company.

Rincover, A. and Devany, J. (1982) The application of sensory extinction procedures to self-injury. *Analysis and Intervention in Developmental Disabilities*, **2**, 67–81.

Saunders, R.R. and Spradlin, J.E. (1991) A supported routines approach to active treatment for enhancing independence, competence and self-worth. *Behavioral Residential Treatment*, **6**, 11–37.

Wilcox, B. and Bellamy, G.T. (1987) *A Comprehensive Guide to the Activities Catalog: An Alternative Curriculum for Youth and Adults with Severe Disabilities*. Baltimore, MD: Paul H. Brookes.

Winterling, V., Dunlap, G. and O'Neill, R.E. (1987) The influence of task variation on the aberrant behaviors of autistic students. *Education and Treatment of Children*, **10**, 105–19.

Zirpoli, T.J., Snell, M.E. and Loyd, B.H. (1987) Characteristics of persons with mental retardation who have been abused by caregivers. *Journal of Special Education*, **21**, 31–41.

# 11

# Maintaining local residential placements

*Jim Mansell, Heather Hughes and Peter McGill*

## Introduction

A characteristic of community-based residential services set up to replace institutions is the breakdown of some placements and the re-admission of individuals to institutional care. The most commonly cited reason for placement breakdown given in studies of community services is challenging behaviour (Pagel and Whitling, 1978; Sutter et al, 1980; Thiel, 1981; Intagliata and Willer, 1982). Breakdown incurs costs for service agencies in finding new placements, often at short notice, as well as in dealing with the crisis and its aftermath. Alternative placements are usually hospitals, which impose costs on the individual person with learning disabilities in terms of fewer opportunities for meaningful activity, less staff help available and greater restrictiveness (Felce *et al.*, 1980a, b; 1986; see also Chapter 1) as well as the practical and emotional disruption involved. Family members and staff may also experience placement breakdown as failure.

People at risk of placement breakdown because of challenging behaviour are not a clearly delimited group. Studies of population characteristics show marked variation in the overall rates of challenging behaviour, not least because of the variations in definition and methodology, and rates vary widely over small areas (Chapter 2) and probably reflect different expectations and tolerance of staff as well as real variation in characteristics. Agencies providing community services must therefore meet the needs of a group of people, some of whom will present a clear and continuing challenge but others of whom will have less obvious or less difficult problems at this point in time. The size of the group who might potentially produce a challenge to services will be a significant proportion of the whole client group.

Expectations that simply transferring people from institutions to community placements will lead to reductions in challenging behaviour may be overoptimistic. Some studies tracking individuals from institutions to community placements show no change in level of challenging behaviour (e.g., Conroy *et al.*, 1982) or even higher rates of challenging behaviour after transfer (de Paiva and Lowe, 1990; Fine *et al.*, 1990; see also Chapter 5). Since the function of much challenging behaviour appears to be demand avoidance (Chapter 3), enriched environments may set the occasion for more problems than the barren, undemanding regime of many institutions.

Nor can treatment interventions yet play much part in responding to the needs of people with challenging behaviour. Although there is an extensive literature demonstrating at least short-term effectiveness of treatment techniques (particularly behavioural techniques), many problems remain intractable because of insufficient knowledge (see for example the discussion of covariation by Schroeder and MacLean, 1987). Just as important, most services are not in practice able to deliver the sophisticated intervention necessary to apply what knowledge there is. A recent survey by Oliver *et al.* (1987) of people with self-injury as well as learning disability in the south-east of England found that only 2% had written psychological treatment programmes. Nor is it the case that when programmes are developed they are used by staff: there is evidence (Emerson and Emerson, 1987) that staff do not understand the methods involved, do not themselves feel part of the programme design process and do not believe that any results would be sustained because of other problems in their service.

Since challenging behaviours are unlikely to spontaneously disappear after transfer to care in the community, nor to be readily resolved through short-term treatment programmes, the task facing services is in practice that of continuing management, in the sense of supporting the individual in achieving as good a quality of life as possible in spite of his/her problems. While some individuals may show less serious problems at some times, the services which support them will always need to be able to respond to recurrence of the problem behaviour. This is not to rule out the prospect of genuine reductions in challenging behaviour through better treatment or better applications of existing treatments, but to acknowledge the practical task services need to address now.

The challenge facing community services at the organizational level is to maintain enough capacity in the whole service system to cope with widely differing levels of challenging behaviour presented by different individuals in different places at different times. Far from being a discrete problem affecting a small minority of people, to be dealt with by making special provision without reference to the organization of other services, difficult behaviour is a system-wide challenge to the capability of service agencies (cf. Chapter 4).

This chapter uses a project carried out in partnership with a whole system of community-based services to illustrate how placement breakdowns are a symptom of wider problems of organization and competence in the agency. It builds on Chapter 10 by relating placement organization to the managerial and organizational framework within which placements exist.

In 1989 the authors began to work with the Learning Difficulties Care Group of Camberwell Health Authority in London. The Care Group provided about 100 residential places in a mixture of staffed houses in the community and a 40-place campus-style residential centre (about 20 homes in all); all the services had been provided since 1983 as part of a large-scale de-institutionalization project (Korman and Glennerster, 1990). By mid-1989 the Care Group reported major difficulties in maintaining placements for people with challenging behaviour. Increasingly and unpredictably, crises were occurring in residential placements which led to the removal of an individual due to their challenging behaviour, usually to a private institution at much higher cost than all but the most expensive local services.

## What causes placement breakdown? A case study

Despite believing at first that breakdown was due to challenging behaviour which was itself entirely unpredictable, detailed review of sample cases with a cross-section of Care Group staff showed that there were clear predisposing factors which involved the planning of the service and the way it was currently managed (i.e. they did not just reflect problems between the staff and residents in the house concerned).

For example, in one instance the placement of a young woman with a history of aggression failed despite meticulous preparation, including a stay in a special assessment unit where a successful approach to working with her during difficult periods had been developed. The breakdown occurred at a weekend, when police were called to remove the woman, initially to a ward in a local psychiatric hospital. Within 24 hours the woman had been transferred to a large private hospital in another Region. Review of this event (over a year later) identified factors predisposing towards breakdown (summarized in Figure 11.1).

When the service was first planned to bring the woman out of a closing long-stay hospital, the Care Group operated a general recruitment policy for all houses together, which failed to give specific information about the individuals being served. Staff were therefore recruited without knowing what to expect and

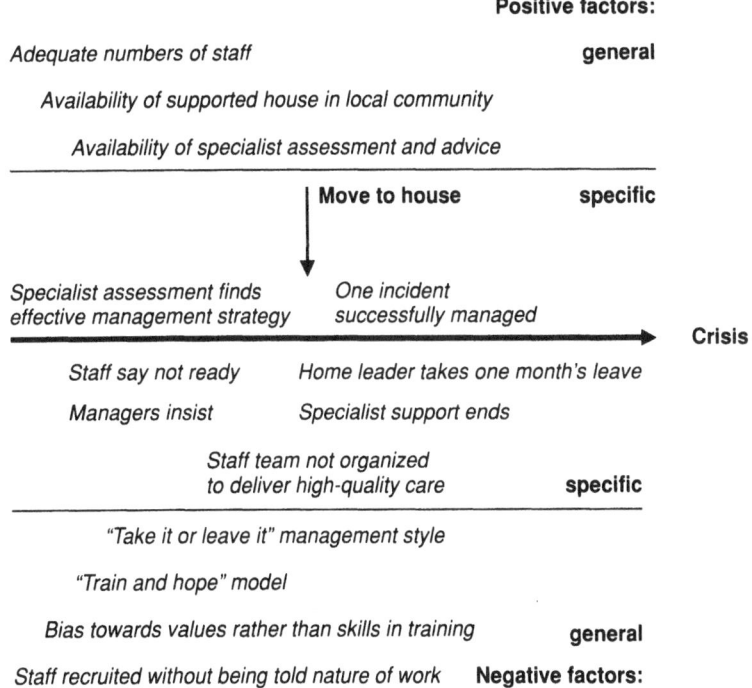

**Figure 11.1** Summary of factors predisposing towards placement breakdown in the case study.

managers reported that staff had been anxious from the moment they discovered that they were to serve someone with problems.

The model of staffed housing used at that time focused on stated adherence by staff to normalization principles (i.e. what staff say) rather than on how these principles were carried through into practice (what staff do). Training for staff was not followed through to make sure that it was put into practice once the house had opened, so that even though there was very specific and tested guidance for staff as to how to respond to particular challenges the main focus of training was outside the real work situation – the 'train and hope' model of generalization (Stokes and Baer, 1977).

When staff repeatedly argued that the young woman's transfer to the house should be delayed because they were not yet ready, managers interpreted this as lack of motivation rather than lack of skill and eventually insisted that the move take place.

After two months, the professional support provided from the special assessment unit was withdrawn as planned (the unit did not offer an outreach service). In this first spell there had been just one instance of the most important challenging behaviour, which had been successfully managed by staff in the house.

Although the whole responsibility for maintaining good working practices now devolved on the Care Group, managers agreed that they had really offered staff ground-rules for working with people with challenging behaviour on a 'take it or leave it' basis. In practice, the staff team were not well organized. Opportunities for participation in household and community activities were not systematically created by staff and service users were often left with relatively little to do. After working very long hours for many weeks since the transfer, the home leader (with management encouragement) took a month's leave. This coincided with the withdrawal of specialist support.

It was during this period that the placement ended in crisis. The young woman became aggressive but, instead of following the guidelines agreed, the staff on duty (neither of whom had actually dealt with the problem before) locked themselves into an upstairs room. After calling for help from a window, police were called and the woman was removed, first to the local psychiatric hospital and then to the private hospital.

Managers agreed that they had not known what was happening in the house, either in terms of day-to-day practice over the period before the crisis or when it occurred. Their first involvement was after the police had arrived. Even if they had known, they felt that they would not have had any options available for supporting staff on the spot nor for respite in or out of the home, although they had found money to pay for a place in an institution once the placement had broken down. They spent time counselling staff immediately after the breakdown, but felt after the event that they had inadvertently confirmed the staff assessment that the woman could not live in the community.

The consequences of this breakdown for the woman concerned had been transfer to a large private hospital a long way from her family; the break-up of the staff team and the resignation within a year of most of them; and much higher revenue costs for the Care Group. This had led to increased pressure to develop a local institution which made no pretence of treatment or high-quality of care, but which was cheap.

The striking feature of this kind of review is that it so readily identifies factors which led, more or less directly, to the placement breakdown. The challenging behaviour is not, in itself, the reason for breakdown (in this example the most difficult behaviour was understood and could be managed); rather it represents extra vulnerability to problems of service (dis)organization. Since staff were appointed without knowing the kind of work they would be expected to do, were given the choice of whether or not to use the only effective management technique and were left without their leader at a key point in the transition from external support to local responsibility, it is hardly surprising that the placement should break down.

### A systems perspective on placement breakdown

In Chapter 4, it was suggested that it is useful to conceptualize service provision as it relates to challenging behaviour as four subsystems, concerned with prevention, specialized long-term support, early detection and crisis management. Using this perspective, a programme of work was planned by Camberwell to tackle the problems faced by the residential service. This began with an external evaluation (Hughes and Mansell, 1990) and was followed up by a wide range of interventions across the whole service (Hughes and Mansell, 1992).

## Prevention

In terms of prevention, almost all the services in the care group were providing 'minding' rather than active support. Despite adequately high staffing levels and much investment of training in 'normalization' the common picture was that staff did not know how to help the people they served to participate in everyday activities, gain independence and overcome their problems. Levels of client participation in activities of everyday living inside the home, and the help and other contact received from staff, were low by comparison with exemplary services (Figure 11.2), and staff themselves complained of false impressions being given in recruitment and training of the needs of the people with whom they would work.

This meant that challenging behaviour was more likely to arise anywhere in the service because of unskilled support, more likely to be a problem when it did occur, and more likely to become more serious over time. It also meant that those houses providing more sophisticated help for people with serious and persistent challenging behaviour were more isolated and less able to call on help or understanding from the rest of the service when they experienced particular periods of stress.

## Early detection

Early detection of problems was made less likely because neither managers nor front line staff discriminated between 'minding' and 'active support' models of care. The evaluation showed that very little useful information about how each placement was doing week-by-week got to decision-makers in senior positions in the care group. Despite many meetings, neither first-line nor middle managers spent much time in services where they might gain direct experience for themselves of levels of performance. The only formal information about performance came in the form of individual programme planning reviews, but these were so time-consuming and complex that not many happened and there were in any case no mechanisms for aggregating information to look at service-wide management issues.

This meant that emerging crises took managers by surprise, so that they were ill-prepared, but it also meant that the organization's 'theory of action' (Patton, 1986) – its understanding

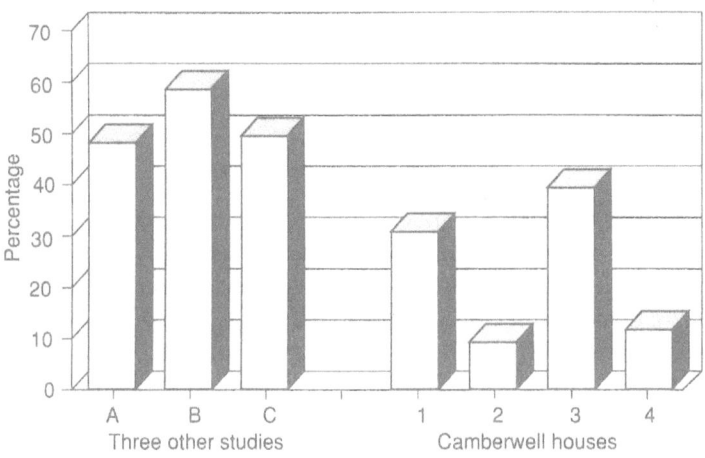

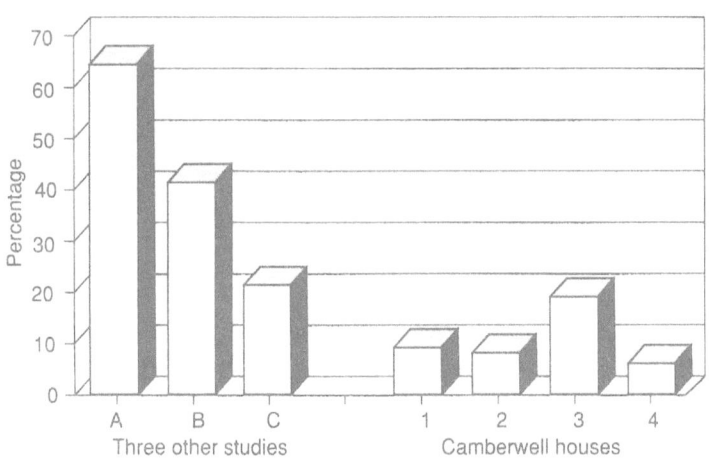

**Figure 11.2** Levels of client participation and staff contact in Camberwell houses compared with other studies. (a) Client participation in activity. (b) Contact received by clients.

of the links between what was done in one area and what happened elsewhere – was poor, as for example in arranging that the home leader should go on a month's leave just when the placement might be most vulnerable to the withdrawal of specialist support.

## Long-term specialized support

This service agency had invested in developing long-term specialized support for people with the most serious and persistent challenging behaviour known to the service. Using the resources of two Regional Health Authority initiatives, the Special Development Team (Chapter 6) and the Mental Impairment Evaluation and Treatment Service (Murphy *et al.*, 1991; Murphy and Clare, 1991), several placements had been set up where much more attention had been given to good practice in face-to-face work with clients and the managerial and planning background to support this quality of service. But, as the example above illustrates, the different perspective of local managers and staff from those of the specialist agencies made it hard for them to take the required methods on board, and the specialized placements remained rather isolated from the mainstream of community services, making them more vulnerable than they might otherwise have been. Both placements set up with the help of the Special Development Team broke down, although one has since been successfully re-established.

## Crisis management

When major problems did occur, the care group's approach to crisis management was largely reactive. There were no arrangements already worked out to supply the extra practical and emotional support people would need to cope with a problem in the placement, and in particular there was no capacity to sustain this kind of support over the days and weeks it might take to develop constructive responses to problems. Whereas a crisis in some areas of public life (such as transport disasters) is addressed by (1) putting into action well-rehearsed and understood contingency plans, (2) gathering resources needed and putting extra resources on standby and (3) bringing in the most senior and experienced decision-makers to manage the response, in this situation it was met with no plans, no reserves and the only option which the care group could deliver was transfer to an expensive private institution.

## Shaping up the service system

The intervention adopted by Camberwell took as its initial focus the model of care provided in all of the houses. The aim was to improve the quality of care in each house, by replacing 'minding' with skilled support to facilitate the involvement and independence of service users, and thereby to increase the resilience of the whole service and reduce the likelihood of placement breakdowns.

The 'active support' model of care was derived from earlier work in services for people with challenging behaviour (Emerson *et al.*, 1987; see also Chapter 6), and on staff training (Brown and Bailey, 1986a, b; Brown and Brown, 1989a, b; Brown *et al.*, 1987; 1988; 1990a, b), building on work by Mansell *et al.* (1987a) and Felce (1989). The key characteristics of this model are that service users experience a rich and varied lifestyle in which their participation and independence is directly facilitated by the help and encouragement provided by staff; as well as skills in facilitating participation in activity, incidental teaching and the constructive management of challenging behaviour, staff work is characterized by being carefully organized to provide choice and minimize times when users are unable to do anything; this is accomplished both through individual programme planning mechanisms and also through planning work as a group on a shift-by-shift basis (Chapter 10).

Often there are major obstacles to providing this model of care because services are poorly designed (too institutional) or under-resourced (too few staff). In this case, all the houses (even on the campus unit) met minimum criteria for introducing the model: the resources were available but were not being properly used.

The introduction of the new model of care was organized as a 'whole environment training' intervention (Whiffen, 1984; Mansell *et al.*, 1987b), in which 12 days' hands-on training was given to each staff team in working with the people they served. The authors and their colleagues took the lead in designing this training and in delivering it to the first eight houses, although training was jointly provided with the middle managers of the service in order to strengthen their competence and role in providing practice leadership. A second group of eight houses received training from managers with support and advice from the consultants and then managers took responsibility for completing the training in all houses in the Care Group.

This approach was chosen because practical training has consistently been shown to be superior to classroom training in producing changed performance on the job (Anderson, 1987); training *in situ* should increase the likelihood of maintenance and generalization; and supporting managers to do the training rather than using external trainers exclusively was intended to strengthen the managers' role in providing leadership in quality of care and their ownership of the intervention.

In addition there were many administrative changes to emphasize the importance of active support by care staff and leadership in quality of care by first-line and middle managers. These dealt with issues like recruitment practice, the content of induction training, the job descriptions used and the way staff were deployed. The whole environment training programme was backed up by a series of orientation workshops on issues such as challenging behaviour, communication skills and teaching; sending four key care staff on a University Diploma course in working with people who have challenging behaviour, two staff on a Trainers' Development Programme and one trainer on an MA programme in learning disability.

The third component of the intervention to improve services in the Care Group was improvement in information about the quality of service received by clients and those features of the Care Group's organization which were most directly related to quality. The aim here was to correct the imbalance in management information that existed because there was so much less information about quality than finance or personnel, and to increase the extent to which management decisions were evaluated against their impact on quality.

The basic building block of the Quality Management Information System was information collected by front-line staff as a routine part of their work with the people they served. This covered participation in household and community activities; the holding of monthly keyworker reviews; and samples of direct observation of client engagement in activity using the method adopted (Beasley *et al.*, 1989) in the earlier evaluation. As well as being used by the staff team in reviewing and planning their work, this information was collated centrally each month. To it was added some information about the number of staff who had received training and a 'Quality Capability Index' – a rating of whether each house had in place five key features needed to provide the 'active support' model, based on earlier work by Boles and Bible (1978).

Finally the Care Group reviewed how it managed crises which did occur. The aim here was to develop a process for predicting which services were most vulnerable, for gathering the resources necessary to help people manage through a difficult period and for avoiding emergency transfers to institutional care. The products were written procedures for use within the service and initiatives to explain clearly what the Care Group wanted from the two other agencies most involved when crises did occur – the mental health services and the police.

## The impact of the intervention

The impact of whole environment training allowed dramatic improvements to be made with existing resources. Many service users were assisted to participate in everyday activities for the first time since their move to the Care Group. In seven of the eight houses where whole-environment training was first carried out, the trainers' report indicated greater levels of involvement in a wider range of activities by service users. Staff became more skilled at sharing activities and responded enthusiastically to the extra help they were getting. For some of the house managers, the clear priority given to achieving client outcomes and the leadership role taken by their own managers made them more confident in asking for help.

One result of the training was a marked shift in reputation for a small but significant number of individuals with special needs. For example, a deaf and blind client in one house with whom staff had been at a loss to know how to work was, by the end of the training period, being helped to prepare meals. In another house a person with severe self-injury defeated most attempts by staff to involve her in any activity. The training helped introduce a number of reactive management strategies to enable staff to work through difficult situations and also a 'positive programming' intervention which made the young woman's environment more predictable and understandable to her through the presentation of similar requests and activities at pre-arranged times. The outcome of this was that for the first time, staff could interact with her in such a way that she would not injure herself. This allowed her to go out shopping and to cafes, activities she particularly enjoyed, as well as participate in everyday activities around the house.

These individual examples challenged any complacency about previously acceptable levels of staff and managers' performance and achieved wide currency in the service as they happened, producing optimism and enthusiasm in the Care Group's managers.

The number of people in the Care Group who have taken part in the whole-environment training has steadily increased (Figure 11.3), as have the number of houses meeting the criteria of the Quality Capability Index (Figure 11.4).

Figure 11.5 shows the number of placement breakdowns before and after the intervention. There have been no out-of-area placements since August 1990. The last four people who were transferred out of the area have been brought back to local services. In the main, this has been achieved by making within-agency transfers, so it is too soon to say that the competence of services has increased enough to avoid placement breakdowns. Rather, what

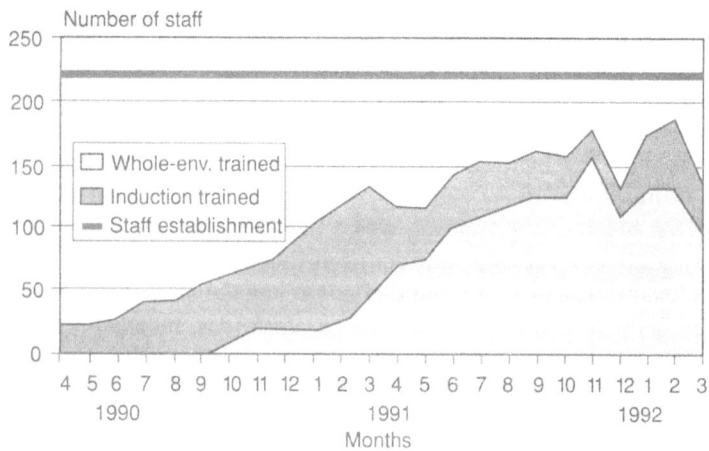

**Figure 11.3**  Number of staff in post who have received induction training and whole-environment training.

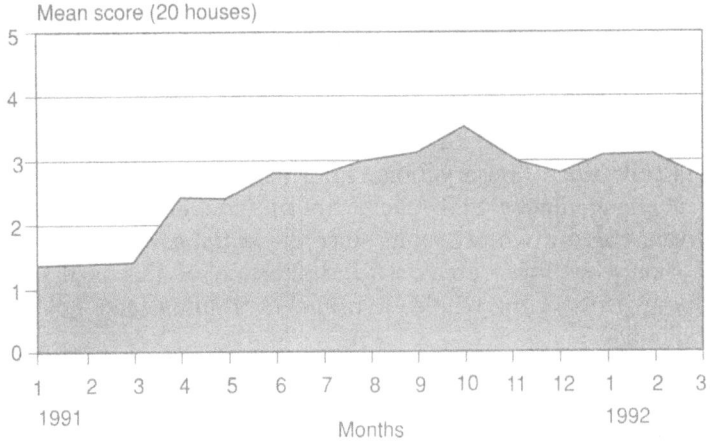

**Figure 11.4**   Mean score on Quality Capability Index.

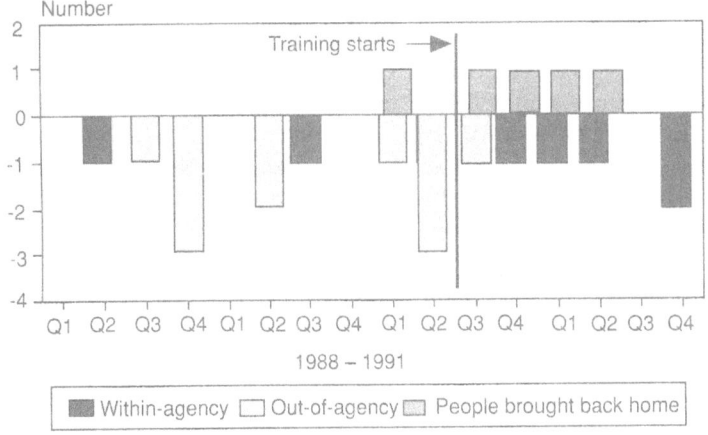

**Figure 11.5**   Placement breakdowns.

seems to have happened is that changed perceptions by managers and staff have made them take different decisions in advance of sufficiently improved front-line staff performance. Managers of the service say that the knowledge that there is a workable alternative to the 'minding' model of care, coupled with the evidence of what was achieved in the whole-environment training, has made them determined to develop better services and not necessarily to respond to crises by seeking out-of-area placements.

In terms of the outcomes experienced by clients, the Quality Management Information System shows mixed results. There has been an increase in community contacts (Figure 11.6) but the Care Group's management have found it impossible to establish sufficient collection of observational information to examine levels of client engagement or staff–client contact. Independently collected information on two occasions since the initial evaluation shows no change in these areas. The implication of this is that the achievements of the whole-environment training have not been maintained.

In terms of attributing those changes that have occurred in the performance of this service to particular interventions it is important to recognize that the project took place against a background of wider change. There have been some new senior and middle managers and increased staff turnover, which have probably helped the process of change as people who were not prepared to take part left the organization. Less helpful changes have been cuts in staffing as the Care Group has borne a share of National Health Service underfunding and the uncertainty generated by the reorganization of health and social services following the 1989 NHS and Community Care Act. The extent to which managers have been able to maintain a clear focus on quality has reflected the relative lack of priority given by their superiors to improving

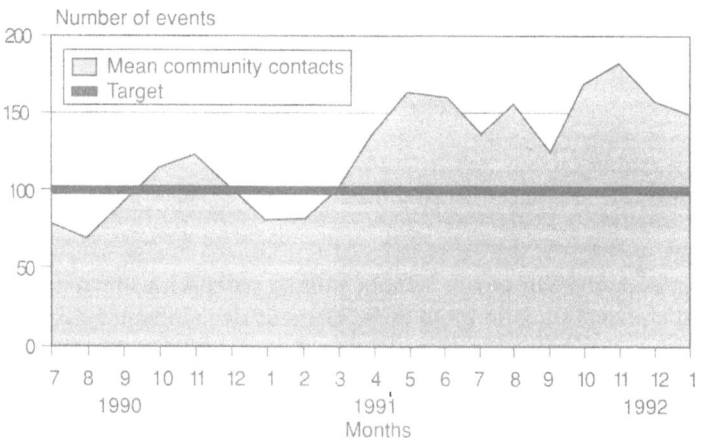

**Figure 11.6** Mean number of community contacts per month.

quality compared with attending to the competing demands of reorganization. Finally, the unbending bureaucracy of large organizations has also played its part: compared with the kind of employment practice which underpins much American work on staff performance, these managers faced very time-consuming and difficult procedures to deal with middle managers or staff who failed to improve their performance, and extremely limited opportunities for differentially rewarding and supporting good work.

Nevertheless, the service has learned to cope with the problems posed by challenging behaviour without recourse to expensive placements in institutional surroundings, and it has embarked on a process which should yield improvements in quality for all the people it serves. The 'blame' for placement breakdown is now taken by the managers of the service rather than by the service user.

## Implications for service organization

This concluding section aims to draw out some of the implications for service organization of the approach described above. These are, first, implications for the model of care adopted throughout the residential service; second, implications for training and the role of front-line and middle managers; and finally implications for decision-making by senior managers.

The first point which needs to be drawn out is that the fortunes of special placements for people with challenging behaviour are closely linked to the way other residential services are organized. Although often set up with special resources and attention to their planning and management, they should not be seen as separate or fundamentally different from other residential services. They should attend to the full range of needs of the people they serve, so that in many respects they will be organized like other placements (paying as much attention to participation in household and community activities, to personal growth and development, to friendship and networks, and so on). Other placements should at least not exacerbate the less serious challenging behaviours of some of the people they serve, and should have the capability to manage and work through most of these problems when they become more serious (lest everyone end up needing a specialized service). And if these things are true, then when an individual placement enters a period of exceptional difficulty, where the practical, technical and emotional resources of the staff are insufficient, other services can help because they share enough of the model of care to be able to do so.

Perhaps the most fundamental common element of services for people with learning disabilities in this respect is that they should embrace a model of care which provides 'active support' rather than 'minding'. There will be many ways of conceptualizing the processes which achieve important outcomes for service users, so the precise specification of a model of care is no more than a starting point. The important issue is that staff, and the managers and professionals who support them, should recognize that they bear the primary responsibility for enabling or facilitating the achievement of desired outcomes by service users. Good results are not accidental; nor, for many people with learning disabilities, will they be achieved by giving people a place in the community and leaving them to get on with it (see also Chapter 10).

The second implication is that, as the project described above shows, adopting the 'active support' model has major implications for training and management. In this example, even to introduce the basic approach, organizing activities and staff allocation at the group level in order to achieve individual goals required retraining of the workforce. This was partly because the content of induction and in-service training had focused on philosophy and principles without helping people turn these into operational practice at the level of direct work with service users, and partly because of the use of classroom-based training by specialist training staff to the exclusion of hands-on practice supervised by more skilled practitioners. The induction training of staff in the Andover project took only two weeks (Mansell *et al.*, 1987a) but met these criteria and undoubtedly contributed to the very good results achieved in this project (Felce 1989).

Perhaps the most difficult part of the intervention was redefining the role of house managers and patch managers as primarily concerned with 'practice leadership' rather than administration. Felce *et al.* (1980b) found that, in some of the first attempts at community-based residential services for people with severe or profound learning disabilities in Wessex, senior staff spent much more time in administration than in work with service users compared with those in hospital. The wider range of demands, and the higher standards of care usually aspired to in community services, make greater demands on managers. If the effect of this is to remove the most skilled, most experienced resource from unqualified staff and the people being served then perhaps the organization of administrative work needs review. But the experience of this project suggests that even more important than re-examining administration are the two areas of improving the expertise of first-line and middle managers so that they have the knowledge and skill base to provide practice-leadership, and re-valuing the achievement of client outcomes as the most important activity in the organization.

This is but one example of how service providers have to tackle organizational muddle, in which activities like staff recruitment or training, or the selection of issues to which to devote management attention, or the staff rotas in use in each house, have to be evaluated in terms of their impact on service users, carers and staff and re-shaped and coordinated towards the goal of achieving good outcomes. Failure to do this is sometimes at root a reflection of the problem of 'technological indeterminacy' (Perrow, 1967) – the lack of knowledge about the precise relationship between inputs, process and outcome in organizations. Thus, for example, in this project the Care Group had invested a great deal of staff time and effort in debating, designing and implementing an individual programme planning system; yet, as de Kock *et al.* (1988) point out, there is no clear evidence that such systems result in improved client outcomes – their development rests on a belief that this is so. It is very difficult, therefore, to see how the managers of the Care Group could make a well-founded decision to invest resources in individual programme planning rather than (say) organization of staff as a group.

The problem of developing ways of working which actually turn out to be less than optimal in terms of achieving desired outcomes becomes more complicated in large organizations which have standardized (or institutionalized) procedures, especially in areas like recruitment practice or financial management, developed in response to other concerns. The example from the project that illustrates this is the way in which managers could find extra money for out-of-area placements but not for local initiatives; in part, at least, this reflected the health authority's policy of tight cost control combined with special funds only for the most serious emergencies (of course it was also due to lack of understanding of the possibilities).

Finally, it may also be important to consider the extent to which this kind of mismatch between what the organization says it wants to do and how it actually conducts itself is functional for decision-makers (especially the most senior managers in the organization). It allows them to espouse progressive values and goals and to state these as expectations of staff without necessarily providing the managerial support and resources needed to realize them in practice. This may not be an explicit policy, in that it may reflect the once widely held view that general managers do not need to know anything about the working methods of the people they manage. But just as it is important to understand what function is served by the behaviour of individual clients who challenge services, so it should not be assumed that weaknesses in the way services work are accidental or simply the result of ignorance.

If this is an important part of the problem then it is not likely to be a sustainable strategy by decision-makers. In the short term, stating high ideals without ensuring staff have the support and skill to deliver them might be sustained by quietly placing people whose services can no longer cope in out-of-area placements. Over time, the lack of competence in local services will manufacture more and more placement breakdowns and the trickle will become a rush which threatens the viability of all community-based services. Designing community-based service systems which can meet the needs of everyone in the client group is therefore the appropriate goal.

## References

Anderson, S.R. (1987) The management of staff behaviour in residential treatment facilities: a review of training techniques, in *Staff Training in Mental Handicap* (eds J. Hogg and P. Mittler). Beckenham: Croom Helm, pp. 66–122.

Beasley, F., Hewson, S. and Mansell, J. (1989) *MTS: Handbook for Observers*. Canterbury: Centre for the Applied Psychology of Social Care, University of Kent.

Boles, S.M. and Bible, G.H. (1978) The student service index, in *Current Behavioral Trends for the Developmentally Disabled* (ed. M.S. Berkler). Baltimore, MD: University Park Press, pp.153–95.

Brown, H. and Bailey, R. (1986a) *Working with Families*. Bringing People Back Home Series of Video-assisted Training Packages. Bexhill-on-Sea: South East Thames Regional Health Authority (available from Outset Publications, St. Leonards).

Brown, H. and Bailey, R. (1986b) *Designing Services to Meet Individual Need*. Bringing People Back Home Series of Video-assisted Training Packages. Bexhill-on-Sea: ESCATA/South East Thames Regional Health Authority (available from Outset Publications, St. Leonards).

Brown, H. and Brown, V. (1989a) *Building Social Networks*. Bringing People Back Home Series of Video-assisted Training Packages. Bexhill-on-Sea: South East Thames Regional Health Authority (available from Outset Publications, St. Leonards).

Brown, H. and Brown, V. (1989b) *Understanding and Responding to Difficult Behaviour*. Bringing People Back Home Series of Video-assisted Training Packages. Bexhill-on-Sea: South East Thames Regional Health Authority (available from Outset Publications, St. Leonards).

Brown, H., Toogood, S. and Brown, V. (1987) *Participation in Everyday Activities*. Bringing People Back Home Series of Video-assisted Training Packages. Bexhill-on-Sea: ESCATA/South East Thames Regional Health Authority (available from Outset Publications, St. Leonards).

Brown, H., Bell, C. and Brown, V. (1988) *Teaching New Skills*. Bringing People Back Home Series of Video-assisted Training Packages. Bexhill-on-Sea: South East Thames Regional Health Authority (available from Outset Publications, St. Leonards).

Brown, H., Ferns, P. and Brown, V. (1990a) *Supervising Staff*. Bringing People Back Home Series of Video-assisted Training Packages. Bexhill-on-Sea: South East Thames Regional Health Authority (available from Outset Publications, St. Leonards).

Brown, H., Szivos, S., Keyhoe-Clarke, A. and Brown, V. (1990b) *Developing Communication Skills*. Bringing People Back Home Series of Video-assisted Training Packages. Bexhill-on-Sea: South East Thames Regional Health Authority (available from Outset Publications, St. Leonards).

Conroy, J., Efthimiou, J. and Lemanowicz, J. (1982) A matched comparison of the developmental growth of institutionalized and deinstitutionalized mentally retarded clients. *American Journal of Mental Deficiency*, **86**, 581–7.

de Kock, U., Saxby, H., Felce, D., Thomas, M. and Jenkins, J. (1988) Individual planning for adults with severe or profound mental handicaps in a community-based service. *Mental Handicap*, **16**, 152–5.

de Paiva, S. and Lowe, K. (1990) *The Evaluation of NIMROD, a Community Based Service for People with Mental Handicap: The Incidence of Problem Behaviours*. Cardiff: Mental Handicap in Wales Applied Research Unit.

Emerson, E. and Emerson, C. (1987) Barriers to the implementation of habilitative behavioral programs in an institutional setting. *Mental Retardation*, **25**, 101–6.

Emerson, E., Barrett, S., Bell, C., Cummings, R., McCool, C., Toogood, A. and Mansell, J. (1987) *Developing Services for People with Severe Learning Difficulties and Challenging Behaviours*. Canterbury: Institute of Social and Applied Psychology, University of Kent.

Felce, D. (1989) *Staffed Housing for Adults with Severe or Profound Mental Handicaps: The Andover Project*. Kidderminster: British Institute of Mental Handicap.

Felce, D., Kushlick, A. and Mansell, J. (1980a) Evaluation of alternative residential facilities for the severely mentally handicapped in Wessex: Client engagement. *Advances in Behaviour Research and Therapy*, **3**, 13–8.

Felce, D., Mansell, J. and Kushlick, A. (1980b) Evaluation of alternative residential facilities for the severely mentally handicapped in Wessex: Staff performance. *Advances in Behaviour Research and Therapy*, **3**, 25–30.

Felce, D., de Kock, U. and Repp, A.C. (1986) An eco-behavioral comparison of small community-based houses and traditional large hospitals for severely and profoundly mentally handicapped adults. *Applied Research in Mental Retardation*, **7**, 393–408.

Fine, M.A., Tangeman, P.J. and Woodard, J. (1990) Changes in adaptive behavior of older adults with mental retardation following de-institutionalization. *American Journal on Mental Retardation*, **94**, 661–8.

Hughes, H.M. and Mansell, J. (1990) *Consultation to Camberwell Health Authority Learning Difficulties Care Group: Evaluation Report*. Canterbury: Centre for the Applied Psychology of Social Care, University of Kent.

Hughes, H.M. and Mansell, J. (1992) *Consultation to Camberwell Health Authority Learning Difficulties Care Group: Intervention Report*. Canterbury: Centre for the Applied Psychology of Social Care, University of Kent.

Intagliata, J. and Willer, B. (1982) Reinstitutionalization of mentally retarded persons successfully placed into family-care and group homes. *American Journal of Mental Deficiency*, **87**, 34–9.

Korman, N. and Glennerster, H. (1990) *Hospital Closure*. Milton Keynes: Open University Press.

Mansell, J., Felce, D., Jenkins, J., de Kock, U. and Toogood, S. (1987a) *Developing Staffed Housing for People with Mental Handicaps*. Tunbridge Wells: Costello.

Mansell, J., Brown, H., McGill, P., Hoskin, S., Lindley, P. and Emerson, E. (1987b) *Bringing People Back Home: A Staff Training Initiative in Mental Handicap*. Bristol and Bexhill-on-Sea: National Health Service Training Authority and South East Thames Regional Health Authority.

Murphy, G. and Clare, I. (1991) MIETS: a service option for people with mild mental handicaps and challenging behaviour or psychiatric problems – 2. Assessment, treatment and outcome for service users and service effectiveness. *Mental Handicap Research*, **4**, 2, 180–206.

Murphy, G., Holland, A., Fowler, P. and Reep, J. (1991) MIETS: a service option for people with mild mental handicaps and challenging behaviour or psychiatric problems – 1. Philosophy, service and service users. *Mental Handicap Research*, **4**, 1, 41–66.

Oliver, C., Murphy, G. and Corbett, J. (1987) Self-injurious behaviour in people with mental handicap: A total population study. *Journal of Mental Deficiency Research*, **31**, 147–62.

Pagel, S. and Whitling, C. (1978) Readmission to a state hospital for mentally retarded persons: Reasons for community placement failure. *Mental Retardation*, **16**, 25–8.

Patton, M.Q. (1986) *Utilization-Focused Evaluation*. Beverly Hills: Sage

Publications.

Perrow, C. (1967) A framework for the comparative analysis of organisations. *American Sociological Review*, **32**, 194–208.

Schroeder, S.R. and MacLean, W. (1987) If it isn't one thing, it's another: Experimental analysis of covariation in behavior management data of severe behavior disturbances, in *Living Environments and Mental Retardation* (eds S. Landesman and P. Vietze). Washington, DC: American Association on Mental Retardation, pp. 315–37.

Stokes, T. and Baer, D. (1977) An implicit technology of generalization. *Journal of Applied Behavior Analysis*, **10**, 349–67.

Sutter, P., Mayeda, T., Call, T., Yanagi, G. and Lee, S. (1980) Comparison of successful and unsuccessful community placed mentally retarded persons. *American Journal of Mental Deficiency*, **85**, 262–7.

Thiel, G.W. (1981) Relationship of IQ, adaptive behavior, age, and environmental demand to community-placement success of mentally retarded adults. *American Journal of Mental Deficiency*, **86**, 208–11.

Whiffen, P. (1984) *Initiatives in In-service Training: Helping Staff to Care for Mentally Handicapped People in the Community*. London: Central Council for Education and Training in Social Work.

# 12

# Assessing costs and benefits

*Martin Knapp and Jim Mansell*

## Introduction

For most of the period in which community-based services have been proposed as complete alternatives to institutional care, the main focus of debate has been their feasibility. With the widespread development of supported housing in the 1980s, attention has been concentrated on people with special needs, and particularly people with challenging behaviour. Even here, the development of working models of supported housing has gone a long way to demonstrate that, given adequate commitment and investment of time and effort, these services are a feasible and desirable alternative to hospital care (Chapters 5 and 6).

But while experience and confidence about feasibility has grown, cost constraints have become more important. It could be argued, for example, that local and central government expenditure on health and social services has not kept pace with need in learning disability services (for example in the underfunding of pay awards and the pursuit of 'efficiency savings'), and that, within health authorities and social services departments, priorities have shifted away from learning disability to other services. The introduction of general managers in the health service and the growth of the 'new managerialism' in social services (involving heightened resource consciousness, performance reviews and devolved budgets) have introduced more 'business-like' attitudes, and the encouragement of a mixed economy of community care has ushered in contracts of greater specificity.

These factors may have encouraged policy-makers and practitioners to pay more attention to costs, but they are not the only reasons for doing so. Increasing expectations mean that there have never been, and will never be, enough resources to meet all of society's wants or needs, so that choices must always be made within a cost constraint. Making the best use of resources therefore requires careful evaluation of both the benefits and the costs of particular policy decisions and practice decisions. As Griffiths (1988) remarked: 'To talk of policy in matters of care except in the context of available resources and timescales for action owes more to theology than to the purposeful delivery of a caring service' (Griffiths, 1988, para. 9).

For all these reasons, decisions about making community-based services available to people with challenging behaviour in the future are increasingly likely to involve arguments about what these services cost and whether the benefits they provide justify the cost. This need not engender pessimism among the proponents of community services; the American experience shows that, when both are expected to achieve the same quality standards, community services can demonstrate their cost effectiveness compared with institutions (e.g., Conroy and Bradley, 1985). The important issue is not whether a cost focus is justified, but whether costs are appropriately defined and utilized.

This chapter therefore introduces the basic principles of applied cost analysis in social and health care contexts, and then employs them to examine some of the key cost issues concerning provision for people with severe learning disabilities and challenging behaviours. The research, and indeed the service development which it would require, remains to be done to provide anything approaching definitive answers about the costs and benefits of services for people with learning disabilities and challenging behaviours: the purpose of this chapter is rather to clarify the arguments and issues which need to be considered and, where possible, to illustrate them in so far as evidence makes that possible.

## The principles of applied cost analysis

In costing health and social care, whether for research, policy formulation or practice guidance, there are four main principles to employ (Knapp, 1993; Knapp and Beecham, 1990). These are that (1) costs should be measured comprehensively, (2) cost variation should be explored for the insights it offers rather than ignored through averaging costs, (3) the effect of confounding factors in cost comparisons should be minimized and (4) outcomes for users and carers should be considered at the same time as costs.

1.  **Costs should be measured comprehensively.**
    This means that all relevant service components of care 'packages' will need to be included. Most discussions of the costs of services deal with the costs actually reported by service-providing agencies, typically as cost per place. These costs are likely to need adjusting to reflect indirect and hidden resource implications. For example, the unit costs of residential and day services should not overlook the costs of the service agency bureaucracy, the capital investment and the services provided by other agencies, most notably social security, day care, general health care and adult education. Where services are supported by specialist teams, the costs of these need to be included. Similarly, the additional cost to generic services of meeting the needs of particular individuals should be taken into account (for example, there may be a special dental health clinic for people with challenging behaviour, or the training of ordinary health, education and social welfare professionals may need to be adapted to reflect the needs of people with learning disabilities). In the context of increasing numbers of adults with learning disabilities and challenging behaviour continuing to live at home with their families it is also important to include the costs falling on carers, difficult though they may be to measure in practice.

2.  **Cost variation should be explored for the insights it offers.**
    Quite wide variations in cost between users, facilities and areas of the country are likely to be revealed in any examination of these services. The second principle is not to ignore them by restricting discussion to averages, but to examine the policy and practice insights which they can offer. As services become more closely tailored to individual needs, policy-makers and practitioners need to know, not simply that one service is cheaper (or more cost-effective) than another, but **for whom** and **in what circumstances**. Of course, average costs help assess the resource implications of different options, but there is generally a need to go beyond them in discussing and assessing policies and practices.

3.  **The effect of confounding factors in cost comparisons should be minimized.**

In making comparisons between policies, users, services or facilities, only like-with-like matches have full validity. Although insights can usually be retrieved from less than perfect comparisons, policy prescriptions are too often built on erroneous deduction. This is a familiar problem in the comparison of the costs of hospital and other provision, for often the residents of the former are considerably more disabled, so that any cost differences reflect individual disability levels as well as place of residence; disentangling the two is possible, though not straightforward.

4. **Outcomes for users and carers should be considered at the same time.**
   Finally, cost information should not be employed in isolation from information on outcomes for users and carers. Since the goal of decision-making should be to secure the best value for money, information about the effects of services on those they are supposed to help needs to be weighed against information about the costs of those services. This task is not made any easier by the multidimensional nature of outcomes and the impossibility of reducing most of them to monetary magnitudes. Note that in considering outcomes negative effects might just as well be relevant as perceived improvements: in general in the field of community care there is evidence of increasing burdens being placed on carers, for example (see Dalley, 1988, pp. 5 *et seq.*), as well as of some improvements for clients in community services.

These four principles are widely accepted as the basic requirements for constructing, employing and interpreting costs. In the remainder of this chapter they will be used to examine four of the resource questions which surface with some regularity in the discussion of services for people with severe learning disabilities and challenging behaviours: (1) What is the cost of community care? (2) How large are hospital-community cost differences? (3) Will community care costs decrease over time? (4) Are higher costs explained by better outcomes?

## What is the cost of community care?

There were 18 000 fewer in-patient beds occupied by people with learning disabilities in England in 1989 than ten years earlier. The scale of this exodus is such that it includes many people with severe learning disabilities, and in the attempt to develop high-quality alternatives 'in the community', much of the debate concerning support of people with severe learning disabilities and challenging behaviours has focused on costs. Agencies responsible for the support of people in the community need to know their own and (perhaps with less urgency) other people's costs of this shift in the balance of provision. This is partly so that they can budget properly for what might be needed and demonstrate their good management of resources. But it is also necessary to estimate likely costs in order to devolve some spending powers to care managers, and to inform any decisions about contracting-out services to other agencies with an accurate understanding of their own expenditure patterns.

In moving to a broad view of costs – the search for comprehensiveness as urged by the first principle – it is not expected or even necessary that each agency involved in the care of people with learning disabilities will use these comprehensive costs in their decisions, but they need some appreciation of them in order to understand the incentives and disincentives at work within the care system. Most care agencies will find it hard to expand provision without financial compensation, and it was arguably the inability and unwillingness of health authorities to transfer some of the funds tied up in hospitals to local authorities and voluntary organizations which delayed the rundown of long-stay provision for many years. Failure to recognize and act upon the costs of informal care has resulted in a shift in the balance of care towards sometimes inappropriate private and voluntary sector residential placements, facilitated by the availability of social security funding. The joint community care planning and joint working required by the 1989 NHS and Community Care Act may not be enough to persuade many statutory bodies to establish single budgets for services for people with learning disabilities (or more specifically for those with challenging behaviours) but it demands a broader view of costs than has been conventional practice.

The cost figures most readily obtained are accounting costs based on reported, audited expenditures. These do not necessarily give all the information needed for the evaluation or planning of health or social care programmes. Economic theory would advocate using **long-run marginal opportunity costs**, which are not necessarily the same as accounting costs. By 'marginal' is meant the change in total cost attributable only to the policy or practice change under consideration. For example, if six people leave long-term hospital for community-based accommodation, the reduction in hospital cost will be less than the average cost per in-patient because the small decrease in in-patient numbers will not allow much or any reduction in staffing or overhead costs. By 'long-run' is meant the move beyond the small-scale and immediate development of community care (which might be achieved by using present services more intensively at very low marginal cost) to take account of the need for sustainable patterns of service. Since national policy intentions are to substitute community services for most long-term hospital beds, it would hardly be credible to measure only short-run cost implications. By 'opportunity cost' is meant the measurement of opportunities forgone rather than amounts spent. Opportunity cost measures the true private or social value of a resource or service, based upon its value in its best alternative use. In a freely operating market, this 'best alternative use value' would be identical to the price paid, but for most services a rather different measure is needed. For example, capital may be zero-priced or measured by the recorded depreciation payments, which will not usually reflect the opportunity costs of using them. The (zero) payments to volunteers and informal carers do not usually indicate their social value. This is not the place to delve further into these topics; it is simply enough to recognize that the costs appearing in an agency's annual accounts may need to be adjusted and employed cautiously (for further explanation and discussion of these points see Allen and Beecham, 1993; Knapp, 1993).

The evaluation of the Care in the Community demonstration programme (Knapp *et al.*, 1992) illustrates the range of costs to be covered. In 1983, the then Department of Health and Social Security announced a fund of £25 000 000 (at today's prices) for a programme of pilot projects to explore different ways of moving people and resources into the community. Twenty-eight pilot projects were launched under the initiative, each funded for three years, 11 of them for people with learning disabilities (a small proportion of whom exhibited challenging behaviours). Hospital and community costs were examined in the evaluation. The former were based on average revenue expenditures for whole establishments, disaggregated down to the ward level where possible, plus a capital element based on an annuitized valuation of site and durable resources, and an element for service inputs from outside the hospital budget, such as social work, education or volunteer visiting. The costs of community care were calculated from information on service utilization gathered in interviews with staff (often case managers) nine months after each client was discharged from hospital. Social security payments were used as proxies for living expenses (a common assumption), and were of direct interest in the examination of the distributional consequences and funding of community care.

Comprehensive community care costs, arranged by type of accommodation, are summarized in Table 12.1. The largest single component of cost is accommodation, which often includes much of the staff support needed by clients. But as the table illustrates, 'community care' does not stop with the place of residence. Comprehensive costing is needed to gauge the respective implications of community care for public, voluntary and private agencies and for the personal resources of clients: the table shows that significant costs would be overlooked by a narrower approach. It also helps illustrate how consistency of definition is needed when making comparisons with long-stay hospitals, since most of the community services have already been subsumed within hospital budgets (the third principle identified at the beginning of this chapter). Finally, it is worth emphasizing that comprehensive costing is feasible; that it is possible by the methods used to identify reasonably accurately the real costs falling on the different participants in the provision of services.

Applying the fourth principle of applied cost analysis, it is relevant to ask, what did these costs buy? Improvements in quality of life after leaving hospital were very marked for most of the people with learning disabilities in the demonstration programme (Knapp *et al.*, 1992). Statistically significant improvements were found along many dimensions. The cost of community care was higher than the cost of hospital for more than half the sample, but higher costs bought better quality care and better quality of life (see below). Smaller and more domestic accommodation in the community was associated with better client outcomes: in other words, there was some support for services based on ideas of normalization. The policy question raised by these results is whether local agencies are able or prepared to incur the higher costs of community care in order to reap these marked improvements in client outcomes; this question is returned to later in the chapter.

**Table 12.1** Community care costs, by place of residence, for people with learning disabilities. Percentage of total package cost by place of residence in the community. RES = residential home; HOST = hostel; SGH = staffed group home; SHELT = sheltered housing; USGH = unstaffed group home; INDEP = independent accommodation; FOST = adult fostering

| Community care component | RES (%) | HOST (%) | SGH (%) | SHELT (%) | USGH (%) | INDEP (%) | Cost (%) | All (%) |
|---|---|---|---|---|---|---|---|---|
| Accommodation and living expenses[1] | 62 | 75 | 58 | 50 | 33 | 36 | 42 | 63 |
| Project overheads[2] | 26 | 8 | 22 | 29 | 33 | 34 | 31 | 18 |
| General practitioner | 1 | 0 | 0 | 1 | 1 | 0 | 0 | 0 |
| Day activity services | 2 | 10 | 4 | 5 | 4 | 8 | 12 | 7 |
| Education | 2 | 5 | 8 | 3 | 0 | 7 | 7 | 6 |
| Hospital in-patient | 1 | 0 | 1 | 0 | 5 | 0 | 0 | 1 |
| Hospital day and out-patient | 0 | 0 | 0 | 1 | 1 | 0 | 0 | 0 |
| Community health care[3] | 2 | 0 | 3 | 2 | 1 | 0 | 4 | 2 |
| Community social care | 4 | 0 | 3 | 10 | 22 | 14 | 3 | 3 |
| Other[4] | 0 | 1 | 0 | 0 | 0 | 0 | 1 | 0 |
| Total (%) | 100 | 100 | 100 | 100 | 100 | 100 | 100 | 100 |
| Sample size | 6 | 86 | 67 | 14 | 6 | 6 | 9 | 194 |

1. Includes staff costs where staff are employed solely at place of residence and included in accommodation budget
2. Inclusions vary from project to project, usually covering some immediate managerial support and some peripatetic staff support
3. Includes community nursing, medical practitioners not attached to hospital or family practices, miscellaneous community health paramedic services (chiropody, dietary services, incontinence service, etc)
4. Includes police, travel not covered elsewhere and miscellaneous minor services

A good community care plan will include a comprehensive range of services targeted at the needs and wants of users and families; a good community care **costing** should be similarly comprehensive. In this way, the full resource needs of policy options can be recognized, and the combination of services used by any one person can be carefully and jointly planned by case managers, users and others in cognizance of their funding implications.

### How large are hospital–community cost differences?

An immediate corollary is to ask whether the costs of community care are 'too high', particularly in relation to the costs of hospital accommodation. Two common arguments which regularly peppered policy debates in the 1970s and early 1980s were that community care is either more or less expensive than hospital provision of equivalent standard. These simple, and usually untested, comparative cost arguments have given way to more complex, searching and – eventually – illuminating questions concerning the distribution of the community and hospital cost burdens, and the incentives and disincentives therein to well-funded, high-quality provision.

One approach has been to present costs for alternatives to hospital which are incomplete. These are employed to appeal to local or national decision-makers so as to substitute for or bolster other arguments for shifting the locus of care from institutions. The obvious danger inherent in this well-meaning ploy is self-fulfilment: so successfully is the case made that community care is allocated exactly the (low) costs which its proponents claim. The consequences of such underfunding follow in terms of poor facilities, non-existent support, empty lives for people denied access to day care or education classes, and under-supervision.

The underestimation of community care costs not only results from omitting some indirect or hidden components – it has been common to overlook the housing, personal and informal care costs of families caring for disabled relatives as an alternative to hospital or residential accommodation – but also stems from the comparison of two quite different populations. The costs of service packages are rarely invariant with respect to the characteristics of service users, and so comparisons between care settings should take account of any differences between client populations. For example, the first groups of people to leave hospital under closure programmes are generally less 'dependent' in terms of skills, challenging behaviours and other characteristics than those who remain behind. Their hospital care will therefore be costing rather less than the hospital average, yet they are probably more costly to support than the typical client living with the family. An important task in the examination of community costs, therefore, is to make like-with-like comparisons.

Most proponents of community-based services for people with learning disability and challenging behaviour recognize their high costs, but claim that a true estimate of the costs of institutional care would show that the difference between institutional and community care is not as great as is often believed. This argument depends on correctly attributing the costs of caring for individuals with challenging behaviour within institutions and also on identifying other costs which arise as a consequence of this model. It is assumed that the correct attribution of costs would show that the expense of higher staffing and equipment costs associated with caring for people with challenging behaviour are hidden by being averaged across ward or hospital costs that include the much lower costs associated with people of lower dependency. In-patient hospital costs are known to vary with patient characteristics. Wright and Haycox (1984), for example, reported wide cost differences between wards, and Johnes and Haycox (1986) used these same data to demonstrate links between costs and levels of disability. These are certainly not isolated findings, nor would one expect them to be. The reduction in hospital in-patient numbers has been accompanied by a rapid increase in average hospital costs (a 73% increase in the ten years since 1979), predominantly because it is usually the more dependent/disabled people who remain to be resettled in the community towards the end of hospital closure programmes (for example, see Korman and Glennerster, 1990; Knapp *et al.*, 1992).

Other costs which might need to be included are, for example, the costs of placement breakdown in mainstream services. Here the issue is that if the whole range of services is divided into community services which are not organized to cope with challenging behaviour and institutions which are, costs will arise from the care of people whose problems are no longer severe in the institutional settings and from the breakdown of community services as people enter crisis. Since the population of people with challenging behaviour is not clearly delimited (up to 40% of the population in residential care having potentially serious challenging behaviour) these costs might not be insignificant.

A major policy challenge is therefore to ensure that the fragmentation of responsibility and funding in the support of people with challenging behaviour does not create incentives for decision-makers to choose options which minimize their own costs whilst raising other people's. This was, of course, precisely the issue which so exercised the Audit Commission (1986) in its influential report, *Making a Reality of Community Care*. The slow progress towards a consolidated community care system in many parts of the country, and the failure to deal with uncontrolled social security funding with the speed really needed have meant that those perverse incentives remain. Families facing the discharge from hospital of a disabled relative, and with little idea how local or health authorities are going to provide support in the community, have strong incentives to encourage the development of village communities without information about the full costs and benefits involved.

### Will community care costs decrease over time?

Proponents of community-based services for people with challenging behaviour have argued that higher costs of community care reduce as the results of better care in the community change individual client behaviour, and that once novel service models are set up among more supportive 'mainstream' services, their costs will reduce. The claim that community care costs will fall because better care will change individual client behaviour reflects beliefs about the general therapeutic effect of better quality of care as well as the impact of specific treatment or therapy, where this is provided.

The main problem with finding evidence for this assertion is that services for people with challenging behaviour are still sufficiently new that there are not yet studies of costs and benefits which would link any reduction in costs to changes in client characteristics, rather than to reduced quality of care. In the *Care in the Community* study already cited, it was found that for nearly 400 people with learning disabilities, leaving long-stay hospitals to move into a variety of planned and well-supported community settings, community care improved their quality of life in the first year, reduced skills deficits and demonstrated how staffing levels and costs could fall as a result (Knapp *et al.*, 1992, Chapter 13). However, only a small number of these people had challenging behaviour: in general, there is not yet the same evidence for services which include substantial numbers of people with challenging behaviour.

However, the provision of community services does not in itself appear to reduce the incidence of challenging behaviour. The experience of the NIMROD service was that levels of challenging behaviour did not reduce after transfer to community settings (Chapter 5). There is also evidence to suggest that community services are often not yet well enough organized or resourced to deliver anything resembling treatment. For example, in their study of self-injury among people with learning disabilities in south-east England, Oliver *et al.* (1987) found that only 2% of people had written psychological treatment programmes. An evaluation of community services in south-east London (Hughes and Mansell, 1990; see also Chapter 11) found that typically staff and their managers did not know how to work with the people they served to promote client engagement in meaningful activity. Against this, though, is the evidence from the Special Development Team project (Chapter 6) of reduced levels of major and minor problem behaviours. These differing findings emphasize the importance of distinguishing between services which, although they are of broadly the same type, are organized differently and produce different results.

The related question is to what extent higher costs of community services for people who have challenging behaviour are due to the novelty of the service model. Once established among more supportive 'mainstream' learning disability services, it may be that their costs will fall. For example, the Special Development Team project involved extra training for staff, extra specialist input and extra management support, all provided by the team. At least part of this extra support was necessitated because the 'mainstream' learning disability services were not nearly geared up to provide the required levels of input. If all learning disability services were better organized to meet the needs of their own clients, the gap between them and specialist services for people with challenging behaviour would be less and the cost of providing the extra help that challenging behaviour requires would be less. In the long-term, 'steady state' situation, when new community services have worked through the transitional phase and are established within local service systems, costs should be significantly lower than in the transition period itself.

## Are higher costs explained by better outcomes?

Community–hospital cost differences might not be as great as some people have maintained, and community care costs may well fall as their users attain a greater degree of independence and as agencies learn from their innovative programmes, but it seems unlikely that community care will in practice ever cost less than long-stay hospital provision. Higher-quality community care will be demanded by users, relatives and providing agencies in order to achieve some of the improvements in quality of life which have been denied long-stay hospital residents, and local and central government politicians, even if they wanted to, will find it impossible to resist the well-organized lobbying of user groups, parents and voluntary agencies working in this field. Are, then, higher costs of community care explained by better outcomes?

In so far as community-based services for people with challenging behaviour do cost more than institutions it may be argued that this is because they both provide a wider range of services than hospitals and achieve higher quality than hospitals. The range of services may include education or work where none was provided before (a significant minority of the hospital population in England receives no day care; see also Chapter 7) as well as treatment and care of problems of physical and mental health (e.g., remedial intervention on sensory handicaps, bereavement counselling, psychological or psychiatric treatment, mobility aids) which apparently went unrecognized in hospital. The higher quality of services includes principally the kind of extra assistance and facilitation described elsewhere in this volume, provided to enable client participation in everyday household and community activities in spite of problem behaviours (Chapter 10). Some authors argue that in practice it would not be possible to provide these services in institutions and that the argument over the relative benefits of community versus institutional services is in practice resolved (Conroy and Feinstein, 1990).

These arguments point to the need to examine a wider range of costs and benefits than is often considered, the correct attribution of costs to the care of individuals with challenging behaviour and the closeness of the relationship between costs and benefits. Again, the evaluation of the *Care in the Community* demonstration programme, while not focused on people with challenging behaviour, does provide evidence of a positive link between costs and outcomes: other things being equal, higher-cost community care 'packages' result in better outcomes for users.

The second relevant issue is that of the extent to which the cost-incurring service components in each model are essential. For example, there is some suggestion from the study of houses supported by the Special Development Team that placements in private institutions achieve no better outcomes than placements on the wards of long-stay NHS learning disability hospitals yet cost as much as specialized placements in community group homes; one might therefore imagine that market forces are more responsible for their prices than any therapeutic component of their service.

## Conclusion

From the earliest beginnings of the post-war development of community care, assertions about the relative costs of hospital and community services have been based largely on over-simple and untested assumptions. In recent years there has been a much greater attempt to unravel and clarify the relationship between costs and benefits in all health and social services, and the new purchaser–provider split resulting from the community care reforms is an attempt to institutionalize this scrutiny in the process of service provision. This process should begin to yield more and better information with which to assess the propositions explored in this chapter.

## References

Allen, C. and Beecham, J. (1993) Costing services: Ideals and reality, in *Costing Community Care: Theory and Practice* (eds A. Netten and J. Beecham). Aldershot: Ashgate, pp. 25–42.

Audit Commission (1986) *Making a Reality of Community Care*. London: HMSO.

Conroy, J.W. and Bradley V.T. (1985) *The Pennhurst Longitudinal Study: A Report of Five Years of Research and Analysis*. Philadelphia, PA, and Boston, MA: Temple University Developmental Disabilities Centre and Human Services Research Institute.

Conroy, J.W. and Feinstein, C.S. (1990) A new way of thinking about quality, in *Quality Assurance for Individuals with Developmental Disabilities* (eds V. Bradley and H. Bersani). Baltimore, MD: Paul H. Brookes, pp. 263–278.

Dalley, G. (1988) *Ideologies of Caring: Rethinking Community and Collectivism*. London: Macmillan.

Griffiths, R. (1988) *Community Care: Agenda for Action*. London: HMSO.

Hughes, H.M. and Mansell, J. (1990) *Consultation to Camberwell Health Authority Learning Disabilities Care Group: Evaluation Report*. Canterbury: Centre for the Applied Psychology of Social Care, University of Kent.

Johnes, G. and Haycox, A. (1986) Cost structures in a large hospital for the mentally handicapped. *Social Science and Medicine*, 22, 605–10.

Knapp, M.R.J. (1993) The basic principles of applied costs research, in *Costing Community Care: Theory and Practice* (eds A. Netten and J. Beecham). Aldershot: Ashgate, pp. 61–72.

Knapp, M.R.J. and Beecham, J. (1990) Costing mental health services. *Psychological Medicine*, 20, 893–908.

Knapp, M.R.J., Cambridge, P., Thomason, C., Beecham, J., Allen, C. and Darton, R.A. (1992) *Care in the Community: Challenge and Demonstration*. Aldershot: Ashgate.

Korman, N. and Glennerster, H. (1990) *Hospital Closure*. Milton Keynes: Open University Press.

Oliver, C., Murphy, G. and Corbett, J. (1987) Self-injurious behaviour in people with mental handicap: a total population study. *Journal of Mental Deficiency Research*, 31, 147–62.

Wright, K. and Haycox, A. (1984) *Public sector costs of caring for mentally handicapped persons in a large hospital*. Discussion Paper 1. York: Institute for Research in the Social Sciences/Centre for Health Economics, University of York.

# 13

# Policy and policy implications

*Jim Mansell*

The purpose of this final chapter is to review some of the policy implications of the approach set out in the earlier part of the book, drawing particularly on the recent report of a Department of Health Project Group (Department of Health, 1993). After explaining the context in which this latest policy initiative developed, the main features of the report are described (with emphasis on severe learning disability) and its implementation discussed. The report refers only to England: the strategy for service development in learning disabilities is different in Wales (Welsh Office, 1991) and there is no comparable Scottish guidance, and of course the structure and organization of services in the UK is quite different from the other countries which have set out to replace institutional care. Nevertheless, visits to services in these countries suggest that the main issues raised in the English report are probably present in all these service systems.

## The policy context

The making of policy in learning disabilities by the English Department of Health has been dominated since the Second World War by three general contextual factors. First, the structural split between nationally funded and controlled hospitals and local government social services has led to repeated (failed) attempts to divide people with learning disabilities into separate groups who could be the primary responsibility of each agency. Second, professional, parental and lobby opinion has been split between pro- and anti-hospital positions, particularly since 1970 when the then Campaign for the Mentally Handicapped was set up to promote community services for everyone, whatever their level of disability (Campaign for the Mentally Handicapped, 1972). Third, the Department of Health has, compared with other central Government departments, adopted a *'laissez-faire'* model in its relationship with local authority social services authorities, so that most guidance is permissive; apart from a short period in the early 1970s no serious attempt has been made to shape local action into a national strategy.

Most recently, these factors found expression in the health service and community care reforms of 1989–93. The White Papers and associated documents restated the separation of health care and social care roles, ignoring the practical difficulties this separation brings for people with long-term disabilities where health and social care needs seem inextricably intertwined. In learning disability, this distinction was partly elaborated in special guidance (Department of Health, 1991), though with the exception clause which has appeared in some form in all policy since 1970: that where the degree and complexity of individual social care needs make it reasonable, the health service can take over the social care function. The groups of people specifically mentioned in this connection are those with major multiple handicaps or behaviour disturbance.

The split between those who favour retaining hospital provision (often in some other guise, such as 'village communities') and those who want its orderly replacement with small-scale services in the community, coupled with the Department's *laissez-faire* style, has led to a pluralist framework in which hospital-type services have continued to be developed in both public and independent sectors while elsewhere hospitals have been closed down and there are large-scale developments of community services.

In addition to these general issues, the other main contextual factor of the 1980s and 1990s has been the sustained attempt to use costs, or 'value for money', as the yardstick by which policy measures should be judged. One of the main ways of doing this has been to stimulate the delivery of existing public services by independent and therefore commercially accountable, providers.

Within this broad framework, policy-making relating to people with challenging behaviour or mental health needs at the beginning of the 1990s faced some specific constraints and opportunities. The constraints were that new guidance should not re-open the policy debate about models of care, but should live within the framework offered in the most recent advice; that the style of any guidance should be minimalist rather than comprehensive (in the reported words of a previous Secretary of State, it should not be 'nannying field agencies'); and that it should not require extra money. Failure to work within these limits would have made any report vulnerable to pressure within and outside the Department of Health and would have risked having it 'buried'.

There were, however, also important opportunities. Within the Department, there was a long-standing recognition that services for people with challenging behaviour or mental health needs were problematic for local service agencies. There were problems of very poor-quality provision, of expensive arrangements being resorted to in crises and of the general policy of developing community-based services being put at risk by weak management of this issue. Among people actually working in services there was expressed demand for guidance and fear that services for this client group were likely to slip between their respective responsibilities as perceived by health and social services authorities.

The Department had already recognized that some health authorities appeared to have misunderstood the community care reforms to mean that they would have no continuing role in the care of people with learning disabilities beyond what they provided in general and psychiatric hospitals, and that as a result no further investment (perhaps even asset-stripping) was taking place in health authority learning disability services. Specific guidance had been issued to correct any misunderstanding (Department of Health, 1991):

> There has been much concern that, with local authority social services departments becoming the main statutory agency for providing services for people with learning disabilities, the NHS would have no role. This would be a complete misunderstanding. We see the NHS having an important long-term role, as well as what is best viewed as the transitional responsibility for the remaining specialist mental handicap hospitals. (Department of Health, 1991, para. 26)

In terms of the style of any policy guidance, opportunities were also presented by the community care reforms and by the Department's previous experience. The reforms placed a clear emphasis on the individual and on the quality of service the individual receives. Since quality and individualization are also central themes in the recent development of learning disability services there were clear possibilities for linking specific guidance about challenging behaviour to the main policy initiative. The Department had made two previous attempts to issue guidance in this area (Department of Health and Social Security, 1984; Department of Health, 1989). In both cases they had produced reviews of all possible options without drawing any conclusions. Perhaps not surprisingly, therefore, these reports had sunk without trace. Now the Department was ready for a more direct approach.

### Key themes in the report

In setting up the Project Group, the Department of Health framed its task in these terms:

> We believe that the time has come to offer health authorities and social services authorities something more specific in the way of guidance, and we propose to do this by seeking to build on the achievements of a very small number of local services we judge to be operating with some success. In essence, the aim is to analyse how four local services approach the task, and to synthesize the findings into practical guidance from which local services might be constructed elsewhere, with the likelihood that they too will be successful. (Department of Health, 1993, section 1)

The four services were the Additional Support Team, Exeter (Williams *et al.*, 1991); the Special Projects Team, Sunderland ((Johnson, 1990; Johnson and Cooper, 1991); the Mental Impairment Evaluation and Treatment Service, South East Thames Region (Dockrell *et al.*, 1990; 1992; Murphy and Clare, 1991; Murphy *et al.*, 1991); and the Special Development Team, also for the South East Thames Region (McGill *et al.*, 1991; Emerson and McGill, in press; Mansell and Beasley, in press; see also Chapter 6).

The report considers the definition of the client group, their numbers and needs; describes the key elements of the exemplary services; comments on the most appropriate models of care; and then details guidance for commissioning authorities, contrasting examples of good with weak practice. Rather than summarize its content in this chapter, five themes which pervade the report are discussed below.

*The social context of challenging behaviour*

In common with several contributions to this book (for example, Chapters 2, 3, 4 and 10), the report emphasizes the social context of challenging behaviour: that it is the product of both individual factors and the circumstances in which the person lives (Table 13.1).

One implication of this is that people with learning disabilities who have challenging behaviour form an extremely diverse group, including individuals with all levels of learning disability, many different sensory or physical impairments and presenting quite different kinds of challenges, ranging from chronic self-injury by people with profound learning disability to law-breaking by people whose learning disability is mild but who have mental health problems. Services themselves therefore need to be highly individualized. Although acknowledging that people have special needs, the point is made at the outset that people with challenging behaviour have the same needs as anyone else and that issues of 'double discrimination' on grounds of race and gender are likely to be particularly important. The report also identifies the needs of carers and staff as important considerations. Noting that the failure of community services to keep pace

Table 13.1 Factors contributing to challenging behaviour (Source: Department of Health, 1993)

| The individual | Their circumstances |
| --- | --- |
| • the degree of learning disability<br>• a mental illness<br>• a physical disability, e.g. epilepsy<br>• a sensory impairment<br>• absence of adequate verbal communication<br>• age<br>• physical illness | • history of neglect<br>• history of sexual abuse<br>• history of physical abuse<br>• a reputation for challenging others in the past<br>• restrictive home or daytime environment which maximizes confrontations<br>• surroundings which an individual dislikes<br>• lack of understanding of the **meaning** of non-verbal behaviour by carers<br>• low expectations of carers<br>• overemphasis on risk reduction |

with hospital closure is imposing a greater burden on families, and that working with people who present major challenges involves a great deal of stress, the report says that services should not be provided by exploiting the personal commitment and dedication of carers and staff.

The other major implication of recognizing that challenging behaviour is the product of a complex mix of individual and environmental factors is that an exclusive focus on the people who have the most challenging problems is not likely to be sufficient:

> the proper role and characteristics of specialist services can only be achieved by attending to the competence of 'mainstream' learning disability services. The priority is to improve the capability of mainstream services to prevent problems arising in the first place, to manage them when they occur and to implement relatively sophisticated long-term arrangements for management, treatment and care. In so far as this can be achieved, specialist services will be able to concentrate on people with the most complex and difficult needs. At the moment, even moderate levels of challenging behaviour are not being appropriately managed in mainstream learning disability services and specialist services (including some of dubious quality) face apparently unlimited demand. (Department of Health, 1993, covering letter)

In this way the report identifies the competence or capability of local 'mainstream' services for people with learning disabilities as an important factor determining the number of people defined as presenting a serious challenge:

> Whether these services continue to get better depends in part on how they respond to challenging behaviour, not just in the small number of people who present exceptional problems at any one time, but throughout their service. If they develop the capacity to work with people who present challenges in small, local services they will keep the size of the problem to a minimum and they will provide a good service to individuals in both their mainstream and specialized services. ... If local services are not developed then a trickle of expensive out-of-area placements will become a rush as more people are excluded from mainstream community services by being defined as un-

manageable in the community. Large amounts of money will be tied up in buying less good services. The policy of community care will be said to have failed. (Department of Health, 1993, section 6)

### *Importance of management commitment*

The second strand in the report is the belief that, in policy terms in the middle part of the 1990s, weakness of management commitment may be a more important limiting factor in improving services than knowledge and experience of models of service. A key observation made to the Project Group was that the senior managers of local service agencies could be classified by their intentions in relation to services for people with challenging behaviour, and that this helped explain different approaches to service development for this client group.

'Removers' do not wish to develop locally the competence to serve people with challenging behaviour (perhaps because they perceive the task as too difficult, or not worth the effort). Instead, they seek to place people who cannot be served locally in out-of-area residential placements, often at considerable expense. 'Containers' do attempt to provide local services (perhaps because of the cost of out-of-area placements) but seek only to contain people in low-cost (and therefore poorly staffed) settings. 'Developers' try to provide local services which really do address individual needs, and therefore give higher priority to funding services which, with more staff and more training and management input, are more expensive than ordinary community services.

The report suggests that reasons for this include beliefs that nothing much can be achieved and so it is not worth spending the money, or that the numbers concerned are so small that the effort of developing services is not worth it, or that cheap, low-staffed institutional care is really providing the quality its proponents claim. It restates the reasons why priority should be given to these services.

1. **People with challenging behaviour have the greatest needs.** People with learning disabilities and challenging behaviour present the most complex and difficult problems, both at clinical and service organization levels. Although their numbers may be relatively small, unless services respond well

they occupy disproportionate amounts of time and money. (Department of Health, 1993, section 5.1.1)

2. **Good-quality services achieve results.**

   Current research suggests that good quality services already make a substantial difference to the quality of life of individuals with challenging behaviour, and therefore by implication to their carers and staff. If the characteristics that make these services work were more widespread and better supported by management it would be possible to apply even more of the available knowledge at the clinical level and to achieve even better results for individuals. (Department of Health, 1993, section 5.1.2)

3. **Failure to develop services threatens the policy of community care.**

   Doing nothing locally is not an option. Out-of-area placements will 'silt up' and reinstitutionalization (through emergency admissions to psychiatric hospitals or via the prisons) will occur. Special institutions and residential homes for people with challenging behaviour will be expensive but of poor quality and will attract public criticism. Overall, the efficiency of services will decrease because of the widespread lack of competence in working with people who have challenging behaviour. Commissioners will have less control over and choice of services. Individual service users, carers and staff will be hurt and some individuals with challenging behaviour will be at increased risk of abuse. Staff will be at increased risk from the consequences of developing their own strategies and responses and managers will be held accountable where well-intentioned staff operate illegal or inappropriate procedures. (Department of Health, 1993, section 5.1.3)

This leads to the conclusion that:

the key to the development of better services is management commitment. We are confident that there is now sufficient knowledge and practical experience to substantially improve services, given the kind of sustained commitment from policy-makers and managers that the services we studied had enjoyed. Many people we met expressed anxiety that this commitment was diminishing. We think that the Department of Health could usefully re-emphasize the priority these services should command. (Department of Health, 1993, covering letter)

*The service development process*

The Project Group faced the problem of how to respond to demands for clarity in dividing responsibility between health and social services authorities and in choosing between community or institution-based models of long-term care, given the constraints of wider national policy. The main vehicle it uses to address these problems is the idea that the development of services is a process in which different arrangements might be justified at different stages.

Constrained by the wider framework of defining needs as either health or social care responsibilities, the report does not attempt to define a boundary. It offers chapter and verse to correct any misapprehension among health authorities that the community care reforms might mean that they would have no continuing responsibility for services for people with learning disabilities (Department of Health, 1991), and suggests that where the boundary between different agencies is set will depend more on the relative skills and experience of each agency locally than on artificial definitions of what tasks might be health or social care. It offers the experience of the Special Development Team in South East Thames Regional Health Authority (Chapter 6), where the same type of highly staffed and organized house is provided in some places by local authority social services departments and in others by health authorities, depending on the stage of service development reached locally.

Although the report is clear that community-based residential and day care services are the option preferred by members of the Project Group, the guidance to health and social services authorities commissioning services for their local populations recognizes that some will continue to need to use poorer-quality services while they develop the local infrastructure and expertise needed:

Commissioners with no experience of local community-based services for people with challenging behaviour should begin developing these to gain information about local need and the expertise to improve services; continued use of poor quality services (usually large institutions or residential homes) to provide long-term residential and day care should only continue to give a breathing-space for local service development. Service development should be planned on an iterative, incremental basis so that plans can be adapted in response to individual needs and as local expertise and confidence grows. (Department of Health, 1993, section 5.3)

This is also the place where the report focuses on staffing, saying that if the opportunities provided by community-based models of care are to be realized in practice, commissioners should have clear strategies for ensuring that providers have adequate numbers of suitably trained staff over the longer term, avoiding the perverse incentive for individual providers to rely on 'poaching' staff.

### Empiricism and cost constraints

Having recognized that one motive for commissioners to purchase poorer-quality services was their lower cost, the Project Group had to produce a report which addressed the problem of resources. It approached the issue partly by looking at resources as a question of priorities, partly by taking into account a wider range of costs and partly by focusing on 'value for money' as the yardstick by which service development choices should be made.

The report points out that the services represented on the Project Group were all developed within the existing resource framework available to their host agencies and suggests that resources are therefore as much a question of priorities as of the amount of money available.

Turning to costs, the report says that commissioners should take care to identify all the current expenditure. The report says that, although adequate services for people with challenging behaviour will probably take more resources than currently allocated (since there is no logical basis to existing resource levels), there are probably more resources in use than is apparent at first. It gives the example of some agencies which spend substantial amounts of contingency reserves held at agency level on this group, while failing for want of money to develop the local capacity to serve.

Commissioners are also advised to take account of the hidden costs of failure to develop local services (Figure 13.1), such as the costs of handling crises and placement breakdowns, and the financial and other costs borne by carers, to avoid increasing the burden on carers by reducing levels of service. Echoing Knapp and Mansell (Chapter 12), the report calls for increasingly individualized costs to remove the confounding effect of averaging

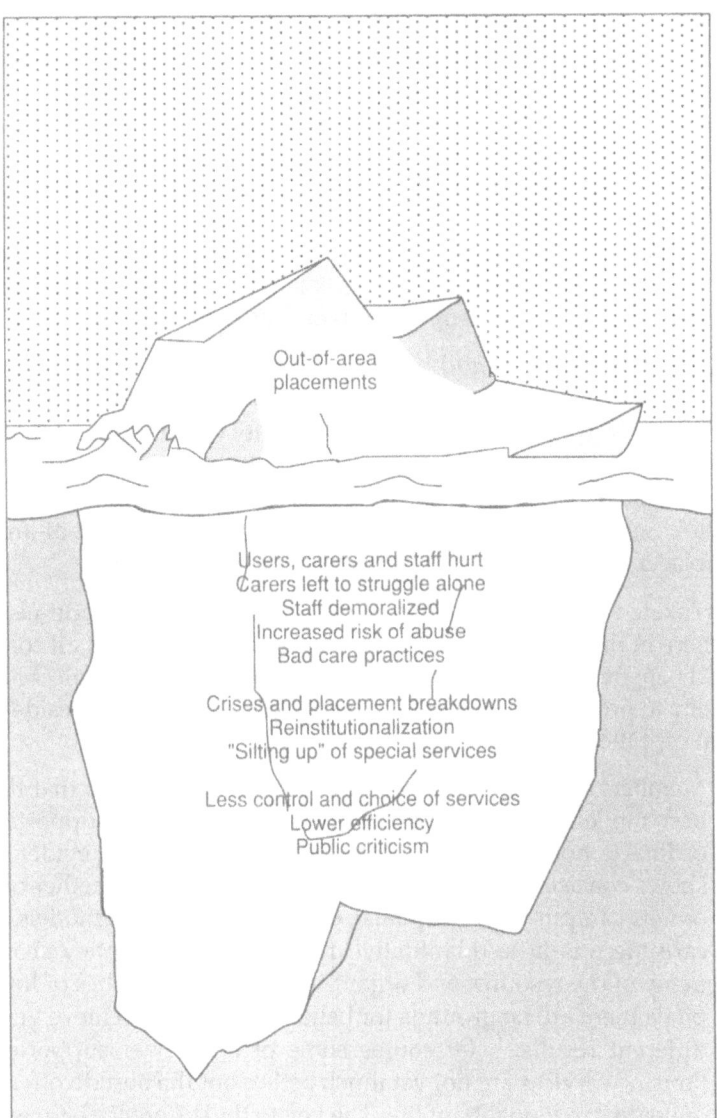

Out-of-area placements

Users, carers and staff hurt
Carers left to struggle alone
Staff demoralized
Increased risk of abuse
Bad care practices

Crises and placement breakdowns
Reinstitutionalization
"Silting up" of special services

Less control and choice of services
Lower efficiency
Public criticism

**Figure 13.1** The hidden cost of failing to develop local services (Source: Department of Health, 1993).

across clients and settings. In the short term, the report suggests that commissioners should certainly look to redirect resources from relatively expensive out-of-area placements to local service development, although it also acknowledges that a very small number of individuals will be very expensive to serve wherever they live and it would be naive to expect cost savings as a matter of course.

The report also focuses on 'value for money', pointing out that value for money cannot be judged solely on the basis of costs but requires an assessment of the benefits and outcomes produced.

> Commissioners should have equal regard for the value of services (the benefits they offer to the service user) as for their cost. They should attend to the general quality of life ... in addition to the specific treatment of challenging behaviour. At service system level, value for money needs to be demonstrated by the low number of placement breakdowns and of out-of-area placements. (Department of Health, 1993, section 5.4)

Taken with the comments about models of care made elsewhere in the report, this embodies the assumption that if all costs and benefits are taken into account community-based services are likely to prove the best choice. For example, in relation to residential care the report says:

> Members of the Committee are themselves persuaded that the best model of residential care is likely to be the supported ordinary housing model. The available research evidence shows consistently poor quality of life in hospital (whether old or new campus-style hospitals); on other large-group models of care there is little quantitative research but since they share many of the resource and organizational characteristics of hospitals there are no grounds for believing they will achieve very different results ... Of course some of the newer supported housing services are not yet much better: but the best do offer a quite different quality of life. The key to the difference between good and indifferent community services lies not in resources, but in the quality of management (especially first-line management). (Department of Health, 1993, section 4.1)

In this sense the report adopts a confidently empiricist approach to the debate about models of care. This reflects something of a change in the debate over models of care, which was characterized in the 1970s and early 1980s by the question 'Are community services feasible?'; with more widespread development and clear demonstrations of success in community services, there is now more pressure for institutional models to demonstrate what they really achieve.

In this last connection the report calls for a critical appraisal by those purchasing services; referring to the example of the services represented on the Project Group, it says:

A crucial difference between these services and some others is that management can evaluate whether what the service claims to do it really achieves. Since virtually all services claim to provide individualized care based on the latest assessment methods it is essential that service managers and purchasers can really discriminate between good and mediocre performance. This can be a particular problem for services providing long-term residential or day care, where a successful service looks like an ordinary home or occupation, when in fact it is a carefully designed and organized service dependent on a great deal of skill and management. (Department of Health, 1993, section 3.4)

*Comprehensiveness*

The fifth strand which runs through the report is also one which figures largely in this book. It is that individual components or parts of the whole service system often depend on the existence of many other components working well, and that good services for individuals require the integration of different aspects or parts of services into an effective whole.

At the broadest level, this is a point the report makes in considering relationships between different agencies. It suggests joint commissioning as a possible way for health and social services to work together, but also calls for good working relationships between these and other agencies such as housing, education and the police.

At the service system level, the report calls for the required range of service types (for example, for the provision of good quality work or education placements as well as support for life at home) as well as the different functional elements needed (for prevention of challenging behaviour, its identification, assessment and treatment, see Chapter 4).

Finally, within the individual components of services the report emphasizes the planning and management needed to routinely deliver high quality service to people.

> Good understanding of the reasons for an individual's challenging behaviour and of how this interacts with the everyday organization of the service . . . requires a greater degree of skill among staff and particularly good management (especially first-line management) to keep the service on track. Management is also crucial in ensuring that professional specialists and front-line staff work together; that specialist advice is practicable and sensible and that staff follow it. . . . In particular, managers need to distinguish the middle ground between pessimism about models of care ('you can't do anything with these people') and naive misinterpretations about normalization ('only values matter – all structure is oppressive'); life for people with major disabilities in good services will often look quite ordinary, but this ordinariness will be the product of a great deal of careful planning and management. (Department of Health, 1993, section 3.4)

## Implementation

The task facing those responsible for services for people who have learning disabilities and challenging behaviour is clear, if difficult. They have to build on the work they did to introduce new values into services by turning those values into practice, i.e., they have to bring 'mainstream' community services up to the level of the models which inspired their development. They have to do this while continuing to make an orderly transition from institutional to community-based service models, and against a background of many other claims on their time and resources (whether generated directly by the needs of clients or due to administrative change and reorganization).

A report alone, even if backed up through official circulars, is not likely to produce change on the required scale, primarily because management attention and commitment from all members of the local service-providing coalition will need to be sustained beyond the period surrounding publication to carry out the improvements required. Commitment is required from managers of different agencies, not all of whom come into the category of 'developers'; new services and new ways of working have to be introduced and then sustained throughout learning disability services and beyond, among those generic services which include people with learning disabilities among their clients, and this will require strategic planning, especially in relation to developing a skilled workforce, as well as the diversity and competition a mixed economy of welfare is supposed to bring.

If this is left to the formal review mechanisms which operate through Regional Health Authorities and the Social Services Inspectorate there is the risk that poor performance in this area will be 'traded-off' against work on other issues, since these reviews necessarily focus on a very small number of major priorities. What is needed is a process of implementation which targets the operational managers responsible for commissioning local services and their counterparts in provider agencies: a process which can facilitate local action without obstructing the main priority-setting pathway (which is often likely to be preoccupied with other matters).

There is a parallel here with hospital closure, as in the well-documented example of Darenth Park. There, little progress was made in developing local replacement services while the formal relationships between the Regional and District Health Authorities were used; it was only when the Regional Health Authority developed new links directly with local operational managers that real progress began to be made (Korman and Glennerster, 1990; Mansell, 1988a). These included forums to work collaboratively and to bring people together to learn from each other and a central task force which acted in part as interpreters and facilitators of local action within the framework of a regional project.

One example of this way of working was the use of a 'learning set' to enable local teams to develop staffed housing as their main form of residential care at a time when the prevailing climate had favoured institutional solutions (Mansell, 1988b; 1989). The teams, drawn from health and social services (and sometimes the voluntary sector too), met every six to eight weeks over a period of 18 months to work through the practical problems of implementation. As well as effective dissemination of the best available knowledge and experience, they derived support and credibility from working together and they produced a rapid expansion in community-based services.

A similar model is needed here. A national initiative, embracing enough field authorities to make a significant impact in services, through which the experience of existing examples of good practice can be securely put into practice. Regional initiatives like that in the south-east of England and national publications and networks promulgated by the King's Fund have made a start, but these have mainly focused on an already committed, and largely professional rather than managerial, audience. The commitment required of senior managers can only be sustained by government leadership.

## References

Campaign for the Mentally Handicapped (1972) *Even Better Services for the Mentally Handicapped*. London: Campaign for the Mentally Handicapped.

Department of Health (1989) *Needs and Responses: Services for Adults with Mental Handicap who are Mentally Ill, who have Behaviour Problems or who Offend*. London: HMSO.

Department of Health (1991) *Stephen Dorrell's Mencap Speech: Statement on Services for People with Learning Disabilities – Tuesday 25 June 1991*. London: Department of Health.

Department of Health (1993) *Services for People with Learning Disabilities and Challenging Behaviour or Mental Health Needs: Report of a Project Group* (Chairman: Prof. J.L. Mansell). London: HMSO.

Department of Health and Social Security (1984) *Helping Mentally Handicapped People with Special Problems: Report of a DHSS Study Team*. London: HMSO.

Dockrell, J., Gaskell, G. and Rehman, H. (1990) Challenging behaviours: Problems, provisions and 'solutions', in *Treatment of Mental Illness and Behavioural Disorder in the Mentally Retarded* (eds A. Dosen, A. Van Gennep and G.J. Zwanikken). Leiden: Logon Publications.

Dockrell, J., Gaskell, G. and Rehman, H. (1992) *A Preliminary Report of the Evaluation of the Mental Impairment Evaluation and Treatment Service (MIETS)*. Departmental Research Report 92–42. London: Department of Social Psychology, London School of Economics.

Emerson, E. and McGill, P. (in press) Developing services for people with severe learning disabilities and seriously challenging behaviours: South East Thames Regional Health Authority, 1985–1991, in *People with Severe Learning Difficulties who also Display Challenging Behaviour* (eds I. Fleming and B. Stenfert Kroese). Manchester: Manchester University Press.

Johnson, D. (1990) Steps to a better service. *Health Service Journal*, **7 June**, 844–5.

Johnson, D. and Cooper, B. (1991) The Special Projects Team, Sunderland, in *Meeting the Challenge: Some UK Perspectives on Community Services for People with Learning Difficulties and Challenging Behaviour* (eds D. Allen, R. Banks and S. Staite). London: King's Fund

Centre, pp. 36–40.

Korman, N. and Glennerster, H. (1990) *Hospital Closure*. Milton Keynes: Open University Press.

McGill, P., Hawkins, C. and Hughes, H. (1991) The Special Development Team, South East Thames, in *Meeting the Challenge: Some UK Perspectives on Community Services for People with Learning Difficulties and Challenging Behaviour* (eds D. Allen, R. Banks and S. Staite). London: King's Fund Centre, pp. 7–13.

Mansell, J. (1988a) Training for service development, in *An Ordinary Life in Practice: Lessons from the Experience of Developing Comprehensive Community-based Services for People with Learning Disabilities* (ed. D. Towell). London: King's Fund Centre.

Mansell, J. (1988b) *Staffed Housing for People with Mental Handicaps: Achieving Widespread Dissemination*. Bexhill-on-Sea: South East Thames Regional Health Authority.

Mansell, J. (1989) Evaluation of training in the development of staffed housing for people with mental handicaps. *Mental Handicap Research*, **2**, 137–51.

Mansell, J. and Beasley, F. (in press) Small staffed houses for people with a severe mental handicap and challenging behaviour. *British Journal of Social Work*, (in press).

Murphy, G. and Clare, I. (1991) MIETS: A service option for people with mild mental handicaps and challenging behaviour or psychiatric problems – 2. Assessment, treatment and outcome for service users and service effectiveness. *Mental Handicap Research*, **4**, 180–206.

Murphy, G., Holland, A., Fowler, P. and Reep, J. (1991) MIETS: A service option for people with mild mental handicaps and challenging behaviour or psychiatric problems – 1. Philosophy, service and service users. *Mental Handicap Research*, **4**, 41–66.

Welsh Office (1991) *Challenges and Responses: A Report on Services in Support of Adults with Mental Handicaps with Exceptionally Challenging Behaviours, Mental Illnesses, or who Offend*. Cardiff: Welsh Office.

Williams, C., Hewitt, P. and Bratt, A. (1991) Responding to the needs of people with learning difficulties whose behaviour we perceive as challenging. The past, present and future: A perspective from Exeter Health Authority, in *Service Responses to People with Learning Difficulties and Challenging Behaviour* (ed. J. Harris). Kidderminster: BIMH, pp. 20–4.

# Afterword

The central argument of this book has been that it is a mistake to construe challenging behaviour as an entirely clinical problem. Instead, it is a complex phenomenon which has to be addressed as the outcome of many individual and environmental factors, including, among others, the biological effects of specific syndromes, the detailed organization of support for the person and the way service systems are set up and run.

Once such a conceptualization is accepted, the task of providing services for people with challenging behaviour becomes both more difficult and more interesting. It cannot be left in the hands of 'specialists' such as psychologists or psychiatrists, since even their best efforts will be limited by the contexts within which they work. Rather, the entire system of supports surrounding the individual needs to be developed and designed using the best knowledge we have about their effects, both generally and specifically for the individual concerned. A decision by a senior manager who has never met the person may have more impact on the latter's quality of life than anything that the 'specialist' can do.

Service managers, then, have a powerful and important role. By the kinds of services which they purchase, by the parameters they set for the operation of existing services, by the attention they give to staff training and support, and so on, managers can have a major impact on outcomes for people with challenging behaviour and their carers. If the potential of their role is to be fulfilled they need both an understanding of the nature of challenging behaviour and a commitment to providing quality services to those with the greatest needs.

They cannot do this, however, by decree. Good services **develop** and it is crucial that managers provide the necessary culture for this to happen. There is a danger that the attention given to service development in recent years may wither as new community-based services become established and less susceptible to scrutiny. As in the best commercial organizations the manager's role here is to facilitate and sustain the pursuit of excellence.

Of course, managers can only develop services in the context of cost evaluation and control. Such a context should not be seen as necessarily constraining but rather as providing an incentive to carefully evaluate both the costs and benefits of services and to strive towards better services. Tight cost control is only a problem when outcomes are ignored.

Finally, for all of this to happen, it is crucial to take a systemic view of the inputs, processes, outputs and outcomes of services for people with challenging behaviour. Such services are complex systems in which change at one point can have unpredicted effects on change at another. While we do not yet understand the system fully it is clear from the chapters in this book that we know something about the most important variables and their interrelationships. By using what we know, we can create better services for people with severe learning disabilities and challenging behaviours.

# Index